MICROBIOLOGY

An Introduction For The
Health Sciences

MICROBIOLOGY

An Introduction For The
Health Sciences

Val Ackerman
Royal North Shore Hospital Sydney

Gloria Dunk-Richards
Caroline Chisholm School of Nursing Melbourne

W. B. Saunders
Baillière Tindall

Harcourt Brace Jovanovich, Publishers
Sydney   Philadelphia   London   Toronto

W.B. Saunders/Ballière Tindall

An imprint of
Harcourt Brace Jovanovich Group
(Australia) Pty Limited
30-52 Smidmore Street
Marrickville, N.S.W. 2204

Harcourt Brace Jovanovich Limited
24/28 Oval Road, London NW1 7DX

Harcourt Brace Jovanovich, Inc.
1250 Sixth Avenue,
San Diego, California 92101-4311

Printed in Australia

National Library of Australia Cataloguing-in-Publication Data

Ackerman, Val.
  Microbiology, an introduction for the health sciences.

  Includes index.
  ISBN 0 7295 0352 6.

  1. Medical microbiology. I. Dunk-Richards, Gloria. II.
Title.

616.01

CONTENTS

LIST OF TABLES AND FIGURES

TABLES

FIGURES

LIST OF COLOUR PLATES

1 Culture of throat swab on blood agar
2 Gram stain of pus (staphylococci)
3 Gram stain of pus (Gram-positive cocci in chains and pairs)
4 Cerebrospinal fluid from a case of meningitis
5 Cerebrospinal fluid (provisional diagnosis: *Cryptococcus neoformans* meningitis)
6 Cerebrospinal fluid containing large numbers of 'pus cells' (provisional diagnosis: *Neisseria meningitidis* meningitis)
7 Two API galleries
8 Sputum: 'pus cells' and Gram-positive cocci mostly in pairs (provisional diagnosis: pneumococcal pneumonia)
9 Roche blood-culture device
10a-e White cells found in normal blood: (a) Two neutrophils and one large lymphocyte, (b) 2 small and 1 large lymphocyte, (c) a monocyte, (d) an eosinophil (e) a basophil
11 Representation of the antibody molecule
12 Immunofluorescence (a schistosome larva outlined in green)
13 Gram stain showing *Streptococcus pneumoniae*, pneumococci singly and in pairs
14 Corynebacteria, 'diphtheroids', on and around an epithelial cell from the mouth
15 Ziehl-Neelsen stain of sputum (tubercle bacilli)
16 A tick (in transillumination)
17 Adult female louse, *Pediculus humanus*
18 A 'nit' (louse egg) attached to a hair
19 Shingles (due to recurrence of Herpes zoster)
20 Inclusion body in cytomegalovirus-infected epithelial cell in urine
21 Chronic *Candida* infection of finger-nails showing destruction of nail tissue
22a Snails, *Bulinus* species (intermediate host of *Schistosoma*)
22b Paddy field (typical environment in which the *Schistosoma* finds its intermediate host)
23a 'Hydatid sand', unattached protoscolices of *Echinococcus*, from a cyst
23b Scolex of *Echinococcus granulosus* in urine, showing crown of hooklets
24a *Plasmodium vivax* (female gametocyte)
24b *Plasmodium falciparum* (ring forms)
25 Scabies on a baby's foot
26 *Candida vaginitis:* vaginal swab showing lactobacilli and yeast cells and hyphae
27 Nurse collecting blood for culture
28 Nursing sister adjusting flow of intravenous infusion
29 Intensive care patient: a 'compromised' patient
30 Technologist inoculating a blood-agar plate with a swab in a safety cabinet
31 Technologist using replicator to inoculate large number of different cultures onto one plate
32 Agar dilution susceptibility plates inoculated with replicator illustrated in Plate 31
33 Selective medium used for detection of intestinal pathogens *(Salmonella typhi)*
34 Technologist using inverted microscope to check cell cultures for evidence of viral growth
35 Unloading drapes from an autoclave after sterilisation
36 Reproduction in fungi (showing zygospores)
37-44 Fungal spores. (Plates **37-41**: environmental saprophytes; **42** species of *Alternaria* isolated from a corneal ulcer; **43** *Microsporum gypseum;* **44** *Penicillium* species)
45 Mycelia of yeast *Candida albicans* in urine

Cover photo *Pseudomonas* growing in lung tissue of a mouse.

PREFACE

Microbiology — the study of microbes — is a science which is becoming increasingly relevant. Even in the so-called 'developed countries' there is more to infectious disease than getting a cold and going to a doctor for an antibiotic that you don't need. The old infections are still with us — diphtheria and whooping cough are kept at bay only by vaccination, and influenza continues to return every year or two. Moreover, new infections are being recognised with disturbing frequency — AIDS and Lyme disease are striking examples.

In the Third World infectious disease is uncontrolled and responsible for millions of deaths every year. 'Third World' did we say? — modern travel ensures that in fact we all live in *one* world; any one of us may today encounter infections that were once labelled 'tropical diseases'.

There are also other reasons for microbiology's relevancy: any understanding of the ecological unity that is Earth must start with microbes.

In this text we have therefore tried to offer an overview of microbiology in all its aspects. Our main emphasis has inevitably been on microbes which cause disease, because that is the aspect which will most concern students of the health sciences. But we have also tried to show that microbes play other roles and that, far from being harmful to humans, their activities are *essential* to us — and to all travellers onboard planet Earth.

In writing this work, our aim has been to combine an authoritative scientific text with a conversational and 'non-threatening' style which will extend the book's use to students with a limited scientific background. We have deliberately taken a different approach from the usual rigorous one of organisation via body systems or types of organisms, believing a thematic approach is friendlier and more useful to our intended readers. To this end, the book also incorporates numerous boxed studies (under such headings as Milestones, In the Lab, and In the Ward), and examples from many areas of microbiology. Specific nursing applications are likewise included, as are short review tests at the end of each chapter. Finally, the text is complemented with over 120 line drawings and photos, and 16 pages of full-colour plates. We are confident that health science students will find this book a valuable and friendly companion, and wish them well with it in their intended studies.

V. A.
G. D.-R.

Note: All names used in case histories are fictitious and no reference is made to any person, living or dead.

ACKNOWLEDGMENTS

We thank our editor, Paul Cliff — if the book is as readable as we hope it is, a lot of the credit goes to him. Maureen Ackerman read the text several times and pointed out most of the obvious errors; for those that remain we must take responsibility.

ILLUSTRATIONS

We acknowledge with gratitude the help of all our colleagues who provided illustrations. The individual sources are as follows.

Colour plates:

1, 6, 7, 8, 9, 14, 26, 30–34, 47–54, 57 Dept of Microbiology, RNS Hospital, Sydney.

2, 3, 4, 13 Dept of Bacteriology, Royal Alexandra Hospital for Children, Sydney.

5, 21, 36–45, 56, 58, 59, Kaminski's Teaching Slides in Medical Mycology, ed. D. Ellis, Adelaide Children's Hospital, 1987.

10 Dr Kam Sing Lau, Dept of Haematology, RNS Hospital.

11 Concept from *Essential Immunology*, Ivan M Roitt, Blackwell Scientific Publications, 6th ed, 1988; fingers by MA, orange by Prizzi's Fruit Palace, photo by VA.

12, 22a 23a, 46, 61 Dr J Walker, Dept of Parasitology, Westmead Medical Centre, Sydney.

15 Dr B Hudson, Dept of Microbiology, RNS Hospital, Sydney.

16, 17, 18, 24a, 24b, 60, 62–71 Parasitology Slide Sequence, ed. S.A. Neville, Dept of Microbiology, The Liverpool Hospital, Sydney, 1987.

19, 25 Reeves, JT and Maibach, H (1884), *Clinical Dermatology Illustrated*, Adis Health Science Press (McLennan & Petty), Sydney.

20, 23b *Urine under the Microscope*, Editiones ‹Roche›, Hoffman La Roche, Basle, 1978.

22b P Cliff.

27 Dept of Haematology, RNS Hospital, Sydney.

28 Sr Cathy Dawkins, Nursing Unit Manager, RNS Hospital, Sydney.

29 Courtesy Dept of Intensive Care, RNS Hospital, Sydney.

35 Sterile Services Dept, RNS Hospital, Sydney.

55 Dr RC Pritchard, Dept of Microbiology, RNS Hospital, Sydney.

72, 73,74 Boehringer Ingelheim International GmbH (photos by Lennart Nilsson).

API Gallery: Carter-Wallace (Aust) Pty Ltd, Frenchs Forest, NSW.

Figures:

4.10, 4.11, 4.12, 4.13, 4.15 Abbott International Ltd, North Chicago, Illinois.

4.12 Dr David Silverman, University of Maryland at Baltimore, School of Medicine, Baltimore Md, 21201, USA.

Poster ('Universal blood and body fluid precautions') Sr Ailsa Ritchie, Infection Control, RNS Hospital.

6.8 Today's Life Science magazine.

13.2a & b Millipore Pty Ltd, Lane Cove, NSW.

13.3 Ward 7C, RNS Hospital.

16.2a, 16.3a, c & d, 16.4a, 16.5b, 16.6a, 16.7a, 16.8, 16.9, 16.10, 16.11 Zaman, Viqar (1983), Scanning Electron Microscopy of Medically Important Parasites, ADIS Health Press (McLennan & Petty), Sydney.

2.5, 4.6, 4.10, 10.3a, 12.3a and b, 14.13, 14.14 Klainer, AS & Geis, I (1973) Agents of Bacterial Disease, Harper & Row, Maryland.

Cover photo: Tap Pharmaceuticals Inc , Deerfield, Illinois, USA.

Photo, p. 89: 'T-Cells recognise antigen on surface of a macrophage' (published *Scientific American* vol 261 no 5 1989); courtesy Morten H Nielsen/Ole Werdelin, University of Copenhagen, Denmark.

Cover and internal design: Tania Edwards; *Illustrations:* Maggie Renvoize; *Technical illustrations:* John Cleasby

Part One
General Microbiology

INTRODUCTION

In 1981 the Centers for Disease Control USA noted that two unusual diseases were being reported more frequently. These were pneumonia due to *Pneumocystis carinii*, and Kaposi's sarcoma. Hitherto *Pneumocystis* pneumonia had occurred typically in people whose immune system was depressed (for example by drugs given to prevent the rejection of a kidney transplant). And Kaposi's sarcoma was a slow-growing tumour in the old. These disorders were now occurring in younger men, in whom the underlying disease was found to be an infection with *human immunodeficiency virus (HIV)*, a virus which kills by undermining the body's immune defences so that other common microbes can no longer be resisted. These were the first recorded cases of what we now call AIDS — the acquired immune deficiency syndrome.

Within the past 20 years, AIDS has been the most spectacular example of a new or newly-recognised infection. But there are other examples — Legionnaires' disease, toxic shock syndrome, Lyme disease. Although many common infections, such as pneumonia, tuberculosis, meningitis and urinary tract infection can now be successfully treated with antibiotics, infectious disease remains a common problem. (If you have a cold when you read this, you won't need convincing that this is true!) This book will show you how microbes are studied, how they live and multiply, how a few cause infections, and how such infections are diagnosed and treated.

MICROBES IN NATURE

Infectious diseases are caused by *microorganisms* (microbes); the study of these creatures is called *microbiology*. The largest microbe is only just visible to the naked eye and most are much smaller. Though small, they are numerous — there are more microbes in and on each human being than there are human beings currently alive on the planet. They are ubiquitous; microbes can be found on and in animals and plants, in the soil, in the air and in the seas and lakes. If water temperature is somewhere between 0^0 and 98^0C some microbe will be able to survive and probably multiply.

We tend to associate 'germs' with disease and unsanitary conditions, but only a small number of the known microbes can harm us. Most are actually beneficial or indifferent. Microbes perform numerous functions essential to the survival of 'higher' life forms. In the seas and rivers, microbes are the first link in the food chain (see p36); many other creatures depend on them for nourishment. Microbes break down dead plants and animals, so that their constituents can be reused. Without the activities of microbes all life on earth would rapidly cease, because the chemicals essential for growth would be locked up in dead bodies and unavailable. Some soil bacteria 'fix' nitrogen from the air, i.e. convert it to a chemical form that can be used by plants. Many can use solar energy for photosynthesis, i.e. to produce from the air the chemicals needed for growth. Many of the foods we eat are produced by the activities of microbes: cheese, yoghurt, beers and wines, bread, soy sauce, sauerkraut and vinegar. Microbiologists and chemical engineers use microbes to prepare drugs and organic chemicals more easily and more cheaply than the chemist can synthesise them in the test-tube. Of course not all microbial activities are beneficial or desirable. Some cause disease of humans, animals or plants, with consequences that may be unpleasant, lethal or economically disastrous. When food spoils or bread goes 'mouldy' this is due to microbes.

A BRIEF HISTORY OF MICROBIOLOGY

As has been mentioned, microbes are generally too small to be visible to the naked eye. The first person to actually observe microbes was a Dutchman — Antonie van Leeuwenhoek — who in 1674 began to report to the Royal Society of London his observations with a simple microscope. He examined pond water, scrapings from teeth and other materials. The diagrams he drew show the same basic microbial forms we know today: rods, spheres and spirals (Fig. 1.1). Nearly 200 hundred years later — in 1857 — Louis Pasteur (1822-1895) showed the importance of these tiny creatures, and proved that microbes called 'yeasts' were responsible for the fermentation of sugars into alcohol in wine or beer, and other smaller organisms bring about the fermentation of milk. Pasteur also settled the controversy about the origin of microbial life. (See 'Milestones', following.)

MILESTONES

Pasteur's broths lay the myth of 'spontaneous generation'

For centuries people had believed that living creatures could be

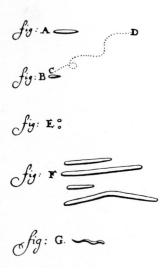

Fig. 1.1 Antonie van Leeuwenhoek's drawings. In letters to the Royal Society of London he described 'animalcules' (little animals) which he saw with his primitive microscope in material from the human mouth. He observed spheres, rods and spirals and noted that some were motile (moving). These sketches are from a letter of 1683.

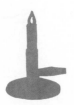

produced by 'spontaneous generation' — that flies appeared spontaneously from manure, frogs from moist soil and maggots from decaying meat. In 1668 the Italian physician Francesco Redi showed that when the meat was covered with gauze to exclude flies, maggots did *not* grow — but belief in spontaneous generation of microbes persisted.

John Needham showed in 1745 that even if you *boiled* a meat broth, it would soon afterwards teem with microorganisms. If you sealed the container from the air this did not happen, but Needham claimed that this kept out the 'vital force' necessary for spontaneous generation — a vital force which some later associated with oxygen, when Antoine Lavoisier (1743–1794) had shown the importance of oxygen for life.

It was Louis Pasteur (1822–1895) who showed that microbes actually entered the heated broths from the *air*. He heated broths under three conditions: in a flask open to the air, in a flask immediately sealed after heating and in a flask with a long S-shaped neck (Fig. A).

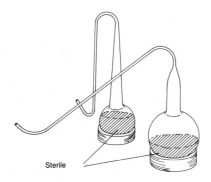

Sterile

Fig. A Pasteur's broths. In swan-neck flasks such as these, Pasteur heated broth so that organisms contained in it were killed. He then left the flasks exposed to the air, the necks remaining open. Because air movements could not carry bacteria down the long curved neck, the broth remained sterile, although the flask was open to the air and to the 'vital force' that many still believed responsible for 'spontaneous generation'.

The open flask soon became turbid from the growth of bacteria which had fallen in from the air. The sealed flask remained clear. *But the S-necked flask also remained clear, despite the fact that it was open to the air and presumably to the 'vital force':* bacteria floating in the air could not be carried down the long thin tube by random air movements and so no bacteria entered the broth in this flask.

The conclusion from these studies was that microbial life, like other life-forms, arose from *living creatures* and could not be 'generated' spontaneously from dead matter, such as meat broth or horsehairs in pond water.

GERM THEORY OF INFECTIOUS DISEASE

People had long been familiar with the results of microbial activity. They had fermented beer or wine, used yeast to leaven bread, and made sauerkraut. And they had likewise encountered the less pleasant effects of microbes — ever since they had gathered in villages and towns, humans had been afflicted by plagues, the contagious nature of such epidemic infections being obvious to ancient observers. Nevertheless epidemics were ascribed to 'poisonous vapours' (*malaria* in fact means 'bad air') — and the 'germ' theory, (i.e. that infections were spread by seeds or 'germs' transmitted from one person to another) was not accepted until late into the nineteenth century, although evidence in favour of it had steadily accumulated.

In the 1830s, microbes were shown to cause an infection of silkworms. In the next 40 years a number of diseases were shown to be caused by or associated with microbes: ringworm, tuberculosis, trichiniasis (an infection by a parasite), anthrax, and leprosy. Louis Pasteur's ideas on the importance of microbes in decomposition and putrefaction led Joseph Lister (1827-1912) to attempt to prevent infection in surgical wounds by the use of antiseptics, with great success. Perhaps the clearest confirmation of the germ theory came from studies of anthrax, then an important disease of sheep and cattle. Casimir Davaine (1812-1882) showed that a rod-shaped bacterium caused anthrax. Robert Koch (1843-1910) confirmed this and went on to prove that the bacterium formed spores which resisted drying and could persist in the soil, still capable of causing disease. In 1881 Pasteur succeeded in protecting sheep and cattle against an injection of anthrax by a culture of those bacilli modified so that they no longer caused disease.

Robert Koch developed the methods which we still use in medical bacteriology today. He grew bacteria on solid media such as the agar plate (p.7 and Plate 1) and 'streaked out' materials to produce single colonies. He also developed stains, to make microbes visible under the microscope. By means of these techniques the causes of most of the common infections — cholera, typhoid, tuberculosis, pneumonia, diphtheria and tetanus — were soon identified. However, it became clear that other diseases were caused by organisms much *smaller* than bacteria — organisms small enough to pass through the filters which held back bacteria; these organisms came to be called *viruses*. Foot-and-mouth disease of cattle was recognised as a virus disease in 1898, and yellow fever was attributed to an agent of this type in 1900. Viruses cannot be easily grown, since they require living cells as hosts and knowledge in this field increased slowly until better methods of investigation were developed in the 1930s. Other scientists, the *parasitologists*, studied diseases such as malaria and hookworm and showed the enormous importance of parasitic infections in the Third World.

To conclude, the study of microbiology and of infectious diseases is today one of the widest domains in science, and one which continues to expand at a rapid pace.

CHAPTER REVIEW

1   Name four new diseases that have occurred during the past 20 years.

2   What is *microbiology* and why is it important?

3   What is the *germ theory of infectious disease* ?

4   What roles do microbes play in nature ?

LOOKING AT BACTERIA

Every body surface in contact with the environment is colonised by bacteria — the 'normal flora' of this site. To begin our examination of the bacterial world, we shall look at the flora of the throat.

A THROAT CULTURE

This is achieved by first taking a swab of the throat of a healthy person, i.e. rubbing a stick tipped with cotton wool on the back of the throat and collecting the secretions; and then inoculating a blood agar plate. The swab is rubbed on the surface of the medium and the inoculum streaked out to separate the bacterial cells (Fig. 2.1). 'Streaking out' is done with a wire loop, which is flamed to sterilise it (Fig. 2.2). Then the plate is placed in an incubator which maintains its temperature at 35^0C for 18-20 hours, an 'overnight culture'.

The next day large numbers of 'colonies' have appeared on the plate (Plate 1). Each colony consists of several million bacterial cells. The colonies are of different sizes and shapes, each characteristic of the species that produced it. Some may be translucent, others grey or white, some are smooth, others rough (Fig. 2.3); some are surrounded by a zone of greening (alpha–haemolysis). Our next step is to examine the bacteria in each colony under the microscope (see 'In the lab', p.10). As light shines *through* the material being examined under the microscope, in order to see microbial cells we must spread them out in a thin layer or *film*. We pick off a colony of each type with the loop and emulsify it in a drop of sterile water, spreading the suspension of cells out to cover a circle about 1 cm in diameter. When the emulsion dries it is 'fixed' by passing it rapidly through the Bunsen flame several times (emulsion side up !).

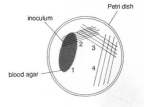

Fig. 2.1 Inoculating a blood agar plate with a throat swab. The bacteriological growth medium, blood agar, is contained in a circular *Petri dish*. After the swab is used to collect the secretions of the throat, it is rubbed on the blood plate at (1). The bacteriological loop is then used to 'streak out' the bacteria deposited, in effect diluting them, so that at (3) and (4) individual colonies are seen. The loop is flamed after streaking out at (2) and at (3), to sterilise it and reduce the numbers of bacteria transferred to the next site.

7

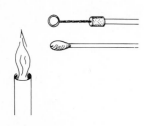

Fig. 2.2 Loop, Bunsen flame and swab — bench tools of the microbiologist.

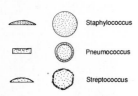

Staphylococcus

Pneumococcus

Streptococcus

Fig. 2.3 Some typical colonies grown from a throat swab. Staphylococcal colonies are 1.5-2 mm across and shiny. Streptococcal colonies are smaller, less than 1mm across, dry and rough. Colonies of *Streptococcus pneumoniae*, the pneumococcus, are flattened and often have a raised edge. Staphylococcal and streptococcal colonies may be surrounded by a clear red zone of beta-haemolysis. Pneumococci and some other streptococci produce alpha-haemolysis (greening).

STAINS

When strongly illuminated by the light passing through them, the cells in such a film appear colourless. Hence we need to colour the cells with a dye — 'stain' them — in order to examine them. A simple stain such as methylene blue, carbolfuchsin or safranin shows us the shape and the arrangement of the cells, but treats all cells pretty well alike. *Differential* stains are often more useful, because they colour some cells but not others, and enable us to distinguish between different sorts of cells. Two differential stains are widely used in microbiology, the Gram stain (see 'In the lab', below) and the acid-fast stain or Ziehl-Neelsen (ZN) stain, which is chiefly used in the detection of tubercle bacilli (p.203). Other stains are used for special purposes, such as the detection of capsules or spores and the examination of fungi and parasites.

IN THE LAB

The Gram stain

This method of staining is named after the Danish bacteriologist Hans Christian Gram (1853–1938) and has nothing to do with the measurement of weight. It is used dozens of times every day in a clinical laboratory. The bacteria to be stained are fixed to a glass slide by heat or alcohol and a solution of crystal violet is applied. This is followed by a solution of iodine, which *mordants* the dye (fixes it more firmly). Then the slide is washed with ethanol or acetone, which removes the dye from some types of bacteria and not from others. Now a *counterstain* (safranin or carbolfuchsin) is applied to dye the cells decolourised by the previous step.

When the slide is examined under the microscope, some sorts of bacteria appear purple/black; these are the ones which have retained the crystal violet and they are termed 'Gram-positive'. Others, from which the crystal violet was removed by the ethanol or acetone, appear orange/red because of the safranin, and are called 'Gram-negative'. The difference between Gram-positive and Gram-negative is not just one of 'complexion', but more importantly reflects fundamental differences in the two types of bacteria (see p.25) — differences which are, for example, reflected in the effect of antibiotics on them.

BACTERIAL SHAPES

Under the microscope bacterial cells are seen to be of different sizes and shapes. Each sphere or rod is an individual organism, capable of growth and division (before heating on the slide), and under favourable circumstances able to give rise to a colony such as we have just picked off the plate. Bacteria have one of three shapes: spheres, rods or spirals (Fig. 2.5). *Cocci* (singular *coccus*, from a Greek word 'berry'), are usually spherical, but can be football-shaped or flattened on one side. Most cocci of medical importance are about one micrometre, μm (or 'micron') in diameter (*micron*, μ = 1/1000 millimetre i.e. one millionth of a metre). Bacterial cells reproduce by dividing into two. If cocci divide only in one plane (direction) they give rise to a chain and are termed *streptococci*. If they divide in more than one plane, they may form sheets or grape-like clusters, *staphylococci*. Some cocci are usually found in pairs (pneumococci and gonococci). Rods are termed *bacilli* (singular *bacillus*). They are commonly 3-5 μm long and usually occur singly, sometimes in chains or side-by-side like a fence. *Spiral* bacteria may have only a gentle curve (*vibrio* type), or up to 20 turns (*spirillum* type or *spirochaete*). Bacteria inherit their shape, which helps to identify them. Some, however, are inherently variable — for example *Haemophilus* usually grows as short Gram-negative rods, but may show occasional long filaments and round forms as well. Growth conditions and antibiotics also influence the shape of bacteria.

MICROBE SIZES

The bodies of all living creatures are made up of cells. A red cell from human blood has a diameter of around 7–8 μm. To cover the full stop at the end of this sentence with a layer of red cells one cell thick would require about 700 such cells. A similar layer of staphylococci would contain 40 000 cells. Figure 2.4 compares the relative sizes of various microbes with a red cell. Again note that microbes are measured in microns — we obviously need to magnify microbes many times in order to see them. A *microscope* is consequently an essential instrument in any microbiology laboratory (see 'In the lab', following).

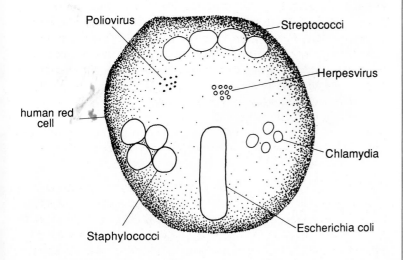

Fig. 2.4 Relative sizes of microbes. The human red cell (see colour plate 10) is 7-8 μm in diameter. Staphylococci and streptococci are about 1 μm in diameter. A Gram-negative rod such as *Escherichia coli* is about 1 μm in diameter and 3-5 μm long. The cells of *Chlamydia* are smaller (0.2-0.5 μm in diameter) and viruses are smaller again. 700 of these red cells side-by-side would cover the fullstop at the end of this sentence.

IN THE LAB

The microscope

The light microscope. The microscope that Antonie van Leeuwenhoek used (p.4) consisted only of a single lens, and the resultant image was unclear. The *modern compound* light microscope, on the other hand, consists of two magnifying systems — the objective lens and the ocular lens (Fig. A & B). Light passes from the light source in the base of the microscope, through the specimen and into the objective lens, where the image of the specimen is magnified. The image is magnified again by the ocular lens.

The usual objective lenses yield magnifications of ×10, ×40 and ×90 or ×100. The ocular lenses magnify ×8 or ×10, so that the final image seen by the observer is magnified from 80-fold to 1000-fold. A magnification of ×80 to ×400 can be used to examine human or animal cells or certain types of (large) microbes. A higher magnification, ×800 to ×1000, is needed to see bacteria. In order to obtain a clear image at high magnification oil is placed on the slide between the specimen and the objective lens. (These lenses are called 'oil-immersion objectives'. The oil prevents scattering of the light and loss of clarity of the image.)

The ability of a microscope to reveal fine detail is termed its 'resolving power'; this is its power to permit the observer to see, as separate objects, two dots very close together. With ordinary light a good microscope can resolve two points 0.2 microns apart. Because resolution is limited by the wave-length of visible light it is impossible to improve on this, except by using a different type of illumination (see *electron microscope*). Other types of microscopes used for special purposes are the *darkground* microscope and the *phase-contrast* microscope, both of which use special techniques of illumination to reveal living organisms without the need for fixation and staining.

The electron microscope. Many of the structures described in microbial cells are too small to be visible with the light microscope, the resolving power of which is limited by the properties of visible light. In order to achieve greater resolution, a 'light beam' of *electrons* is used in the *electron* microscope. A beam of electrons has a wave-length only about 1/100000th that of visible light and can therefore reveal structures down to the size of small molecules. The beam travels in a vacuum and is focussed not by glass lenses but by electromagnetic ones. Magnifications up to ×100000 and beyond are possible. Some electron-micrographs are shown in Figure 2.5.

NAMING MICROBES — GENUS AND SPECIES

Like other living creatures microbes are given two scientific names — genus and species. 'Genus' (plural 'genera') is the larger grouping

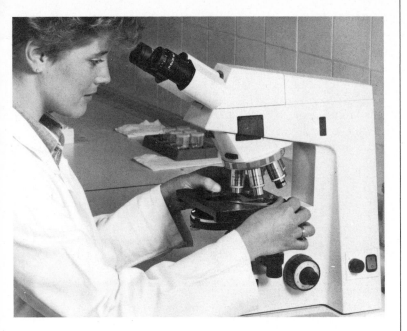

Fig. A A modern light microscope. Note the binocular head (using both eyes reduces eyestrain), the revolving nosepiece bearing five objectives, and the mechanical stage, which enables the operator to move the specimen in any direction.

(b) light microscope   (c) electron microscope

electron source

light source

magnetic
condenser

glass
condenser

(a) human eye

specimen

object

magnetic
objective
lens

glass objective
lens

object

magnetic
objective
lens

intermediate image

intermediate image

magnetic
projector

eyepiece

lens

image on
retina

eye

view screen

eye

Fig. B Optical systems of the eye, the light microscope and the electron microscope. The *eye* has a single lens; light from the object passes through it and forms an image on the light-sensitive cells of the retina. The *light microscope* has an illumination system which directs visible light through the specimen. The image formed by the objective lens is further magnified by the eyepiece. The principle of the *electronmicroscope* is the same. Electrons are generated from a source, pass through a magnetic condenser lens and through the object; an image is formed by the magnetic objective lens and further magnified by the projector lens; the image then appears on an observation screen or photographic plate.

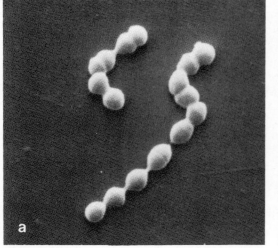

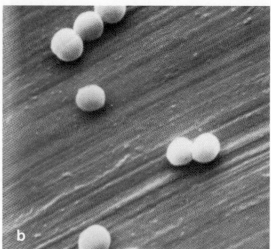

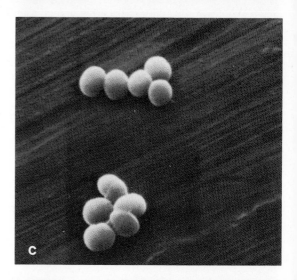

Fig. 2.5 Scanning electronmicrographs of bacterial cells. **(a)** Pneumococci in short chains. **(b)** Streptococci — singles, a pair and a short chain. **(c)** Clumps of cocci. **(d)** Rod-shaped bacteria, a single cell and pairs. **(e)** A spirochete, *Treponema pallidum*.

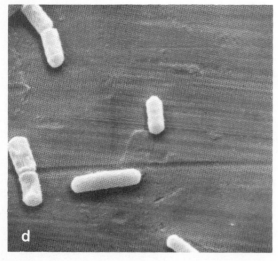

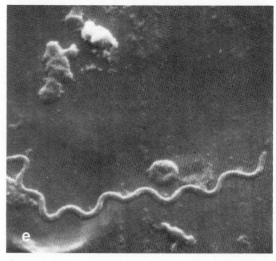

and is written with an initial capital letter. Examples are *Staphylococcus*, and *Escherichia*. There may be many 'species' within one genus. Species are written with a small letter — *Staphylococcus aureus*, *Escherichia coli*. They are modern Latin words and appear in italics. The names are chosen to tell us something about the microbe. For example, the name *Escherichia coli* honours a German scientist named Theodor Escherich and refers to a microbe commonly found in the colon; the cells of *Staphylococcus aureus* form clumps (Greek *staphylos*) of cocci, and the colonies are usually yellow (Latin *aureus*).

CHAPTER REVIEW

1   What is 'normal flora'?
2   How do you inoculate a plate of bacteriological medium ?
3   (a)   What is the Gram stain?
      (b)   Why is it used?
4   What are the shapes and arrangements of bacterial cells?
5   What are *genus* and *species?*
6   How do you make a film from a bacterial colony?
7   (a)   List the different types of microscopes.
      (b)   What are the advantages and disadvantages of the electron microscope, compared with the light microscope?

SOME PRINCIPLES OF CHEMISTRY

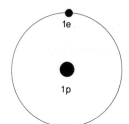

(a) Hydrogen atom

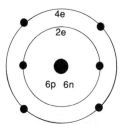

(b) Carbon atom

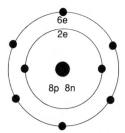

(c) Oxygen atom

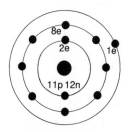

(d) Sodium atom

ATOMS

All matter — whether living or dead, whether animal, vegetable or mineral — is composed of minute particles called *atoms*. We stated in the previous chapter that 700 red cells were needed to cover a full stop. More than a *million million* carbon atoms are required for the same task.

Atoms consist of a nucleus and one or more encircling electrons. The nucleus itself is made up of protons and neutrons. The proton has a positive charge, the electron an equal negative charge, and the neutron is uncharged. The proton and the neutron are equal in weight, and each is nearly 2000 times heavier than the electron. In every atom there are equal numbers of protons and electrons and hence of positive and negative charges. For example, the lightest atom, hydrogen, has one proton in the nucleus and one electron in orbit about it (Fig. 3.1(a)). Carbon has six protons, six neutrons and six electrons; oxygen has 8, 8 and 8; and sodium has 11, 12 and 11 (Fig. 3.1(b)-(d)). The largest naturally occurring atom, uranium, has 92 protons and electrons.

The *atomic weight* almost exactly equals the total number of protons and neutrons (electrons weigh very little). The *atomic number* is the number of protons in the atom's nucleus: hydrogen therefore has atomic number 1, carbon 6, oxygen 8 and sodium 11. An element is made up of atoms all having the same atomic number. The *chemical* characteristics of atoms, i.e. the way(s) in which they react with other atoms, are determined by their number of protons and electrons. Each element has a symbol, usually an abbreviation of the English or Latin name of the element. Thus hydrogen has the

Fig. 3.1 Structure of **(a)** hydrogen atom, **(b)** carbon atom, **(c)** oxygen atom, **(d)** sodium atom.

14

symbol H, carbon the symbol C and iron the symbol Fe (from the Latin word *ferrum* = iron). Table 3.1 lists some characteristics of elements occurring in all living creatures. Only about one fourth of the known elements are found in living matter, and of these hydrogen, carbon, oxygen and nitrogen are the most abundant by far.

TABLE 3.1 CHARACTERISTICS OF SOME COMMON ELEMENTS

Element	Atomic number	Number of protons and electrons	Atomic weight	Symbol
Hydrogen	1	1	1	H
Carbon	6	6	12	C
Nitrogen	7	7	14	N
Oxygen	8	8	16	O
Sodium	11	11	23	Na
Magnesium	12	12	24	Mg
Phosphorus	15	15	31	P
Sulphur	16	16	32	S
Chlorine	17	17	35.5	Cl
Potassium	19	19	39	K
Iron	26	26	56	Fe

MOLECULES

These consist of two or more linked atoms. The unit of weight for molecules and atoms is the dalton (approx. equivalent to the weight of the smallest atom, hydrogen). The sodium atom for instance weighs 23 daltons, i.e. it weighs 23 times as much as a hydrogen atom; the carbon atom weighs 12 daltons and the nitrogen atom 14 daltons. A molecule of NaCl (sodium chloride), common salt, weighs 58.5 daltons, and a molecule of carbon dioxide (CO_2) 44 daltons. Molecules which are characteristic of living tissue have bigger molecular weights than these — often much bigger. Many proteins for instance have molecular weights greater than 100000.

ISOTOPES

Atoms which have the same number of protons in the nucleus — i.e. are the same element — may differ in the numbers of neutrons they possess. For instance carbon (atomic weight 12) usually has 6 protons and 6 neutrons, but a small fraction of carbon atoms possesses 7 or 8 neutrons, and therefore have atomic weights of 13 and 14 respectively. The symbols for these *isotopes* are ^{13}C and ^{14}C. Since the chemical properties of an element are determined by the number of protons and electrons, such isotopes will be indistinguishable in their chemical behaviour, and sophisticated physical methods are needed to detect them. Some isotopes are unstable and break down spontaneously into other elements, giving off rays in the process; these isotopes are said to be *radioactive*. Isotopes are used in biological and medical research and also in the treatment of disease (see Milestones, '*A Phage cocktail*', p.54).

ELECTRONS AND REACTIVITY

The electrons surrounding the nucleus are arranged in *electron shells*: a shell consists of those electrons which are the same distance from the nucleus (see Fig. 3.1). The number of electrons in the *outer* shell largely determines the *chemical properties* of the atom: the way it reacts with other atoms. The maximum number of electrons in the innermost shell is 2, in the second shell 8, in the third 8 (or 18 if there is a fourth shell); we will not be concerned here with atoms larger than these. When the outer shell is filled, the atom does not readily react with other atoms. However, when the outer shell has fewer than the maximum number of electrons, atoms have a greater tendency to react with other atoms, i.e. to lose, gain or share electrons to bring the outer shell up to its maximum number and achieve a stable configuration.

Sodium, which has one electron in its outermost shell, tends to *donate* this electron: this leaves it with an outer shell of 8 (in its second electron shell); see Figure 3.2(a). It thus becomes *positively* charged, since it has one more proton than the number of electrons. The symbol for the sodium ion is Na^+. On the other hand, chlorine, which has seven electrons in the outer shell, tends to *gain* one electron (and one negative charge); symbol Cl^- (Fig.3.2(b)). If the ion has more than one charge this is written in a similar way: Mg^{2+}, PO_4^{3-}.

Fig. 3.2 (a) Sodium atom and sodium ion. The loss of the outermost electron leaves the ion with a stable configuration of 8 electrons in the outer orbit. The result is an excess of one positive charge (11 protons, but 10 electrons). **(b)** Chlorine atom and chloride ion. Gaining one electron gives the chlorine atom the stable configuration of 8 electrons in the orbit and one negative charge in excess.

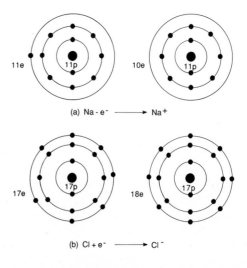

(a) Na - e⁻ ⟶ Na⁺

(b) Cl + e⁻ ⟶ Cl⁻

ATOMIC BONDS

The atoms in molecules are bound together by chemical *bonds*, of which there are several types. Many inorganic molecules are made up of positively and negatively charged particles called *ions* (Fig. 3.2). In the solid state these are held together by the attraction of positive and negative charges: *ionic bonds* (see Fig. 3.3(a)). When dissolved in water, they dissociate into their component ions.

Atoms may also be held together by the sharing of electrons, *covalent bonds*. It is this type of bond which links the component atoms of proteins, carbohydrates and other compounds that make up living cells; such compounds are referred to as *organic compounds*. Sharing one pair of electrons gives rise to a single covalent bond (e.g. C-C); sharing two pairs creates a double covalent bond (C=C) (see Fig. 3.3(b)). Atoms linked by covalent bonds do not dissociate in water to form ions.

Hydrogen bonds are forces of attraction existing between hydrogen atoms and other atoms when hydrogen is linked to oxygen or nitrogen in molecules. These bonds are much weaker than covalent bonds, but between two large molecules many such bonds may form, and the result is a bond of considerable strength (Fig. 3.3(c)).

ACIDS, BASES AND SALTS

As has been stated, substances that are linked by ionic bonds separate into their component ions when dissolved in water. Substances which thus release hydrogen ions and one or more negative ions are called *acids*. Substances which release hydroxyl ions (OH⁻), and one or more positive ions are termed *bases (alkalis)*. A *salt* dissociates into positively and negatively charged ions, none of which are H^+ or OH^- (Fig. 3.4).

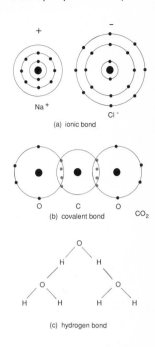

Fig. 3.3 (a) Ionic bond, **(b)** covalent bond, **(c)** hydrogen bond. In an ionic bond, ions are held together by the attraction of positive and negative charges. In covalent bonds, atoms share electrons, so that each has an outer ring of 8. In hydrogen bonds, a force of attraction exists between the hydrogen atom and an oxygen (or nitrogen) atom.

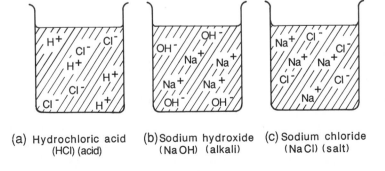

(a) Hydrochloric acid (HCl) (acid)

(b) Sodium hydroxide (NaOH) (alkali)

(c) Sodium chloride (NaCl) (salt)

Fig. 3.4 Solution of **(a)** an acid (HCl), **(b)** an alkali (NaOH), and **(c)** a salt (NaCl). When dissolved in water, acids, alkalis and salts separate into their component ions, which take part in reactions independently.

pH

Living creatures consist largely of water (75% or more) and many ions are present in the intracellular and extracellular fluids. Because the amounts of acid and base in the cell greatly affect its activities, these amounts are carefully controlled. The degree of *acidity* or *alkalinity* is expressed by the *pH scale*, a negative logarithmic scale extending from 0 to 14 (Fig. 3.5); in such a scale an increase or decrease of one unit means a tenfold change. At pH 2, ten times as much acid is present as at pH 3, but only one tenth as much alkali; at pH 9, 100 times as much alkali is present as at pH 7, but only 1/100th as much acid. The more hydrogen ion (H^+) present in the solution, the more acidic it is. The more hydroxyl ion (OH^-) present, the more basic it is. At pH 7, equal amounts of acid and base are present and the solution is *neutral*. The interior of most cells has a pH close to 7. The pH of human blood is 7.4 (7.35–7.45).

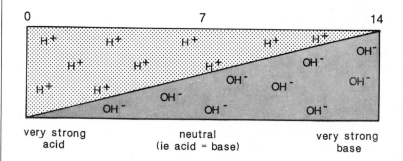

| 0 | 7 | 14 |

very strong acid   neutral (ie acid = base)   very strong base

Fig. 3.5 The pH scale.

CHEMICAL REACTIONS

The energy that takes you up the stairs, the change that comes over the lawn clippings in the compost heap, the smell of the chop that fell behind the fridge last week are all manifestations of *chemical reactions*. Most of the activities of living creatures are chemical reactions.

In chemical reactions, bonds are formed or broken between atoms and molecules. To form a bond requires energy — *chemical energy;* conversely, when a bond is broken, energy is released (usually as heat). Many familiar processes are chemical reactions. Examples are the rusting of iron: iron (Fe) + oxygen (O) →rust (Fe_2O_3), i.e.

$$4Fe + 3O_2 \rightarrow 2\ Fe_2O_3$$

and the burning of methane (a component of natural gas):

$$CH_4 + 2O_2 \rightarrow CO_2 + 2H_2O$$

A further example is provided by the green plant, which traps and uses the energy of sunlight to carry out the following process (the equation summarises a number of reactions): carbon dioxide (CO_2) + water (H_2O) → glucose + oxygen, i.e.

$$6\ CO_2 + 6\ H_2O \rightarrow C_6H_{12}O_6 + 6O_2$$

When an animal consumes the plant, it breaks the glucose down to carbon dioxide and water again and releases the energy, which it uses for its own purposes.

All chemical reactions are *reversible* in theory — in practice most tend to move definitely in one direction or another, and require the input of energy to reverse them (e.g. to reverse the rusting of iron requires the burning of much coke in a smelter.). When wood is burnt the carbohydrates of the wood are converted to energy, just as the carbohydrates of bread are when we eat the bread, or when the blue mould spreads over it. In the fire, the reaction only proceeds at a high temperature.

ENZYMES

In the animal or the microbe, the reaction proceeds at environmental temperatures ($25\text{-}40^0C$ or lower). Living creatures use *enzymes* (Fig. 3.6) to influence chemical reactions in this way. Enzymes are *catalysts* — catalysts accelerate chemical reactions. Enzymes possess an *active site* with which the molecule or molecules combine.

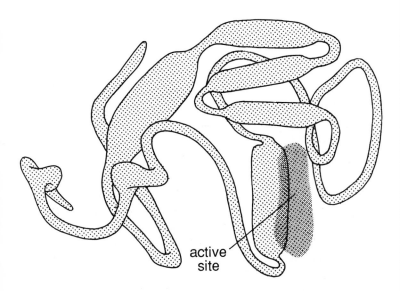

active
site

Fig. 3.6 Lysozyme, an enzyme. Lysozyme consists of a single polypeptide chain. There are four 'disulphide bridges' (i.e. links between two sulphur atoms). The properties of the constituent amino acids and the disulphide bridges bring about the complicated folding, essential for the activity of the enzyme.

Combination with the enzyme alters the shape of the reacting molecule(s) and specifically weakens the chemical bonds involved, so that the reaction is completed more easily, more rapidly and at a lower temperature. A living creature contains anything from several hundred to several thousand enzymes, each of which brings about one specific chemical reaction. In some cases a larger molecule is broken down, as in the digestion of food, in others two smaller molecules are combined. The names of enzymes end in *-ase*; for example, a proteinase breaks down proteins and a DNAase hydrolyses DNA.

We will discuss the types of reactions characteristic of growth, reproduction and metabolism in chapters 5 and 6.

CHAPTER REVIEW

1   Define the following terms:
     (a)   atom
     (b)   element
     (c)   molecule
     (d)   proton
     (e)   electron
     (f)   neutron
     (g)   isotope
     (h)   radioactivity
2   List and describe three major types of chemical bond.
3   Describe the pH scale. What is the pH of blood?
4   What are acids, bases and salts?
5   What does an enzyme do?

MICROBES INSIDE AND OUT: ANATOMY AND STRUCTURE

THE CELL

The cell is the basic unit of life. All living creatures — the whale, the rabbit, the pine tree, the staphylococcus, and the mosquito — despite their superficial differences, are composed of cells. Cells can grow and divide to produce progeny cells which themselves can grow and divide again — these complicated tasks are the essential features of the cell. To perform them the cell must take in *food* — small molecules such as glucose, amino acids, oxygen and carbon dioxide — and convert them into larger molecules that make up the cellular structure and machinery. Cells are chemically very complex; even a bacterial cell weighing only a few million millionths of a gram (say $1\text{-}5 \times 10^{-12}$ g) contains several hundred different small molecules and probably 2000 or more different sorts of large molecules. The small *organic* molecules are amino acids and other nitrogen compounds, sugars, fatty acids and growth factors (vitamins), which are energy sources and building blocks for cellular synthetic processes. The *inorganic* ions (Mg^{++}, Ca^{++}, K^+, Na^+, Cl^-, PO_4^{3-}, SO_4^{2-}) are very important, since they play a major role in maintaining constant the internal environment of the cell. K^+, Mg^{2+} and PO_4^{3-} occur in large quantities inside the cell, even though they may be present only in low concentrations outside; the microbial cell expends energy to accumulate these essential ions and to control the amount of H^+ and OH^-, i.e. the intracellular pH.

The chief large molecules *(macromolecules)* in cells are proteins, carbohydrates, nucleic acids and lipids; they are usually built up of many smaller molecules of the same type.

21

PROTEINS

Proteins make up more than 50% of the cell's dry weight (i.e. the weight after the water is removed). Proteins serve several functions in cells. They form part of the cell wall and of structures inside the cell. They also carry out most of the biochemical processes which provide the cell with energy and enable it to grow and reproduce — the fibres that contract to change the shape of an amoeba, the carriers that transport substances through the cell membrane, and the toxins that sometimes cause illnesses are proteins.

Proteins contain carbon (C), hydrogen (H), oxygen (O), nitrogen (N) and often sulphur (S). They are composed of *amino acids*. There are 20 different amino acids in living matter, all having a similar structure (Fig. 4.1). The skeleton of the molecule contains at least two carbon atoms. To one carbon an oxygen atom and a hydroxyl (OH-) group are bonded: to the other is attached an amino group (-NH$_2$). 'R' in Fig. 4.1 indicates the presence of some other atom or group of atoms: in the simplest amino acid, glycine, R = H, in alanine, R = -CH$_3$; in serine, R = -CH$_2$OH, and in other amino acids the group may be larger and more complex.

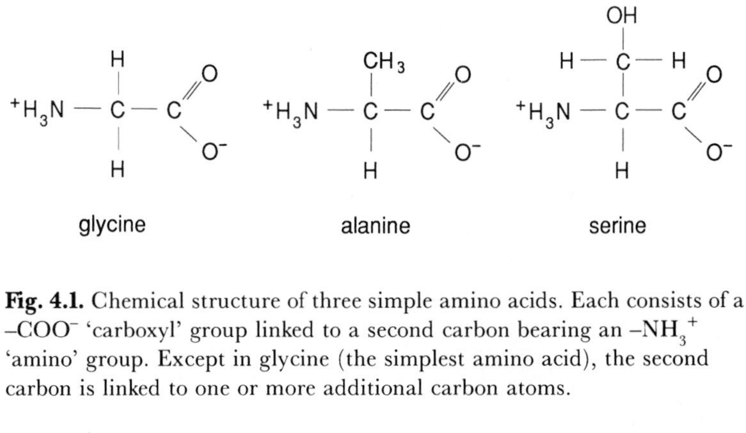

glycine   alanine   serine

Fig. 4.1. Chemical structure of three simple amino acids. Each consists of a –COO⁻ 'carboxyl' group linked to a second carbon bearing an –NH$_3^+$ 'amino' group. Except in glycine (the simplest amino acid), the second carbon is linked to one or more additional carbon atoms.

When two amino acids are joined, a *peptide bond* is formed. Repeating this process creates a peptide chain (Fig. 4.2). The resulting 'polypeptide' may contain hundreds of amino acids. One or more polypeptide chains make up a *protein*. Figure 4.3 shows the polypeptide chains of a small protein: insulin. Although we have drawn them as straight, in truth each peptide chain is a spiral, and both spirals fold to produce a complex three-dimensional structure. Proteins play their biological roles only when they retain their folded structure (Fig. 3.6). The polypeptide chain can be unfolded by heat or certain chemicals (e.g. disinfectants, p.172) and then the protein loses its biological activity. This unfolding is termed *denaturation*.

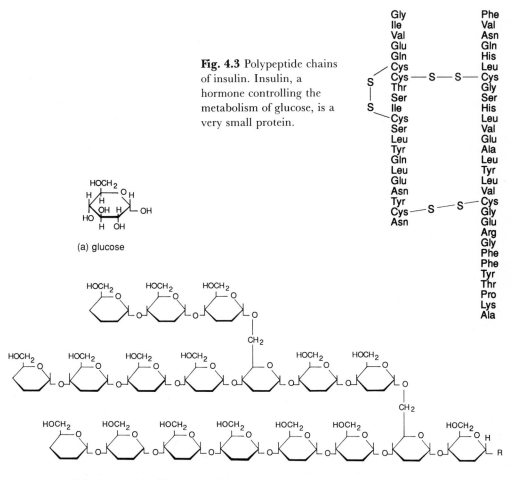

Fig. 4.2 Formation of a peptide bond. A covalent bond is formed between the carbon of the carboxyl group and the nitrogen of the amino group. In the process, a molecule of water is also generated.

Fig. 4.3 Polypeptide chains of insulin. Insulin, a hormone controlling the metabolism of glucose, is a very small protein.

(a) glucose

(b) glycogen (simplified presentation: each unit represents a glucose molecule)

Fig. 4.4 Structure of **(a)** glucose and **(b)** glycogen. Glucose is a '6-carbon' sugar. The polysaccharide glycogen, a storage carbohydrate of animals, is made up of glucose units linked in branching chains. Starch is a similar polysaccharide found in plants.

CARBOHYDRATES

These are so called because they contain hydrogen and oxygen in the same proportions as water - i.e. the carbon is 'hydrated'. The formula of glucose is $C_6H_{12}O_6$ and of ribose, which occurs in nucleic acids, $C_5H_{10}O_5$. Sucrose (cane sugar) and starch are also carbohydrates. In glycogen many glucose molecules are linked together in branching chains (Fig. 4.4(b)). Carbohydrates have many roles. They are 'burnt' to provide energy for other cellular processes, they function as energy stores; they form compounds with proteins and are part of nucleic acids; and they make up part of the bacterial or fungal cell wall.

Fig. 4.5 Structure of **(a)** a phospholipid and **(b)** a fatty acid.

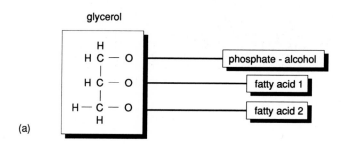

FATS

Lipids (fats) also consist of C, H and O, but the proportion of oxygen in them is less. Lipids are an important component of membranes. They are insoluble in water; because of this they can retain water and thus function as a barrier separating the contents of the cell, the cytoplasm, from the environment. Lipids are compounds of an alcohol (glycerol) with fatty acids and sometimes other compounds. From Figure 4.5(b) we can see that a fatty acid is a long chain of carbon atoms with hydrogens attached, terminated by a carboxyl group (-COOH). *Phospholipids*, which form the major part of cell membranes, contain a phosphoric acid residue as well as fatty acids.

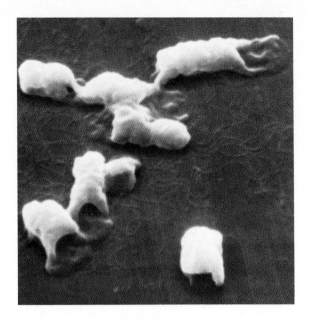

Fig. 4.6 *Proteus mirabilis*, a
Gram-negative rod, with
numerous flagella, seen as
long slender threads
surrounding the cells
(electronmicrograph).

PROCARYOTIC AND EUCARYOTIC CELLS, AND VIRUSES

The cells of living creatures are of two types: *procaryotic* and *eucaryotic* — *caryotic* means 'possessing a nucleus'. Bacteria are procaryotes; many other microbes and the higher animals and plants are eucaryotes. All cells are chemically similar — nucleic acids, proteins, carbohydrates and lipids are found in both types, and the biochemical reactions whereby they obtain energy, grow and reproduce are closely related. It is in *structure* that they differ. Procaryotic cells are in general smaller than eucaryotic ones. The *viruses*, which are not cells, are smaller again. We shall discuss microbial structure within the three diverse groups of procaryotes, viruses and eucaryotes.

1 PROCARYOTES

BACTERIA: STRUCTURE

Bacteria have a relatively simple structure (Fig. 4.7).
Cell wall. The cell wall encloses the *cell membrane* and cytoplasm, with the genetic material (cytoplasm = everything inside the cell membrane). Outside the cell wall is the *glycocalyx*. The cell wall itself is a complex meshwork which determines the cell's shape. As shown earlier, bacteria are classified as Gram-positive or Gram-negative, according to their reaction in the Gram stain (see chapter 2).

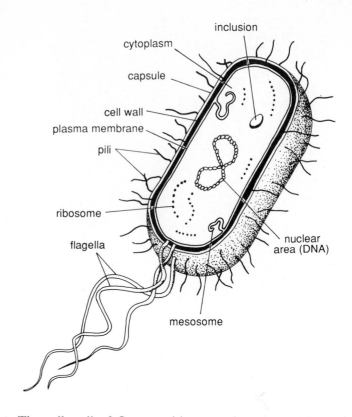

Fig. 4.7 The bacterial cell. The diagram shows a typical cell sliced lengthwise, the main structures labelled.

The cell wall of Gram-positive organisms is made up of carbohydrate chains built up of repeating units consisting of two different sugars. These chains are cross-linked by peptide bridges of several amino-acids linked together, so that the whole cell is enclosed in a single giant molecule (Fig.4.8). This rigid network of carbohydrate and peptide is called *peptidoglycan* and in Gram-positive organisms it is several layers thick. The two sugars forming the carbohydrate chains do not occur in higher animals and plants — the peptidoglycan molecule is unique to bacteria. Another type of carbohydrate, *teichoic acid*, is also present, linked to the peptidoglycan and to the cell membrane beneath. Outside the peptidoglycan layer there is often a layer of protein molecules.

The cell wall of Gram-negative bacteria is more complicated. The peptidoglycan network has the same basic structure as in Gram-positive bacteria, but is not so thick and is sandwiched between the outer membrane (to which it is covalently linked) and the cell membrane (Fig. 4.9). The outer membrane consists of *lipoproteins* and *lipopolysaccharides* and is an important barrier between the environment and the cytoplasm of the cell. Through this layer pass protein channels, along which food, salts (and antibiotics) pass to the interior. Part of the lipopolysaccharide is made up of chains of sugars (the O antigens) by which many Gram-negative rods can be identified. The lipopolysaccharide is called *endotoxin* and has striking toxic effects on humans and higher animals.

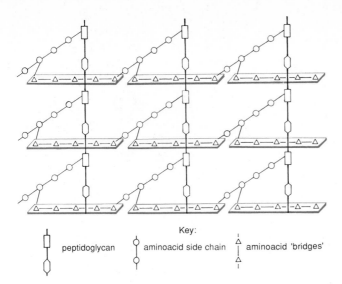

Fig. 4.8 Structure of peptidoglycan. Peptidoglycan is an important constituent of the bacterial cell wall. Long chains of two sugars are linked to each other by amino-acid side-chains and amino-acid bridges. Thus the cell is encased in a single huge molecule.

Key:

peptidoglycan   aminoacid side chain   aminoacid 'bridges'

Outside the cell wall there is usually another layer, the *glycocalyx*. This is made up of carbohydrate or polypeptide or both. It may be closely attached to the cell wall as a capsule, or more loosely as a slime layer. The glycocalyx may play several roles. For instance the capsule of many pathogens is important in their ability to resist phagocytosis and destruction (see p.137). In some habitats, such as on the surfaces of teeth, or on plastic devices inserted into humans, the glycocalyx builds up to form a matrix that secures the adhesion of numerous layers of bacteria and may prevent antibiotics from acting on them.

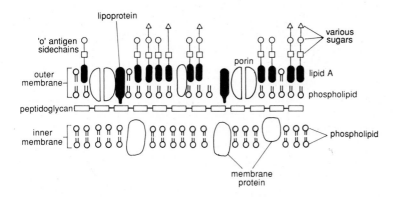

Fig. 4.9 The cell wall in Gram-negative bacteria. Both inner and outer membranes consist of phospholipid layers, in which other molecules are embedded. In the inner membrane are membrane proteins; in the outer membrane are porins (proteins constituting pores through which substances pass to the interior), lipoproteins and lipid A with its attached O-antigen side-chains. Between the inner and outer membranes is the peptidoglycan layer, usually not as thick as in Gram-positive cells.

Flagella (singular flagellum, i.e. 'whip'). These are long filaments which propel bacteria - not by waving back and forth, but by rotating after the fashion of a propeller. Bacteria may have one, several or many flagella, or none at all, according to the species (e.g. Fig. 4.6). Flagella are very fine and are most reliably seen by electron-microscopy. The ability to swim about, *motility*, is a feature used in identification and can be detected by watching the organisms in a drop of medium under the microscope. Staphylococci and streptococci are non-motile, some Gram-positive rods and many (but by no means all) Gram-negative rods are motile.

Cell membrane. Inside the peptidoglycan layer is the cell membrane bounding the cytoplasm of the cell. This membrane is a double layer of phospholipid into which protein molecules are set (Fig. 4.9). The phospholipid molecules are arranged with the glycerol-phosphate 'heads' on the surfaces and the fatty-acid 'tails' extending inwards. Some protein molecules in the membrane are attached to the surface, while others go right through the membrane and provide channels for the transport of substances across it. This membrane is selectively *permeable*; it allows some molecules to pass, while holding back others (p.48).

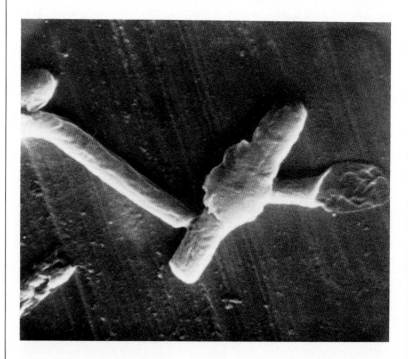

Fig. 4.10 A *Clostridium* species showing a spore, seen distending the middle of the rod (electronmicrograph).

Cytoplasm. The *cytoplasm* of the cell is a viscous mixture of proteins, nucleic acids, carbohydrates, lipids, the smaller molecules from which they are synthesised, and inorganic ions. Within the cytoplasm take place all the biochemical reactions that maintain the living cell and enable it to reproduce. We can distinguish a number of structures in it. In the nuclear area lies the genetic material of the cell, the *chromosome*, a single circular molecule of deoxyribonucleic acid (DNA) in which is encoded all the genetic information of the cell. In procaryotic cells, the nuclear area is not delimited from the rest of the cytoplasm by a membrane (as is the nucleus in eucaryotic cells). In addition, bacteria often carry, separate from the chromosome, smaller circles of DNA called *plasmids*.

Ribosomes. Ribosomes are made up of ribonucleic acid (RNA) and protein, and are involved in protein synthesis (see chapter 6). They are present in thousands in the cytoplasm. Other storage granules, polysaccharide, lipid and phosphate are sometimes present.

Spores. When food is scarce, some bacteria (of the genera *Clostridium* and *Bacillus*) form spores — highly resistant bodies which can survive adverse conditions for years and are very difficult to destroy by heat and chemicals (Fig. 4.10). Under suitable conditions they can germinate to yield actively-growing cells again. In Gram stains, spores appear neither purple-black nor red, but colourless because the dyes do not penetrate them.

OTHER TYPES OF PROCARYOTES

There are a number of procaryotic organisms which do not fully fit the above description of Gram-positive and Gram-negative bacteria. In structure and biochemical activities they are clearly bacteria, containing both RNA and DNA (viruses have only one type of nucleic acid). The *Mycoplasmas* (Fig. 4.11) are the smallest free-living microbes. They resemble most closely small Gram-negative bacteria, but lack a cell wall. While as small as the larger viruses, they do not require intact cells for growth. Most can grow in the presence or absence of oxygen (i.e. they are 'facultative anaerobes'). They reproduce by binary fission (i.e. dividing in two) as bacteria do. On agar they grow slowly, forming tiny colonies, at most 300 microns across and often much smaller. The cells grow down into the agar and produce a 'fried egg' appearance. For growth most require sterols (complex lipids otherwise present only in eucaryotic cells) and use glucose or arginine as energy sources. Some mycoplasmas infect humans.

Rickettsiae. The Rickettsiae (Fig. 4.12) are among the smallest bacteria and are obligate intracellular parasites (i.e they can grow only inside other cells). They are very short bacilli, and very variable in shape. The Gram reaction is negative. Most cannot be grown in the usual bacteriological media, but only in cultured cells, eggs or experimental animals. Culture should only be attempted in specially equipped laboratories, since the organisms are very infectious. Apart from *Coxiella burnetii*, they will survive only briefly outside a host. Rickettsiae are responsible for a number of infections in humans, such as typhus and Q fever.

Fig. 4.11 *Mycoplasma pneumoniae* growing as small spheres on an agar medium (electronmicrograph).

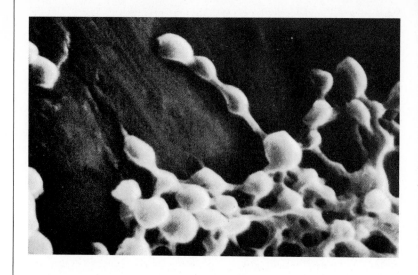

Fig. 4.12 *Rickettsia rickettsii.* This electronmicrograph shows the rickettsial cells in the cytoplasm of an infected epithelial cell. Rickettsiae can only multiply inside eucaryotic cells.

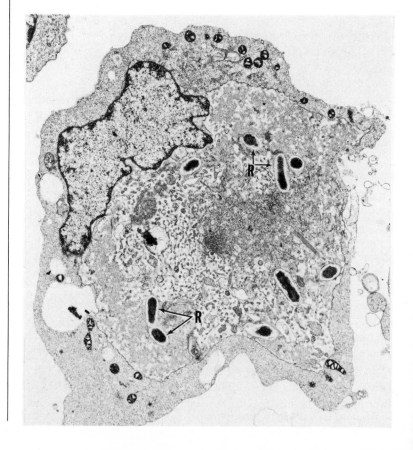

Chlamydiae. The chlamydiae are obligate intracellular parasites of eucaryotic cells (Fig. 4.13). They are small organisms — the elementary body being only 300 μm in diameter. They possess a cell wall of Gram-negative type. They can synthesise protein, but not the energy carrier adenosine triphosphate (ATP), and are thus energy parasites. Their existence was first detected because of the inclusions that they form in infected cells. The chlamydiae do not reproduce by simple binary fission, as do most bacteria, but have a unique developmental cycle within the cell. Again, because of their infectiousness, isolation of these organisms is attempted only in special laboratories.

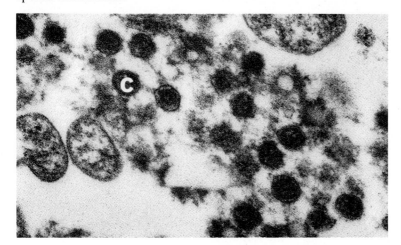

Fig. 4.13 *Chlamydia.* Numerous organisms are seen in the cytoplasm of the host cell, as round to oval structures (labelled 'C') (electronmicrograph).

2 VIRUSES

Virus is a Latin word meaning 'poison' or 'venom'. It has come to be used for a type of microbe different from any we have discussed so far. Historically, the first feature of viruses to be noted was their small size — they could pass through filters which would retain the smallest bacteria. Next it was realised that they could not multiply except inside the appropriate host cell; animal, plant and bacterial cells are all host to some viruses. The study of *bacterial* viruses, bacteriophages, 'eaters of bacteria', has made particularly important contributions to modern biology.

STRUCTURE

A virus is *not* a cell. 'A virus is a piece of bad news wrapped up in protein' (P and J Medawar) — bad news, because the genetic information in the virus may disturb the cell, even to the point of killing it. Outside its particular host cell the virus exists as an infectious particle, the *virion* (Fig. 4.14). This consists of a nucleic acid (DNA or RNA, but not both) whereas all other microbes contain both DNA and RNA. The nucleic acid is enclosed in a layer of protein, the *capsid*; some animal viruses have a membrane outside this coat again, the *envelope*. Thus basically a virus is a bundle of genes

Fig. 4.14 The shapes of viruses. The viruses of animals are naked or enveloped, icosahedral or helical. Poliovirus is a naked icosahedral virus, influenza an enveloped helical one, and herpes an enveloped icosahedral virus

wrapped in a protein coat. Inside the host cell the virus exists chiefly as nucleic acid — which controls the synthesis, by the host cell's enzymes, of more viral nucleic acid and of the protein units that make up its outer coat.

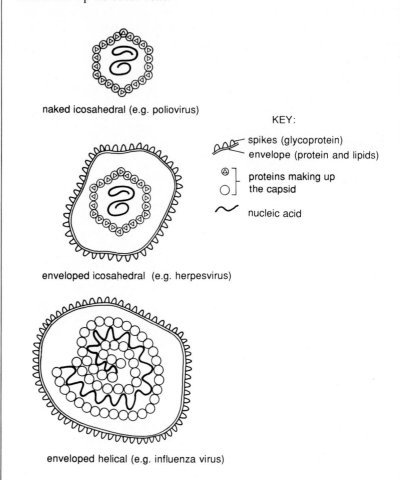

naked icosahedral (e.g. poliovirus)

KEY:

spikes (glycoprotein)
envelope (protein and lipids)

proteins making up the capsid

nucleic acid

enveloped icosahedral (e.g. herpesvirus)

enveloped helical (e.g. influenza virus)

The virion usually contains a single molecule of nucleic acid. Small viruses have nucleic acid comprising as few as 3000 pairs of nucleotides: such a nucleic acid can code for 3-4 proteins, i.e. it consists of 3-4 genes. The largest viruses contain several hundred genes. In addition some virus particles include enzymes essential for the replication of the virus within the host cell. The outer coats of many viruses are made up of identical subunits of one or two types, arranged in a spiral or in a polyhedron. Viruses vary in size and shape a good deal (Fig. 4.15). By electronmicroscopy one can detect viruses in clinical specimens and recognise at least the family to which they belong, thus diagnosing certain types of viral infection. Some bacteriophages are filamentous or polyhedral, others have a complicated structure; in essence each is a 'biological syringe', which adheres to receptors on the surface of the bacterium and injects its nucleic acid.

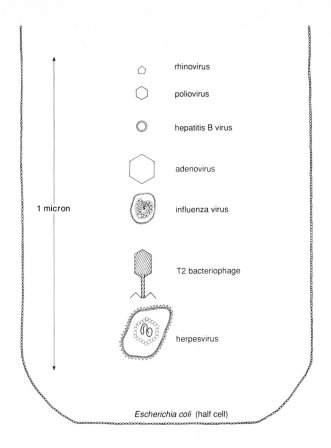

rhinovirus

poliovirus

hepatitis B virus

adenovirus

influenza virus

1 micron

T2 bacteriophage

herpesvirus

Escherichia coli (half cell)

Fig. 4.15 Relative sizes of virions. Several types are compared in size with a cell of *Escherichia coli*. The virions range from 27nm in diameter (rhinoviruses) to 180-200 nm (herpesviruses).

3 EUCARYOTES

Most other microbes (and all higher plants and animals) are classified as *eucaryotic cells* — fungi, protozoa, algae and helminths are the microbial forms. A typical eucaryotic cell is seen in Fig. 4.16. Note that it is more complex than a procaryotic cell. Inside the cell wall is the cell membrane enclosing the cytoplasm. Within the cytoplasm are various structures that do not appear in procaryotic cells: mitochondria, the Golgi apparatus, endoplasmic reticulum, and in photosynthetic cells chloroplasts.

Many eucaryotic cells do not have a cell wall like the one in Fig. 4.16. If one is present, it is simpler in structure than the cell wall of procaryotes and consists of polysaccharide. In algae and plant cells the cell wall is made of cellulose, in most fungi of chitin and in yeasts of glucan and/or mannan. These polysaccharides differ in the sugars that compose them or in the way the sugars are linked together. No eucaryotic cell has a cell wall of peptidoglycan, a fact of medical importance, since penicillin and many other antibiotics act on bacteria by interfering with the synthesis of the cell wall. These drugs leave eucaryotic cells untouched.

The outer boundary of the eucaryotic cell is the cell membrane or the cell wall; in most cases there is no additional coating

Fig. 4.16 A typical eucaryotic cell sliced lengthwise, the main structures labelled.

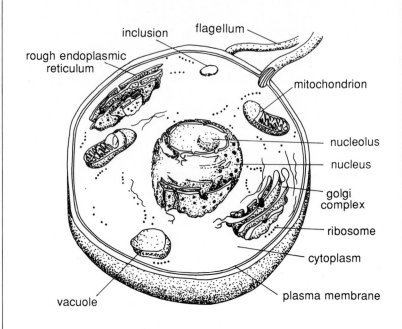

analogous to the capsule of procaryotes. The cell membrane of eucaryotes is very similar in structure to that of procaryotes, though the individual proteins, carbohydrates and lipids differ. Many eucaryotes have organelles projecting from the cell membrane and serving to move the cell or move substances over the cell surface. These are flagella and cilia. They are thicker and more complex structures than the flagella of procaryotes.

CYTOPLASM

Unlike the cytoplasm of procaryotic cells the cytoplasm of eucaryotes has a complex internal structure, a framework of tubules and fibrils (cytoskeleton), which supports intracellular organelles and is involved in the movement of the cytoplasm from one part of the cell to another. This *cytoplasmic streaming* helps the cell to move over surfaces and to engulf materials.

ORGANELLES

In the eucaryotic cell many of the activities of the cell are localised in organelles specialised for one or other task: the nucleus, endoplasmic reticulum, ribosomes, Golgi complex, lysosomes and chloroplasts.

Nucleus. The *nucleus,* the largest organelle, is usually spherical or ovoid. It is bounded by a double membrane, each part of which resembles the cell membrane. Within the nucleus are the fluid nucleoplasm, the nucleoli and the DNA, in which the genetic information of the cell is recorded. The nucleoli synthesise ribosomal RNA, a major component of the ribosomes. The nuclear DNA is almost all the DNA of the cell — a little is present in mitochondria and chloroplasts. It is associated with basic proteins and is organised into a number of individual units. In the resting state, when the cell is not in process of dividing, the DNA is in threads called chromatin. Before the nucleus divides, the chromatin shrinks and forms rods, the chromosomes. The number of chromosomes is characteristic of each microbial, animal or plant species.

Endoplasmic reticulum. The cytoplasm contains a complicated system of membranes in parallel pairs with spaces of various sizes between them. This *endoplasmic reticulum* forms a canal system within the cytoplasm. It is thought to be the framework on which synthesis and transport of proteins, lipids and other products takes place.

Ribosomes. On the surface of the endoplasmic reticulum, and also free in the cytoplasm, are found the ribosomes, the protein factories of the cell. The cytoplasmic ribosomes of eucaryotes are somewhat larger than those of procaryotes; mitochondria and chloroplasts also contain ribosomes, but of procaryotic type.

Mitochondria. These are of various shapes (spheres or rods), and are scattered through the cytoplasm in large numbers (Fig. 4.17). They are bounded by an outer membrane and enclose an inner membrane thrown into complicated folds. The enzymes involved in the synthesis of ATP, the energy currency of the cell, are located on the inner membrane.

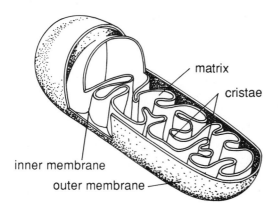

Fig. 4.17 A mitochondrion. The outer membrane is relatively smooth, the inner is thrown into complex folds. The enzymes of the citric acid cycle and of oxidative phosphorylation are located in the inner membrane. Mitochondria generate most of the energy of aerobic cells.

Golgi complex. This is a system of discs and vesicles involved in the secretion of synthesised molecules from the cell. Lipids and proteins synthesised by the endoplasmic reticulum and the ribosomes are conveyed to the Golgi complex and incorporated into vesicles, which then move to the surface of the cell, where the contents are released. *Lysosomes*, also formed by the Golgi complex, are bags of enzymes that can break down foreign materials such as bacteria. The white cells of the blood contain numerous lysosomes. Table 4.1. compares procaryotic and eucaryotic cells.

TABLE 4.1 COMPARISON OF PROCARYOTIC AND EUCARYOTIC CELLS

Feature	Procaryotic	Eucaryotic
cell wall		
peptidoglycan	present	absent
cellulose	absent	present
chitin	absent	present
lipopolysaccharide	present (Gram-ives)	absent
nuclear membrane	absent	present
DNA in distinct units,		
chromosomes	absent	present
DNA-associated proteins	absent	present
Mitochondria	absent	present
Endoplasmic reticulum	absent	present
Golgi complex	absent	present
Ribosomes	70S[1]	80S

[1]S = Svedberg unit, a measurement of size based on the speed of sedimentation in a centrifuge.

EUCARYOTE GROUPS

Eurocaryotic microbes are grouped into algae, fungi, protozoa and helminths. See Figures 4.18(a)-(e).

Algae. The floating green stuff in a pond and the waving fronds of seaweed are *algae*. They are photosynthetic and are a very important element in aquatic food chains. A few algae synthesise toxins. If the algae are eaten by fish, humans may encounter the toxin with fatal results.

Fungi. These are heterotrophs, relying for energy, carbon and nitrogen sources on organic compounds synthesised by plants. Most fungi are saprophytes in soil and water, breaking down plant material and recycling it. They secrete into the environment enzymes that attack proteins, polysaccharides and lipids (including cellulose and pectin, parts of plants indigestible by most animals). Fungi can utilise a vast range of organic compounds, even kerosene or phenol. Of the thousands of fungi, only 100 or so cause disease in man or animals (several thousand are pathogenic for plants). Fungi are unicellular (yeasts) or multicellular (moulds and fleshy fungi). See Plates 36–58. The yeasts are spherical or ovoid and reproduce by budding. An outgrowth (bud) forms at one point and as it grows the cell nucleus divides and one nucleus enters the bud, which eventually separates.

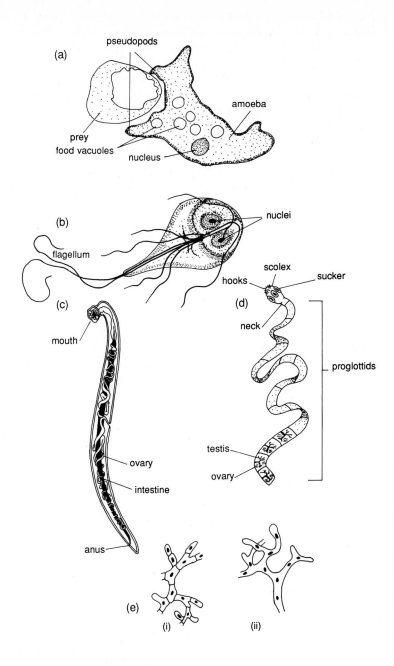

Fig. 4.18 (a) An amoeba engulfs a cell of a green alga **(b)** The trophozoite of *Giardia lamblia*, showing two prominent nuclei and 8 flagella **(c)** A roundworm, *Necator americanus*. The hooks around its mouth enable it to stick to the gut wall and to chew food **(d)** A flatworm, an adult tapeworm, which has both male and female reproductive organs, but no digestive system. It may have as many as 1000 segments (proglottids) **(e)** Fungal hyphae are of two types (i) some are divided by crosswalls into units of cytoplasm, each containing a single nucleus. Others (ii) lack crosswalls and the cytoplasm is in larger masses containing many nuclei.

Moulds and fleshy fungi consist of long filaments, *hyphae*. The hyphae may have cross-walls or be made up of a mass of cytoplasm with numerous nuclei. The hyphae intertwine and branch and the resulting mass of *mycelium* may be easily visible to the naked eye, as a mushroom or a blue patch on bread. Some fungi can grow either as a yeast or a mold; the form usually depends on the environmental temperature. Fungi need only simple media for growth. They grow better in an acid medium, around pH 5, which is unfavourable for most bacteria. Most fungi are aerobic.

Fungi reproduce by means of *spores* and produce many of them. The spores of bacteria are a response to adverse conditions; each bacterium produces one spore. Fungal spores can be of two types: asexual spores are generated by one organism and are genetically identical to it; sexual spores result from the fusion of nuclei from two mating strains and the resulting progeny inherit characteristics from both parents. Spores are borne on a great variety of structures (Plates 36–44) and are important in the identification of fungi, since hyphae and yeasts have few distinctive features.

Parasitic groups: Protozoa and Helminths. We will now look at two types of organisms that are often *parasitic*. These organisms can be made up of one or many cells (unicellular or multicellular organisms).

Protozoa are single-celled eucaryotes - mainly inhabiting soil, water or the intestines of animals, and feeding upon bacteria and other food particles. Some are *parasitic*, causing disease in man and animals, e.g. amoebic dysentery and vaginitis. The *amoebae* are blobs of protoplasm (Fig. 4.18(a)) that move by extending pseudopods (projections of protoplasm) in the desired direction. They engulf food materials by flowing around them and enclosing them in a food vacuole. Another group of protozoa includes *Giardia* (Fig. 4.18(b)) and *Trichomonas*, which move by means of flagella. The active feeding form *(trophozoite)* is often not capable of infecting a new host; some protozoa, e.g. *Giardia* and *Entamoeba*, form *cysts* — these are analogous to spores, and can survive for days or months outside a host. Several *Plasmodium* species (the cause of malaria) have complex life-cycles in which they shuttle between humans and mosquitos (see p.132 and Plate 73). Other protozoan causes of infection in man are *Pneumocystis carinii* (p.247) and *Toxoplasma gondii* (p.246).

Helminths are another important group of parasites. This group is multicellular (the *helminth* worms, Fig. 4.18(c) & (d)). They are considered here because diagnosis of the infections they cause depends on microbiological techniques. The helminths live inside many species of higher animals, including man, and have adapted to this specialised environment. Most have certain features in common: the gut is rudimentary or absent, since the host's tissues or digestive tract provide nourishment, which the parasite absorbs through its body surface; means of locomotion are likewise deficient or absent, since the parasite does not move about and its transfer from host to host does not depend on locomotion; the nervous system is poorly developed, since the creature does not have to respond much to changing situations, because the host provides a constant environment. In contrast, however, the reproductive system of the helminths is often complex and well developed, since the survival of the species depends on its fertility. Some species consist of male and female individuals, others of hermaphrodites (possessing male and female organs in the same animal). Additionally many have life-cycles in which they pass through a number of stages in different hosts. The *definitive host* is the animal in which the parasite spends its adult life; an *intermediate host* is one in which the parasite undergoes one or more stages of development before reaching adulthood.

The helminths are considered in more detail in Chapter 16.

CHAPTER REVIEW

1 In the microbial cell, what are the principal inorganic ions, small organic molecules, and macromolecules?
2 (a) What are DNA and RNA?
  (b) What are their functions?
3 What are the major differences between procaryotic and eucaryotic cells?
4 What are the major differences in cell structure between Gram-positive and Gram-negative bacteria?
5 Briefly describe the following:
  (a) a fungus
  (b) a virus
  (c) an amoeba
  (d) a spore
6 Draw simple diagrams to indicate
  (a) the structure of an amino acid
  (b) a protein
  (c) a carbohydrate
  (d) a lipid.

MICROBIAL GROWTH AND MULTIPLICATION

Bacteria cannot be reliably identified by their appearance under the microscope. To identify them in other ways — such as by their ability to use particular nutrients or to carry out biochemical reactions — we must have large numbers of them. Therefore we need to grow or *culture* them. Culture is also a more effective way of detecting them than microscopy (see following, 'Visible count and viable count').

EXPERIMENT ON PAPER
Visible count and viable count

A colony of *Escherichia coli* (a Gram-negative rod) is picked from a plate and a tube of broth is inoculated. It is incubated at 35⁰C overnight. Next day eight tubes are prepared, each containing 9 mL of sterile broth. 1 mL of the culture is added to the first tube, mixed by filling and emptying a pipette (NB *mouthpipetting is not done in microbiology or in any other clinical laboratory*) and 1 mL transferred to tube 2. This is mixed again, 1 mL transferred to tube 3, and this process is continued. A fresh pipette is used each time, because bacteria stick to glass.

0.1 mL is plated out from each tube onto an agar plate, and spread with a hockey stick (a bent glass rod).

The above process is called a *viable count* or *plate count*: 'viable' because only bacterial cells that are living and can reproduce will form colonies. The plates can now be incubated.

A film is made from each tube by spreading a loopful over an area 1 cm across on a slide. The slides are stained, examined and next day the results are compared with the plates. This will probably show 10-20 colonies on the plate from the seventh tube (one or two on the plate from the eighth tube);

for illustrative purposes we will assume that there are 8 on plate 7. This would indicate the bacterial count in the original broth was 8×10^8, $8 \times 10 \times 10^7$ (we multiply by 10 for each tube used in the dilution, and by 10 because we plated out only 1/10 mL). When the slides are examined it is necessary to hunt very hard to see a Gram-negative rod even in the film from the fifth tube, which contained 10^4 cells/mL. This number of cells would be expected to yield only one Gram-negative rod per 10 oil-immersion fields; i.e. using the oil-immersion lens we would expect to examine 10 fields to find one Gram-negative rod.

There are many situations in medical microbiology where it is important to be able to find one or two bacterial cells per mL, one important instance being meningitis (an infection of the membranes around the brain and spinal cord). A method which detects only 10^4 bacteria per mL is much too insensitive. In the laboratory it is common to grow bacteria from specimens in which no organisms can be seen in the Gram-stained film.

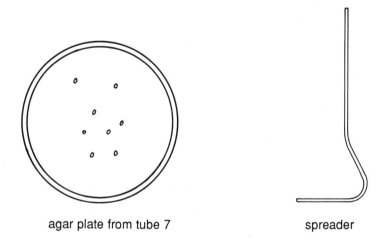

agar plate from tube 7   spreader

Fig. A The glass 'hockey-stick' is used to spread the inoculum on the plate. The agar plate shows the result of this count: 8 colonies after culturing 0.1 mL from the seventh tube.

MEDIA

Microbiologists have spent a lot of time working out *media* to isolate bacteria from infected people or to reveal the characteristics of the bacteria isolated. If a microbe cannot be grown *in vitro* (i.e. in the test-tube, under artificial conditions) it is very difficult to study. One of the features that made Legionnaires' disease mysterious was the reluctance of *Legionella* to grow on the usual diagnostic media.

Interestingly enough, despite all these efforts, the best medium often does not promote growth as well as the usual environment of the bacteria — the numbers of bacteria in the gut or in rich soil are much higher than the microbiologist can usually achieve. We should also remember that in nature mixed cultures are the rule and bacterial *interactions* are common. For example, one species of bacterium may synthesise a vitamin which others use; or organisms that use oxygen may remove it from the environment so that strict anaerobes can grow (strict anaerobes require the complete absence of oxygen for growth).

ENVIRONMENTAL CONDITIONS

To be successful, microbes have to survive, grow and reproduce. Even to survive requires the input of resources. Many of the molecules which form living creatures are unstable, break down and must be constantly resynthesised — to grow demands that the stock of all molecules be increased. Organisms must draw from the *environment* all the substances they require for the synthesis of cell materials and for the generation of energy; all these biochemical reactions are referred to collectively as the *metabolism* of the cell. The organism needs:

- energy sources
- organic nutrients
- vitamins and growth factors
- inorganic salts and trace elements
- a suitable environment

ENERGY SOURCES

Some microbes are capable of photosynthesis. Like green plants they use the energy of the sun to carry out chemical reactions. Most of the others, including those of medical importance, generate energy by burning a carbon compound, a sugar such as glucose or an amino acid. The biochemical processes of energy generation are discussed on p.49.

ORGANIC NUTRIENTS

Because the molecules that make up the microbial body all contain carbon, a source of organic carbon is required for growth. Some bacteria can convert atmospheric CO_2 into the organic compounds they need and with the addition of inorganic salts they can grow and multiply. Such microbes are said to be *autotrophic*. Most other bacteria use an external source of organic carbon. This may be the same compound that is used for energy, e.g. glucose. Such organisms are termed *heterotrophic*. Many components of living cells also contain nitrogen, so a suitable source of this element is needed (NH_4^+ or NO_3^-). The ultimate source of all the carbon and nitrogen in living creatures is the carbon dioxide and nitrogen of the atmosphere. Various inorganic ions must be added.

A very simple bacteriological medium might contain the following:

- glucose — energy source and carbon source
- ammonium chloride (NH_4Cl) — nitrogen source
- Na^+, K^+, Mg^{2+}, PO_4^{3-}, SO_4^{2-}, and Cl^- — inorganic ions
- water

(Certain other elements called trace elements are also required, but in such small quantities that they will usually be present as impurities in other ingredients.)

Many free-living bacteria and even some that live in association with man (e.g. certain strains of *Escherichia coli*) can grow in such a medium. *E. coli* would grow more slowly on this medium than on a complex medium, and most bacteria that cause disease in man would not grow at all. The secretions and tissues of humans contain hundreds of compounds, e.g. amino acids, peptides, sugars, vitamins, that bacteria can utilise for growth. Human beings form a good medium for bacterial growth; many bacteria require such preformed compounds, probably because for millions of years they have been relying on animals and humans to synthesise their requirements.

In order to grow many of the bacteria associated with *humans* we therefore have to provide a rich medium with many preformed compounds. Such complex media are made from the breakdown products of animal proteins, casein (milk protein), meat or yeast. The proteins are hydrolysed into peptones — small peptides usually containing only a few amino acids — which can be utilised by the bacteria.

A typical complex bacteriological medium might contain the following:

- peptone — source of nitrogen compounds, carbon compounds and growth factors
- NaCl — inorganic ions
- glucose — source of carbon and energy
- water

The peptone (protein hydrolysate) would also provide the other necessary salts. However some bacteria (e.g. streptococci) will still not grow, or will only grow very poorly, in such a medium. The usual medium in the hospital microbiology laboratory is blood agar, a medium similar to the above, but to which is added 5-7% of horse, sheep or rabbit blood (treated so that it does not clot). A few species of bacteria (e.g. *Haemophilus* and *Neisseria)* grow better on chocolate agar, blood agar that has been heated at 50-70^{0}C until it has gone brown. This treatment releases haemin, a growth factor, from the red cells and destroys an inhibitor. Other media are occasionally used to grow more unusual pathogens, such as *Legionella*.

VITAMINS AND GROWTH FACTORS

Bacteria which will not grow in a simple chemically defined medium are said to require growth factors. These are substances which are necessary for the growth of bacteria, and which the cell cannot itself synthesise. They are of two types: amino acids, purines, pyrimidines and others are required for inclusion in the cell's structural and other proteins or in nucleic acids — i.e. they represent part of the raw materials used by the cellular machinery. Vitamins are required for incorporation in enzymes involved in the synthesis of these compounds; the cell uses them to make the cellular machinery and they are therefore needed in much smaller amounts. One additional amino acid would permit *Proteus mirabilis* to grow in the simple bacteriological medium above, whereas a streptococcus might require 12 or more amino acids and 20 other growth factors.

INORGANIC SALTS AND TRACE ELEMENTS

The minimal medium set out above contains sodium (Na^+), potassium (K^+), magnesium (Mg^{2+}), chloride (Cl^-), phosphate (PO_4^{3-}) and sulphate (SO_4^{2-}). K^+, Mg^{2+} and PO_4^{3-} are required in fairly substantial quantities, since the functioning of the microbial cell's machinery demands quite high concentrations of these ions. Other metals are needed in smaller quantities — often for incorporation in enzymes: iron (Fe), manganese (Mn), calcium (Ca), cobalt (Co), zinc (Zn), molybdenum (Mo).

ENVIRONMENTAL FACTORS

Apart from the nutrients available, several other environmental factors are important in bacterial growth:
- the availability of liquid water
- the pH of the medium
- the concentration of ions
- the gases present in the atmosphere
- the ambient temperature

Bacteria grow only in *liquid water*; they may survive, but cannot *multiply* in the dry state. Unless they form spores they will die more or less rapidly on drying out.

pH

If we want to grow bacteria which live in association with humans, the pH of the water must be close to neutrality — pH 7.0 — since the pH of human tissues is about 7.4. In a bacteriological medium this is ensured by the mixture of amino acids, ions and other substances present. It may be necessary to add acid or alkali to adjust the pH to a suitable value. All cultures tend to change in pH during growth. If protein hydrolysate is the main component, the pH rises because the removal of NH_2 groups from amino acids yields ammonia (an alkali). If utilisable carbohydrate is present, the pH falls, since the end-product is acid, lactic acid, carbon dioxide and such.

It is necessary therefore to *buffer* the medium — i.e. to add to it chemicals which, because they react with either acid or alkali, can cushion or buffer the effect of an excess of either acid or alkali. The medium itself has buffering activity because of the amino acid content, and the buffering capacity can be increased by the addition of other agents. In the media used in medical microbiology, the buffer used is normally phosphate ions, in the form of Na or K phosphate.

IONIC STRENGTH

The concentration of ions in the medium influences the ability of bacteria to grow. Some bacteria can grow in much stronger salt solutions than others. Staphylococci for example can grow in a medium containing 6.5% NaCl, whereas most other bacteria of clinical interest do not. Certain vibrios, including some that cause diarrhoea in humans, normally live in brackish water and extra NaCl must be added to their media.

ATMOSPHERE: OXYGEN AND CARBON DIOXIDE

The gaseous environment is important for bacterial growth.
Aerobes and anaerobes. Some bacteria will grow only in the presence of oxygen — *obligate aerobes* (aerobic bacteria); others only in the absence of oxygen *(obligate anaerobes)*; some will grow in the presence or absence of oxygen *(facultative anaerobes)*. If it is likely that anaerobes are going to be present and of importance in a clinical specimen, it is essential that the specimen is cultured in the absence of oxygen — preferably in the presence of nitrogen and CO_2. Actually there is a spectrum of oxygen susceptibility — from organisms that are unaffected by the amount of oxygen in the air, to organisms that prefer only a small amount of oxygen, to organisms that can grow in the presence of oxygen, but do better without it, to organisms that will not grow in the presence of oxygen and are killed more or less rapidly by the smallest trace of oxygen.

In order to grow anaerobes, oxygen must be excluded. Liquid media often contain chemicals (such as sodium thioglycollate) that will combine with oxygen dissolved in the medium and remove it. When organisms are to be grown on plates — i.e. on the *surface* of the medium and exposed to any oxygen present — other measures are needed. After inoculation plates are placed in an *anaerobic jar* (Fig. 5.1). When the jar is sealed, oxygen is removed by a chemical reaction, so that the bacteria are exposed only to an atmosphere of nitrogen and carbon dioxide.

The normal flora of the gut and the vagina consists mainly of anaerobes, and anaerobes are present on the skin. Although animals live in air, the sites where anaerobes flourish have very little oxygen; the supply of oxygen is poor there, and the aerobes that are present utilise it and protect the anaerobes.

Carbon dioxide is an essential nutrient for all bacteria and is needed in the synthesis of amino acids and nucleotides. Ordinarily bacteria produce large quantities of the gas themselves when breaking down carbon compounds for energy. Certain bacteria prefer rather more CO_2 than is present in air. Many laboratories use special

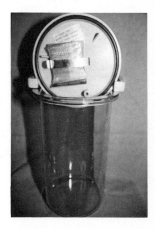

Fig. 5.1 An anaerobic jar. This device provides bacteria with an anaerobic (oxygen-free) atmosphere in which to grow. Water is added to an envelope containing chemicals; the reactions generate hydrogen and carbon dioxide. The palladium catalyst (in the envelope of metal mesh clipped to the lid) brings about the reaction of hydrogen and oxygen to form water, thus removing the oxygen.

incubators for all their primary cultures of specimens; these are gassed with a mixture of 5-10% carbon dioxide and 90-95% air.

TEMPERATURE

In general, bacteria grow best at the temperatures they normally encounter. For instance, *Staphylococcus aureus*, often present in the nose or on the skin, grows most rapidly at temperatures round about 35^0C, whereas a soil bacterium from Tasmania is likely to have its optimum temperature around $15\text{-}20^0C$. This does not mean that *S. aureus* does not grow at 20^0C, but that it grows more slowly; its *generation time*, the time required for one organism to divide into two, will be several times longer. In the clinical laboratory, incubator temperatures are set at 35^0C for most purposes. Bacteria which grow well at refrigerator temperatures can cause problems if they contaminate blood for transfusion, because they might multiply during storage and produce an unpleasant or even fatal reaction, when the blood is transfused.

SOLID VS LIQUID MEDIA

Bacteria will grow in a liquid medium, or broth, or on a solid medium (which might be the broth solidified with a gelling agent). The gelling agent used in media is *agar*, a mixture of polysaccharides made from seaweed (gelatin is unsuitable since it is liquid at 30^0C.). Agar is decomposed by very few bacteria and has the useful property that, once melted, it stays liquid down to a temperature of $45\text{-}50^0C$, so that heat-labile substances such as blood can be added to the medium. The normal procedure for preparing a solid bacteriological medium is to mix the ingredients (e.g. the peptone and salts listed above) with 2% agar and the necessary water. The mixture is then sterilised by autoclaving (see p.170) — usually at a temperature of 121^0C for 15 minutes. Next the medium is cooled — if blood, antibiotics or other heat-labile substances need to be added, this occurs now. The medium is poured into round plastic *Petri dishes*. The agar-containing medium sets in a few minutes. Microbiological media are perishable, and should be made often and stored in the cold.

Solid media have several advantages. Each bacterial species has a typical colony, by which it can be recognised according to size, shape, texture, colouring and the presence of haemolysis around it (Fig. 2.3). If more than one sort of bacterium is present in the *inoculum*, the different colonies can usually be detected. The numbers of each type of colony allow one to estimate their relative proportions in the inoculum. Reagents can be added to the surface of the medium after inoculation and their effect on the growth of different colonies looked for, as an aid to identification.

SELECTIVE AND ENRICHMENT MEDIA

Any medium is selective in that it will grow only a small proportion of the known microbes. Even blood agar is selective for those organisms preferring pH 7, uninhibited by complex media and capable of using glucose or amino acids as energy sources. Microbes can be obtained from natural habitats either by selective isolation or by *enrichment*, i.e. by adjusting the conditions in the medium to favour the growth of some types of bacteria at the expense of others.

Media may be rendered selective by the addition of:
- bile or deoxycholate, which favour the growth of some enteric organisms such as *Salmonella* and *Shigella*;
- dyes such as malachite green or crystal violet, which inhibit Gram-positive species;
- disinfectants such as phenethyl alcohol or cetrimide, which allow *Pseudomonas aeruginosa* to grow at the expense of most other organisms;
- antibiotics: colistin-nalidixic-acid agar inhibits most Gram-negative organisms and allows only Gram-positive organisms to form detectable colonies.

MEDIA FOR GROWING FUNGI

Fungi, like most bacteria, need preformed organic compounds for growth and energy. Most fungi will grow on defined media such as were described above for bacteria. Some fungi will require vitamins, thiamine or biotin, or sulphur-containing amino acids. For most routine diagnostic purposes, as with bacteria, complex organic media are used. A number of fungi cause infections of the skin, hair and nails. These structures are at a lower temperature than the interior of the body and fungal cultures from these sites are incubated at 30^0C.

MEDIA FOR VIROLOGY

To grow viruses in the laboratory we not only need media, but suitable cells, since viruses must be isolated and propagated in living cells. Viral cell-culture media usually contain serum, inorganic salts, buffers, amino acids and vitamins. One called Eagle's medium contains 12 essential amino acids such as lysine, valine, tryptophane, and 9 vitamins, as well as salts. To prevent contamination of the cultures antibiotics are usually added, penicillin plus streptomycin or gentamicin. There is no ideal medium for all cells — some cells will do better in one, some in another. It must also be remembered that some cells will grow only on an appropriate surface, e.g. glass, or treated plastic.

STERILISATION

When we use bacteriological media, we want to grow only the bacteria we are interested in. We must therefore remove all the bacteria which will be present in the materials we use to make the media, in the water and on the glassware. To ensure that the medium contains no living bacteria we must *sterilise* it. Media for growing bacteria and fungi are normally sterilised by moist heat in an autoclave.

Most viral cell-culture media are sterilised by membrane filtration, not by autoclaving, which may render them toxic to the cells. (Sterilisation is discussed in depth in chapter 12.)

DETECTION OF BACTERIAL GROWTH

If we need more accurate information than is provided by streaking out a culture on a plate — if we need to determine how many bacteria are present or how rapidly they have grown — there are several methods available. One is the *viable count* (see box p.40), by which means we determine the number of bacterial cells capable of forming colonies. Another is to count bacteria under the microscope, using a special *counting chamber* which contains a very small volume of fluid. Such a count includes both living, *viable* and dead bacteria. A third method by which the numbers of bacteria in a suspension can be estimated, though more crudely, is by measuring the suspension's *turbidity*, i.e. its capacity to scatter light. The more turbid the liquid, the more bacteria are present. The effect of antibiotics on bacteria can be assessed by comparing the rate of growth (repeated measurements of turbidity) in the presence and absence of the antibiotic. An organism that grows freely in the presence of the antibiotic is resistant to it. Several commercially available devices use this principle.

MICROBIAL METABOLIC PROCESSES

We have seen that the internal structure of microbes is complex and that they require many different substances to grow and multiply. Within the microbe a large number of biochemical reactions take place. Most of these are the same or very similar in procaryotic *and* eucaryotic cells, and in multicellular plants and animals, including humans.

To be utilised for growth the raw materials that the cell requires must enter the cell through the *cytoplasmic membrane*. This membrane is selectively permeable, i.e. some substances can pass through, others cannot. Small molecules such as some sugars, amino acids and water do so; and because the membrane is mostly lipid, substances that are soluble in lipid also pass more readily.

Large molecules, however, such as are present in the tissues and body fluids of animals, *cannot* cross the membrane and must undergo *digestion* before they can be absorbed. For this purpose, microbes secrete into the environment various *extracellular enzymes*, which often constitute part of the invasive machinery of pathogens. These include enzymes capable of breaking down proteins, polysaccharides, nucleic acids and lipids (all of these substances can provide components that the cell can use).

Movement across the membrane may occur by simple diffusion,

facilitated diffusion or active transport. If the concentration of a sugar is higher outside the membrane than inside, then sugar molecules will move across: *simple diffusion*. In *facilitated diffusion* carrier proteins assist in this movement, again in the direction of the concentration gradient. In *active transport* molecules are moved across the membrane even if the concentration is higher at the destination — this means the cell must expend chemical energy to bring about the movement of the molecules.

CELLULAR ENERGY

All living cells need energy — simply to stay alive. All cells have to expend energy to keep the chemical and physical characteristics of their cytoplasm suitable for life, and to maintain their internal milieu at the correct pH and ionic strength. They also require energy in order to grow and replicate themselves.

The ultimate source of all biological energy on earth is the sun. Solar energy can be used by the green plant for photosynthesis (a process which yields carbohydrates). Some bacteria also can use solar energy for photosynthesis, and a few can generate energy by utilising compounds of nitrogen or iron. But most bacteria and all other living creatures, including man and the higher animals, are parasitic on the green plant and ultimately derive all their energy and nutrients from it.

What form does energy take in living cells? The energy is *chemical* energy, i.e. energy in a form which brings about chemical reactions, which may result in: the synthesis of new compounds; the secretion of substances into the environment; locomotion.

Molecules have chemical energy in the bonds which link their atoms. The cell converts this chemical energy into a more readily usable form. It manipulates the molecules by means of enzymes, so that the energy of several bonds is concentrated into one *high-energy* or *energy-rich* bond in a molecule of adenosine triphosphate or *ATP* ('~' symbolises an energy-rich bond).

$$\text{Adenine - ribose - (P)} \sim \text{(P)} \sim \text{(P)}$$

ATP thus serves as the energy currency of the cell — the means whereby the cell channels the energy derived from breaking down sugars and other energy sources into the synthesis of the numerous compounds it needs in order to grow and divide.

The raw material from which microbes generate energy is most often a carbohydrate, but may be an amino acid or other carbon compound. We shall here look at the generation of energy from glucose.

THE GLYCOLYTIC CYCLE AND CITRIC ACID CYCLE

In the glycolytic cycle, glucose is broken down to pyruvic acid; the reactions can be summarised in this way:

$$\text{glucose} \rightarrow 2 \text{ pyruvate} + 2 \text{ e}^- + 2\text{H}^+$$

In these reactions glucose is oxidised. Two electrons and 2 H^+ ions are removed from the glucose molecule (2 e^- + 2 H^+ = 2 hydrogen atoms). The two electrons are passed from molecule to molecule along an electron-transport chain to an electron acceptor, and in this passage two molecules of ATP are generated.

Next, pyruvic acid is oxidised. First one molecule of carbon dioxide is removed and more ATP is generated:

$$\text{Pyruvate} + \text{CoA} \rightarrow \text{Acetyl-CoA} + CO_2 + 2e^-$$

Coenzyme A accepts the 2-carbon acetyl group derived from pyruvate. The acetyl $\sim$ Coenzyme A (acetyl $\sim$ CoA) contains an energy-rich bond. The acetyl group now enters the citric acid cycle, a complex series of reactions in which it is oxidised to CO_2 and its energy converted to ATP via the electron-transport chain. The electrons passing down the electron-transport chain are eventually transferred to molecular oxygen, and this results in the formation of water with hydrogen ions from the medium. During the passage of the electrons down the electron-transport chain, more ATP molecules are generated; this process is responsible for most of the ATP derived from the utilisation of carbon compounds.

In all more than 30 molecules of ATP are produced when one molecule of glucose is oxidised to CO_2 and water. About 60% of the energy locked up in glucose is lost as heat during the process (nevertheless this is nearly twice as efficient as the conversion of gasoline to energy by the motor-car). There are 10 chemical steps between glucose and pyruvic acid, in other words nine other chemicals are successively formed by the enzymes of the glycolytic cycle before pyruvic acid is reached. In the course of the citric acid cycle another nine compounds are formed as acetyl $\sim$ CoA is oxidised. The upshot of these chemical manipulations is that the energy of glucose is released in a step-wise process during which part is trapped in biologically usable form and not lost as heat.

As well as converting sugars to CO_2 and water — a process called *respiration* — the cell may generate energy by *fermentation*. In respiration, electrons are finally accepted by oxygen, the result being water. In fermentation electrons may be accepted by various organic compounds and the end-product of the fermentation may be lactic acid, ethanol ('alcohol'), acetone, glycerol, methanol or other chemicals. Many of the substances produced by fermentations are of considerable industrial importance (see Table 5.1). It is often cheaper to produce a chemical by fermentation than by chemical synthesis, especially since otherwise useless waste products may serve as the starting materials.

TABLE 5.1 SOME PRODUCTS OF FERMENTATION

Lactic acid	yoghurt, sauerkraut, pickles, cheese
Ethanol	beer, wine
Acetic acid	vinegar
Acetone *Butanol* *Glycerol*	} synthesis of many other chemicals
Penicillin *Tetracycline* *Other antibiotics*	} treatment of infection

Not only sugars, but amino acids and fatty acids can be converted to CO_2, water and energy. When amino acids are metabolised the $-NH_2$ group is removed and converted to ammonium ion, which may be excreted or re-used. The carbon chain is modified and enters the citric acid cycle. The carbon atoms of fatty acids are removed in pairs, as acetyl $\sim$ CoA, and enter the citric acid cycle. The cycle functions as the common pathway along which carbon atoms from many different compounds are made to yield energy to the cell.

What happens to the ATP and other types of energy-rich bonds that are generated as we have just described? They are used for several purposes:

- biosynthesis of new cell components
- active transport of substances across membranes
- locomotion — flagellar movement and amoeboid movement
- movement of cytoplasm within the cell

Biosynthesis of new cell components uses the greatest share of energy.

BIOSYNTHESIS

Many cellular components are *polymers*, i.e. they are made up of a number of similar units. Proteins are built up from amino acids; we shall discuss this process in chapter 6. Carbohydrates are put together from sugar molecules. In the synthesis of polyglucan, a storage carbohydrate of microbes, glucose molecules are energised by the attachment of a phosphate group supplied by ATP; in this process ATP becomes adenosine diphosphate (ADP). Enzymes use the energised glucose to form a chain of glucose molecules. The resulting polymer functions as a store of glucose molecules and can be broken down again to glucose as needed. Many syntheses follow this principle: the molecule is first energised and is then linked to another molecule.

$$\text{Glucose} + \text{ATP} \rightarrow \text{Glucose-P} + \text{ADP}$$
$$\text{Glucose-Glucose-Glucose} + \text{Glucose-P} \rightarrow$$
$$\text{Glucose-Glucose-Glucose-Glucose} + \text{P}$$

If necessary the cell can also build the component molecules needed to form the polymers. Thus *Escherichia coli* can synthesise amino acids and then link them together to form proteins. For example, it takes one of the acids of the citric acid cycle, oxalacetic acid, and attaches to it an $-NH_2$ group (derived from ammonia or another amino acid) producing the amino acid aspartic acid (Fig. 5.2(a)). Aspartic acid can then be converted to any one of several other amino acids. An intermediate of the glycolytic cycle is the starting point for the synthesis of other amino acids.

These processes do not go on in 'separate compartments', but are interlinked. Many of the compounds generated during the glycolytic and citric acid cycles and the other degradative pathways are used for the synthesis of chemicals needed for cellular processes or constituents. We can think of the cell's supply of nutrients and

Fig. 5.2 Synthesis of amino acids: examples of two different pathways. The carbon skeleton may be derived from carbohydrates, fatty acids or amino acids and comes via the citric acid cycle or the glycolytic cycle. The –NH$_2$ group comes from an amino-group 'carrier', usually glutamate. The carbon lost by serine in the conversion to glycine **(b)** is transferred to a 'one-carbon' carrier for use in other syntheses.

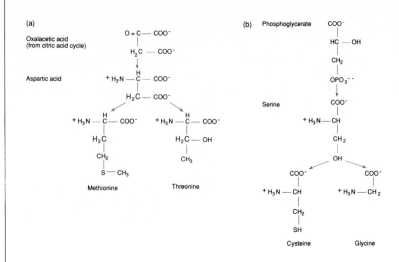

products as forming many different pools. While some molecules in the glucose pool are being 'burnt' to CO$_2$ to provide energy, others are being converted to ribose or to the sugars in the peptidoglycan framework of the cell wall. Molecules of the amino acid aspartic acid are being incorporated into proteins, while others are donating amino groups to form nucleotides or being converted to other amino acids. And if the medium can supply a particular component the cell will not waste energy manufacturing it. Control mechanisms regulate the rate of synthetic and degradative processes to ensure overall efficiency.

CHAPTER REVIEW

1   (a)   Define 'pure' growth.
      (b)   Why is it necessary?
2   List and explain the five major factors necessary for bacterial growth.
3   (a)   Define an anaerobic bacterium.
      (b)   How does this differ from an aerobic one?
4   What are the different growth requirements of:
      (a)   bacteria
      (b)   fungi (e.g. a yeast)
      (c)   viruses
5   (a)   What is the difference between a simple and a complex bacteriological medium?
      (b)   List the constituents of an example of each.
6   (a)   What is a selective medium?
      (b)   When are selective media used in bacteriology?

GENETICS

HEREDITY

We know that characteristics are inherited — children often look like their parents, 'funny' ears run in families, two short-haired grey cats have short-haired grey kittens, and the seeds of yellow daffodils produce yellow daffodils. Similarly, the characteristics of microbes are inherited: their shape, their ability to use certain food or energy sources, to make capsules or flagella, to adhere to tissues, to cause disease and to resist the action of antibiotics. We further know that some characteristics are inherited in an all-or-nothing fashion (e.g. male or female sex, blood group), while other characteristics are inherited in a graduated fashion (e.g. height or hair colour). The study of heredity is termed *genetics*.

Inherited characteristics are carried on *genes*. Genes are arranged on *chromosomes*. Procaryotic cells have a single chromosome, while eucaryotic cells have more. Each gene encodes the structure of a protein; this protein may form part of the cell wall or the intracellular structures, or it may be an enzyme involved in the metabolism of the cell.

DNA

The characteristic feature of living creatures is the ability to reproduce: whether by dividing in two, as many microbes do, or by the complicated rituals of the higher animals (mating displays, discotheques and such). To reproduce means to *copy*: there must be a record from which the copy is made, a formula which sets out what the animal or microbe is made up of. In essence, a living creature

RNA core

Escherichia coli
(a bacterium)

Fig. 6.1 DNA of *Escherichia coli*. The DNA of *E. coli* is about 1mm long, i.e. several hundred times longer than the bacterium. It is coiled into about 60 'domains' around an RNA core and then 'supercoiled' to fit into the bacterial cell.

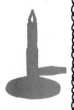

DNA of Escherichia coli

is a collection of complex chemicals. Many of these molecules are very large and are unique to the creature, so that they cannot be obtained from the environment and must therefore be synthesised. Some molecules are required at one point in growth or metabolism, some at another. Many are unstable and must be made repeatedly during life. As most molecules cannot be used as patterns to synthesise copies of themselves, 'blueprints' of each molecule must be 'kept on file'. In the last four billion years a successful method of making such 'molecular blueprints' has been evolved only once. In all living creatures from the earliest bacteria to man, the dolphin and the pine tree, this record is kept in the same fashion — on a 'tape' consisting of molecules of deoxyribonucleic acid (DNA). These enormously long molecules are the biological equivalent of magnetic tape; in the sequence of units along their length is encoded the structure of the organism. This is a long message: if completely unwound, the DNA of *Escherichia coli* is some thousand times longer than the bacterial cell which it encodes (Fig. 6.1).

Experiments in breeding plants, fruitflies and microbes provided a great deal of information about the behaviour of genes before we knew anything about the molecules responsible. It was not until 1944 that DNA was shown by Oswald T. Avery to be able to transfer from one pneumococcus to another the capacity to make a particular polysaccharide capsule. Avery concluded that DNA was able to bring about a *hereditary* change in the pneumococcus. At the time, Avery's conclusion was not accepted, because biochemists did not believe that the DNA molecule was complex enough to carry the necessary information. Eight years later it was conclusively demonstrated that DNA was the genetic material of a bacterial virus: see following, 'A phage cocktail'. This experiment convinced most scientists of the importance of DNA — including James Watson and Francis Crick, who in 1954 worked out how the DNA molecule is put together; this achievement was probably the most important biological discovery of the century.

MILESTONES
A 'phage cocktail'
If we grow *Escherichia coli* in a medium containing an isotope of phosphorus, P^{32}, then the isotope will replace 'ordinary' phosphorus P^{31} in some of the phosphorus-containing molecules, since chemically it behaves exactly as P^{31} does. So nucleotides and DNA will be 'labelled' with P^{32}; since the P^{32} is radioactive, such molecules can be traced. If we provide a medium containing the sulphur isotope S^{35}, the sulphur-containing amino acids will be labelled. Hence any protein made in these cells will likewise be labelled.

A *bacteriophage* is a bacterial virus that multiplies in bacteria, using the host's cell machinery to make its own components. If we grow the bacteriophage T4 in an *E. coli* culture in which the nucleotides have been labelled with P^{32}, the DNA of the phage will be labelled. And in the same way we can prepare phage labelled in the protein coat with S^{35}.

In 1952, Alfred Hershey and Martha Chase infected *E. coli* with phage that they had labelled either in the DNA or in the protein coat. They then put the phage/bacteria suspension in a blender and stirred it violently. They *centrifuged* the suspension and measured the amount of radioactivity associated with the cells and in the supernatant. They found that the DNA label stayed with the cells, while the protein label was mostly in the supernatant. Blender treatment did not alter the numbers of progeny phage particles.

These results showed that:

1   the DNA entered the bacteria, while the protein coat of the phage stayed outside
2   *the DNA contained the genetic information necessary to make phage,* since the bacteria still produced phage particles.

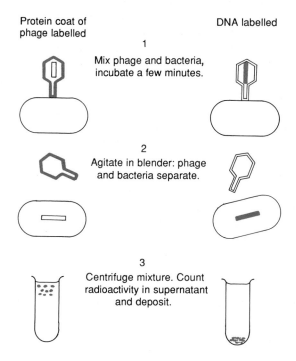

Fig. A A phage cocktail.

STRUCTURE OF DNA

Deoxyribonucleic acid is a long chain built up of nucleotides. Each nucleotide consists of three linked molecules (Fig. 6.2). As can be seen, the backbone of each chain consists of alternating deoxyribose and phosphate molecules (see Fig. 6.3). The carbon atoms of deoxyribose are numbered to distinguish them (Fig. 6.2). In DNA,

(a)   Adenine

(b)   Deoxyribose

(c)   Phosphate group

Fig. 6.2. Constituents of DNA. DNA molecules are made up of 4 nucleotides: a nucleotide consisting of **(a)** an organic base (adenine, guanine, cytosine or thymine), **(b)** a sugar (deoxyribose) and **(c)** a phosphate group. The base and the phosphate are both attached to the sugar.

Fig. 6.3 The DNA double helix. Each chain of the double helix consists of a 'sugar-phosphate backbone'. To each sugar is attached a base. Bases in the two chains are linked by hydrogen bonds, adenine to thymine and cytosine to guanine.

phosphate molecules link the 5' carbon of one sugar to the 3' carbon of another. At one end there is a free hydroxyl (OH) group attached to the 5' carbon of a deoxyribose and at the other end a free hydroxyl is on the 3' carbon of a deoxyribose. Synthesis of DNA takes place only in one direction: from 5' end to 3' end.

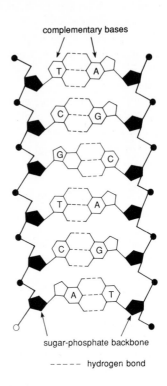

complementary bases

sugar-phosphate backbone

- - - - - hydrogen bond

To each deoxyribose molecule is attached one of the four bases (Fig. 6.3). Notice that the bases do not pair at random: A in one chain pairs with T in the other, C with G. Between A and T two hydrogen bonds form, between C and G three are set up. While hydrogen bonds are weak, there are so many in a DNA molecule that the chains do not separate spontaneously under physiological conditions. Under the influence of heat or high pH, however, the two strands come apart: this is termed *denaturation*. The two strands are complementary: the structure of one decides the structure of the other, and each can serve as a pattern from which the other can be synthesised. This property explains how genes are duplicated — the basis of reproduction.

In the living organism, DNA is double-stranded; two long chains are curled round each other in a *double helix* (or spiral). Inside the *bacterial* cell the DNA is further twisted and coiled, so that it takes up only about 10% of the cell's volume, and it is attached to the cell membrane (Fig. 4.7). All the genetic information of procaryotic cells is encoded in one giant molecule; in *E. coli*, for instance, this molecule contains about 4 million base-pairs (4 million bases on each strand).

In eucaryotic cells likewise, each chromosome is believed to consist of a single huge DNA molecule, which in humans is made up of about 100×10^6 base pairs. This molecule is wound around histones and associated with various other proteins, which probably influence the function of the chromosome and may be involved in regulating the *expression* of genes. When a gene is translated into protein the gene is said to be 'expressed'.

The DNA chain encodes the information which the cell needs to synthesise proteins and other cell constituents, to perform its functions, and to reproduce itself. In order to synthesise a protein, two sorts of information are needed:

- the types of amino acids making up the protein
- the order in which they are linked in the peptide chain

The other features of a protein, how the peptide chains fold and curve around one another to produce the functional three-dimensional structure of an enzyme (Fig. 3.6) or an antibody, are determined by the primary structure.

This information is encoded in the sequence of bases along the DNA strand. This genetic code has only four letters — A, C, G and T — representing adenine, cytosine, guanine and thymine, the four bases in the nucleotides. As there are 20 amino acids in proteins, three-letter words must be used to designate the amino acids (for examples see Table 6.1). If three letters are used, then $4 \times 4 \times 4$, i.e. $4^3 = 64$ words are possible, since there are four ways of filling each position: AAA, AAC, AAG, AAT, ACA, ACC, ACG, ACT and so on. So most amino acids are represented by more than one codon (code word). There are also codons that say 'Stop - this is the end of the polypeptide chain'. Most genes code for proteins, while some code for RNA molecules that have functions in protein synthesis. A protein of average size might have a peptide chain of 400 amino acids and a molecular weight of about 45000. The gene coding for this protein would contain a sequence of 1200 bases in each chain — 1200 base pairs.

TABLE 6.1 EXAMPLES OF 'WORDS' IN THE GENETIC CODE

DNA Sense strand	RNA Codon	RNA Anticodon	Amino Acid
C A C	C A C	G U G	Histidine
C T T	C U U	G A A	Leucine
A A G	A A G	U U C	Lysine
T T C	U U C	A A G	Phenylalanine
T A A	U A A	A A U	Stop signal

(These are examples; most amino acids have more codons than are given here.)

REPLICATION OF DNA

This is the process of making a 'replica' of each strand — an essential preliminary to reproduction. The DNA strands are uncoiled and separated by the untwisting enzymes. Other enzyme systems in the cytoplasm make the deoxyribose and the bases, couple these to phosphate ions taken from the medium, and produce the energy-rich nucleotides necessary to drive the synthetic reaction. DNA polymerases move along each strand, synthesising the complementary strand. Each daughter chromosome consists of two strands, one derived from the parent and one that is freshly synthesised on the template of that parental strand (Fig. 6.4). Each pair of daughter strands is then rewound into a helix. The site where the DNA molecule is untwisted and replication proceeds is called the *replication fork*. In bacteria this site appears to be attached to the cell membrane — this is probably important in ensuring that during cell division one copy of the parental DNA goes to each daughter cell.

Fig. 6.4 Replication of DNA. Each chain of the double helix serves as a template for synthesis of the other. The two daughter strands each contain one parental and one newly-synthesised chain.

	A A A	C A T	T T A	G T T	A A T
	T T T	G T A	A A T	C A A	T T A

↓

old	A A A	C A T	T T A	G T T	A A T
new	T T T	G T A	A A T	C A A	T T A

new	A A A	C A T	T T A	G T T	A A T
old	T T T	G T A	A A T	C A A	T T A

PROTEIN SYNTHESIS

Only one of the two DNA strands — the 'sense' strand — carries the genetic message. The other strand, the *template strand*, exists to make replication of the DNA possible and also functions as the template on which messenger RNA is laid down. The first step in converting the sequence of bases in the DNA into a sequence of amino acids in a polypeptide is to create a messenger ribonucleic acid (RNA) molecule — a process called *transcription* of the DNA. The messenger RNA carries the 'message' of the DNA to the protein factories in the cytoplasm, the *ribosomes*. The nucleotides of RNA also consist of base-sugar-phosphate. The sugar in the nucleotides is ribose, not deoxyribose. Three of the bases are the same as in DNA, but thymine is replaced by a close relative, uracil.

The *template strand* in the DNA of the relevant gene acts as a pattern and a chain of complementary bases is laid down. The result is that, where C appears in the sense strand, C appears in the RNA, G → G, A → A and T → U. The messenger sequence is built up by RNA polymerase from nucleotides in the cytoplasm. The polymerase finds an initiator site, unwinds some DNA and takes instructions from the template strand. The messenger RNA (mRNA) is a single strand; only the sense strand of the DNA is transcribed.

The next step in protein synthesis is to *translate* the message of the mRNA into a sequence of amino acids linked by peptide bonds. Translation is carried out by ribosomes, which abound in the cytoplasm of the cell (Fig. 6.5). Ribosomes consist of two parts, and contain in all about 50 proteins and three RNA molecules. The ribosome 'reads' the message and builds the appropriate amino acids one by one into a chain. Amino acids are synthesised in the cytoplasm or imported from the medium. Before they can be coupled, they must be endowed with sufficient chemical energy to form a peptide bond. This process of activation is accomplished by attaching each amino acid to its own specific carrier molecule of *transfer RNA* (tRNA); this process requires an enzyme and the chemical energy of ATP. Each tRNA carries a recognition sequence, the *anticodon*, by which the amino acid it bears can be recognised. The anticodon is a set of three RNA bases, the RNA complement of the codon in the messenger RNA. When the mRNA binds to the ribosome, the anticodon of tRNA pairs with the codon. If the required amino acid is leucine, the codon that appears in the mRNA is CUU and the anticodon on the leucine-tRNA is GAA (Table 6.1).

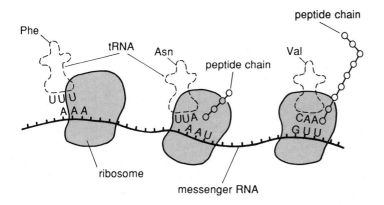

Fig. 6.5 Protein synthesis by the ribosomes. The two parts of the ribosome come together on the messenger RNA. The transfer RNA bearing the anticodon corresponding to the first triplet in the mRNA gives up its amino acid to the ribosome and is released. The second tRNA binds to the ribosome, its amino acid is linked to the first amino acid by a peptide bond, while it is released. The process continues until a stop codon is reached and the peptide chain separates from the ribosome. Several ribosomes can translate the same mRNA molecule simultaneously.

When the two subunits of the ribosome meet a molecule of mRNA, they form a complex with it. The first amino acid tRNA pairs with its codon and is bound, the ribosome moves along the

messenger chain and the second amino acid tRNA pairs with *its*
codon. A peptide bond now forms, the first tRNA is now parted
from its amino acid and is released, the ribosome moves on down
the messenger and a third tRNA is paired. Another peptide bond is
formed, the second tRNA is released and the process continues.
Eventually a STOP signal is reached and the peptide chain is
released from the ribosome. The mRNA detaches itself and the
ribosome separates into its subunits.

REGULATION OF GENE EXPRESSION

The *genome* of the bacterial cell contains all the information
required to do anything the cell needs to do. However, all of the
cell's machinery is not constantly in use. If a particular food
molecule is not available, the enzymes to utilise it are unnecessary.
Synthesising protein is expensive in terms of energy, since to add
one amino acid to the peptide chain demands several molecules of
ATP. Hence there are savings for the cell in being able to regulate
gene translation so that only the proteins needed at a given time
are synthesised. These regulatory processes are termed *induction*
and *repression*.

Enzymes that are produced all the time are termed *constitutive;*
those that appear only in response to the need are *inducible*. An
example of an inducible enzyme found in many bacteria is beta-
galactosidase, which breaks down the sugar lactose to its components — galactose and glucose (lactose has to be hydrolysed before
it can be used by the cell). If no lactose is available, the enzyme
system is not needed and transcription of the beta-galactosidase
gene is shut off. A *repressor protein* is synthesised and this binds to
the operator, the control region on the beta-galactosidase gene
complex; the whole gene complex is called an *operon* (Fig. 6.6).
When lactose enters the cell it brings about a reaction which inacti-
vates the repressor, beta-galactosidase is synthesised and lactose
molecules are hydrolysed and used. Many enzymes that are involved
in metabolism or in the response to environmental conditions are
inducible. For instance, production of beta-lactamase — an enzyme
that destroys penicillin and other beta-lactam antibiotics — is often
induced by the antibiotic.

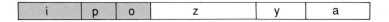

Fig. 6.6 The lactose operon. This stretch of DNA controls the synthesis of
the enzymes involved in the metabolism of lactose. The regulator gene *i*
produces a protein which binds to the operator site *o* and prevents
transcription of the enzyme genes *z, y* and *a*. When an inducer molecule
combines with the repressor, it can no longer bind to the operator site.
RNA polymerase can now attach to the promoter site and initiate
anscription of the DNA. The resulting messenger RNA is translated by the
ribosomes, and the enzymes needed to metabolise lactose are formed.

MUTATION

A *mutation* is a change in the genetic code — the sequence of the DNA bases. Mutations either occur spontaneously, or are brought about by chemicals or radiation — ultra-violet, X-ray or nuclear. In mutation, one base in one chain is replaced by another, or one or more bases are deleted or added. When the DNA is replicated, the other chain is altered correspondingly, so that one daughter cell receives DNA with a new base pair (Fig. 6.7). This will sometimes result in the appearance of a new amino acid in the peptide chain, but not invariably. In the genetic code, all but two of the amino acids are represented by more than one codon — some by as many as six. Alanine is represented by GCT, GCA, GCG, GCC. Obviously a mutation affecting the T of GCT would have no effect on the amino acid encoded, since it would simply replace it with another alanine codon. In the mutation shown in Figure 6.7 thymine is replaced by guanine, the codon CAT is replaced by CAG. When replication takes place, one of the daughter strands has a G-C base pair instead of an A-T, and in the encoded protein glutamine is substituted for histidine.

```
     C C T      T A A      C A T*     C T C      G T T ...
     G G A      C T T      G T A      G A G      C A A ...
     Mutation  T - > G*               |
                                      |
                                      ↓
     C C T      T A A      C A G*     C T C      G T T ...
     G G A      C T T      G T A      G A G      C A A ...

                                      |
                                      ↓
Replication
old  C C T      T A A      C A G*     C T C      G T T ...
new  G G A      C T T      G T C*     G A G      C A A ...
new  C C T      T A A      C A T      C T C      G T T ...
old  G G A      C T T      G T A      G A G      C A A ...
```

Most mutations are neutral, i.e. they do not affect the viability of the cell. Even if the result of the mutation is a replacement of one amino acid by another, the replacement may be sufficiently like the original in chemical nature to have no effect on the protein; or the substitution may be in an unimportant region of the protein and so won't alter its function.

The machinery of DNA replication is very reliable and a mutation in a given gene occurs only once in about a million replications or less. A low level of mutation is desirable from the point of view of the species, since it generates the diversity on which natural selection operates (see following, 'Darwin and natural selection'): without mutation living creatures would not evolve or be able to cope with environmental change; a high level of mutation, however, would be dangerous, since too often it would lead to failure to survive.

Fig. 6.7 A mutation changes a base pair. A mutation, induced by radiation, drugs or other causes, leads to the replacement of T(thymine) by G(guanine). When the DNA is replicated, one of the sets of paired strands contains a G-C base-pair instead of the original T-A; the other set is unchanged.

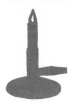

MILESTONES

Darwin and the theory of Natural Selection

During his five year voyage of scientific exploration between 1831 and 1836 aboard *The Beagle*, Charles Darwin observed the enormous variety of living creatures. In the Galapagos Islands he was especially intrigued by the fact that each island had its own varieties of finches, lizards and tortoises. Returning home he continued his biological studies, always pondering on variation and on the processes that yielded so many different species (we now know that there are 20 million or more species of creatures in the world). In his book *The Origin of Species* (1859) Darwin suggested that the two forces responsible were *variation* and *natural selection*.

The numbers of animals inhabiting a region are regulated by competition for food supplies. It is a common observation that the members of a species vary in their characteristics. Those members best suited to the conditions of the region will survive, because they are fleeter of foot, capable of digesting the tougher vegetation or well camouflaged so that they escape observation by predators. Thus, for instance, among the ancestors of the giraffe some had longer necks than others and found more vegetation within their reach. Some of the progeny of such giraffes would inherit a longer neck and, if they continued to live among trees, would have an advantage. Thus each generation would tend to include more long-necked individuals, and eventually, by a process of *natural selection*, the giraffe population would consist of long-necked animals only.

Why do animals vary? Darwin thought that variation was essentially a random process. If the variant was advantageous under the prevailing conditions, it would tend to be retained in the population and eventually to dominate it. Thus, under different conditions, in different environments, the one ancestral form could give rise to two or more different *species*, each adapted to its own environment.

The various processes of mutation (p.61) are now thought to provide the genetic basis of variation.

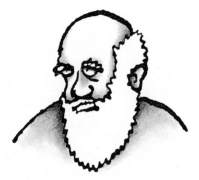

Fig. A Charles Darwin (1809–82).

GENETIC RECOMBINATION

Another way in which organisms can evolve is by acquiring new genes from others. These processes are referred to as *genetic recombination*. In procaryotes, new DNA can be acquired in several ways.

TRANSFORMATION

In *transformation* cells take up naked DNA. Under natural conditions transformation occurs only in a few genera — *Neisseria*, *Haemophilus*, *Bacillus*, *Acinetobacter* being the main ones. However other organisms, e.g. *Escherichia coli*, can be easily manipulated so that they will take up DNA — this is important in genetic engineering (see p.65).

TRANSDUCTION

Transduction is transfer of bacterial DNA by bacteriophages. At a late stage in the replication of phages, phage particles are assembled from the component molecules in the bacterial cytoplasm. Phage DNA is packaged inside the phage head. Sometimes bacterial DNA is included instead of, or as well as, the phage DNA. When such a phage infects another host it injects the bacterial DNA (and usually does not succeed in replicating itself).

CONJUGATION

The large chromosome attached to the cell membrane is not the only genetic information present in procaryotic cells. Many bacteria also carry *plasmids*, small circular double-stranded DNA molecules which are independent of the bacterial chromosome (Fig. 6.8). They range in size from 2000 base-pairs to 150 000 or so (the DNA of bacterial chromosomes contains 2 to 5 million base pairs). They are present in numbers per cell ranging from one to 20 or more depending on the size of the plasmid (small plasmids are usually present in larger numbers).

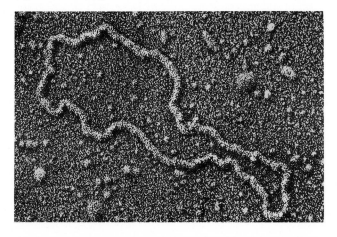

Fig. 6.8 A plasmid: a double-stranded closed circle of DNA.(Electronmicrograph).

The DNA of a plasmid encodes mechanisms that cause the plasmid to replicate within the bacterial cell, thus ensuring that, when the cell divides, each daughter cell receives one or more copies of the plasmid.

Many plasmids bring about their own transfer to other bacteria by means of *conjugation*; these are termed *conjugative plasmids*. For transfer to occur, the two cells must be in direct contact and the plasmid in the donor cell must possess a 'fertility factor' (F factor). A copy of the plasmid is synthesised and transferred to the recipient bacterium. Sometimes the F factor combines with the bacterial chromosome and part of the latter is also transferred. Plasmids that cannot bring about their own transfer may also come across during this process.

Plasmids often confer advantages on the host. They may provide genes which endow the host with the ability to carry out biochemical reactions, e.g. to utilise sucrose or an unusual food source, such as camphor or kerosene. Genes encoding resistance to antibiotics and other toxic substances (e.g. disinfectants) are often carried by plasmids. They may provide the ability to synthesise a toxin or other substance related to *pathogenicity* (the ability to produce disease) — a haemolysin that destroys red cells, or a protein that helps the bacteria stick to the wall of the gut.

Transposons are mobile genetic elements, 'jumping genes', which can move from one stretch of DNA to another and may carry genetic information with them. Transposons consist of two palindromic segments of DNA enclosing a central region which codes for transposition and other functions such as antibiotic resistance ('Madam, I'm Adam' is a palindrome, i.e. a phrase which reads the same forwards and backwards). Transposition can occur from one site to another within a plasmid or chromosome, between plasmid and chromosome or between plasmid and plasmid (several plasmids may be found in a single bacterial cell).

What happens to DNA acquired by transformation, transduction or conjugation? Often it is degraded and its genetic message is lost. Organisms possess enzymes which lyse foreign DNA — these *restriction enzymes* are discussed in more detail shortly. If it escapes the action of the enzymes, the foreign DNA may be integrated into the bacterial chromosome and replace a corrresponding section of the original DNA. For this recombination to occur, the two DNAs must resemble each other closely in one region at least, and the recA (recombination) enzyme must be present.

The DNA of the chromosome is also subject to other changes. A plasmid may integrate itself with (join itself into) the chromosome, and thus import a set of new genes. A transposon may likewise settle down on the chromosome and bring one or more genes with it. If a transposon inserts itself into a stretch of DNA that codes for a protein, it will interrupt the sequence and the protein will no longer be made. The gene is thus lost; this is a form of mutation. As well as bringing in new genes, the insertion sequences of transposons can lead to rearrangement of the order of existing genes or their deletion. Thus the resources of the 'gene pool' available to a procaryote can be varied by acquiring new genes or by 'shuffling the pack' — by re-arranging the available genetic material.

GENETIC ENGINEERING AND CLONING

The chromosome of *Escherichia coli*, just to give one example, contains several thousand genes — so it is obviously desirable to be able to study genes in isolation. In this way we might expect firstly to acquire a lot more knowledge of the fundamental properties of genes, and in addition learn how to manipulate them and to give them more desirable properties. In the last 20 years these things have become possible. The first step was finding out how to cut up the chromosome in a systematic fashion with enzymes.

CLONING DNA

Enzymes that cut the DNA strand, *nucleases,* had been known for a long time, but these had the disadvantage that their action was unpredictable and they reduced the chromosome to short fragments. However there exists another type of nuclease, the *restriction* endonuclease. Living cells apparently need to protect themselves against foreign DNA, which may enter and disorganise their cellular activities. They contain enzymes which label their own DNA, and others which destroy foreign DNA. The latter enzymes — restriction endonucleases — recognise specific nucleotide sequences and cut the DNA chain always at the same point, so that a given chromosome always yields the same fragments. These enzymes cut a DNA chain in only a few sites and do not reduce it randomly to short bits as other cellular nucleases do. Some cut straight through the recognition sequence, others cut it in staggered fashion (leaving single-stranded 'sticky ends'), others cut near it (Fig. 6.9). The recognition sequences are palindromes (see *transposons*). The restriction endonucleases therefore enable us to cut DNA in a predictable fashion, and with their use it has become possible to isolate a given fragment of DNA consistently, and so to *clone* a gene, i.e. to separate it from other genes in the chromosome and propagate it independently of the rest of the genome (see 'Experiment on paper', following).

EXPERIMENT ON PAPER
Cloning a gene
1   The cells are gently broken up and the DNA purified.
2   The DNA is cut into 'gene-size' pieces with a restriction enzyme.
3   The pieces are incorporated into carrier plasmids.
4   The plasmids are inserted into *E. coli* by transformation.

5   The *E. coli* culture is then grown up and the cells that express the desired gene are searched for and propagated.

Let us now apply this method to cloning a gene that makes bacteria resistant to the antibiotic gentamicin. The resistance gene is on a plasmid.

1   An isolate of *Klebsiella pneumoniae* resistant to gentamicin is grown and the plasmid DNA extracted.

2   The restriction enzyme EcoRI is used to cut the plasmid DNA into relatively large pieces — big enough to include one or more genes.

3   The DNA fragments are incorporated into the carrier plasmid pBR322. First, the carrier plasmid is cut with EcoRI, so that it has the same 'sticky ends' as the DNA of the *Klebsiella* plasmid. The DNA fragments are added and the sticky ends joined up again with an enzyme to produce a functioning plasmid containing a piece of foreign DNA. In this way we have, hopefully, included all the DNA fragments of the *Klebsiella* plasmid in carrier plasmids.

4   These plasmids are now introduced into *E. coli* by transformation. *E. coli* is treated to make it easier for DNA to enter.

5   After transformation, the culture is grown and we search for *E. coli* colonies that are resistant to gentamicin: the culture is plated out on medium containing gentamicin, and only those cells that resist gentamicin can grow. Any colony that appears must consist of cells possessing the desired gene.

6   An *E. coli* colony resistant to gentamicin is picked off and grown. The plasmid DNA containing the gentamicin resistance gene can now be extracted and used in other experiments.

Microbial source	Abbreviation	Specific sequence
E. coli	EcoR1	G ^A A T T C
		C T T A A ^G
Bacillus	BamH1	G ^G A T C C
		C C T A G ^G
H. parainfluenzae	Hpal	G T T ^A A C
		C A A ^T T G

(^ indicates point at which the strand is cut)

Fig. 6.9 Restriction endonucleases. These enzymes break down DNA in a very specific fashion, only at points where the specific sequence of base is found. Notice that each upper strand read from left to right has the same sequence as its lower strand, read right to left.

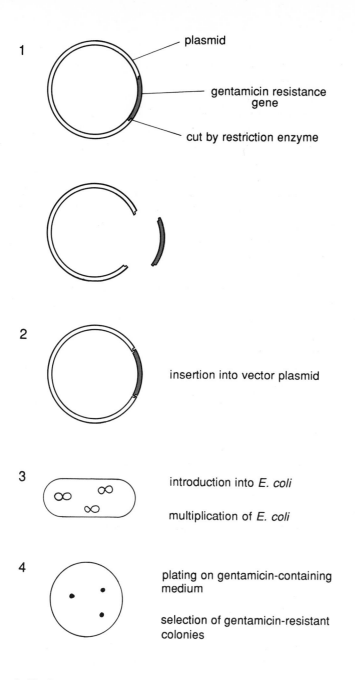

Fig. A Cloning a gene.
1. The plasmid containing the gentamicin resistance gene is digested with a restriction enzyme. The same enzyme is used to cut the vector plasmid.
2. The gentamicin gene is inserted into the vector plasmid.
3. The vector plasmid is introduced into *E. coli* and the bacterial cells grown up.
4 The bacterial cells are spread on gentamicin-containing medium to select those cells containing the resistance gene.

REASONS FOR CLONING DNA

1 FUNDAMENTAL RESEARCH

It has been possible to learn a great deal about the structure of genes, how they are translated and how translation is controlled; many other questions are also being answered. Eucaryotic genes have been found to be unexpectedly complex. They contain *introns*, sequences of DNA which are not translated into messenger RNA and the function of which is not clear. Immunoglobulin molecules contain variable and constant regions (see p.112). These have now been shown to be coded for by separate genes, which have been cloned. Proteins which are to be secreted from the cell have been shown to have 'signal' sequences — the 'signal' sequence binds to the lipid-rich cell membrane and draws the protein through the membrane.

In studying *infectious diseases*, genetic engineering has become very important. By means of probes we can detect the enterotoxin genes found in organisms that cause diarrhoea, we can identify *Legionella* or *Mycobacterium*, we can demonstrate a virus such as cytomegalovirus or herpes simplex in clinical specimens, and we can show that the DNA of hepatitis B virus is present in the cells of a liver cancer (cancer of the liver is known to develop more often in people with hepatitis B infection).

2 MANUFACTURE OF VACCINES AND HORMONES

Cloning methods help us to manufacture substances useful in medicine or industry. Diabetes, for example, is due to lack of the hormone insulin. The gene coding for human insulin has now been cloned into bacteria, which can produce the hormone: genetically engineered human insulin is now replacing insulin extracted from animals. In order to make vaccines, the genes for surface proteins of viruses can be cloned in bacteria or yeasts and large quantities of very pure protein produced, with no risk that it will be contaminated by AIDS virus or oncogenic (cancer-causing) viruses. A vaccine against hepatitis B is now made by means of a gene cloned in yeast (p123). It is also possible to develop organisms with other desirable properties, e.g. bacteria that destroy pollutants.

3 MEDICAL DIAGNOSIS AND IDENTIFICATION

Having cloned the desired gene, we can then make probes, short fragments of the gene — by means of which we can detect the gene with great certainty. The DNA under investigation is immobilised on a nitrocellulose membrane and is denatured by heat or high pH to produce single strands. The probe is then added; if it finds a complementary single strand of DNA, it binds to it and is retained on the filter, where it can be detected by autoradiography or an enzymatic reaction. Probes are now available to diagnose thalassaemia, a hereditary blood disorder, and many other hereditary diseases. Probes made from antibiotic-resistance genes can be used to study the spread of resistance.

CELL DIVISION

Almost all bacteria multiply by dividing in two (Fig. 6.10). Under favourable conditions, the bacterial cell acquires all it needs for growth from its environment, and enlarges. At some point the chromosome duplicates itself by the process just described. Then the *cell itself* divides. The cell wall and cell membrane grow inwards all round the circumference of the cell to form a cross wall. When the cross wall separates the cytoplasm into two equal halves, each with its own chromosome, the cross wall itself splits and two complete cells result. If the cells do not separate after the cross wall forms, chains or clumps of cells will result (streptococci and staphylococci).

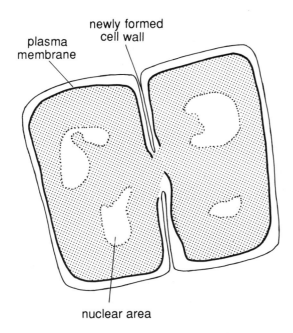

Fig. 6.10 Bacteria dividing. A partition forms across the parent cell and divides it into two daughter cells.

MITOSIS AND MEIOSIS

Cell division in eucaryotes is more complicated — eucaryotes do not have one chromosome, one unit of DNA, but *many* (Fig. 6.11). The number of chromosomes is characteristic of the species. Human beings have 46; and the tobacco plant 48. Each chromosome consists of two long unbranched strands of DNA, as does the bacterial chromosome, but in addition they are paired. Cells containing two of each chromosome are termed *diploid*. In general the chromosomes are duplicates of each other, i.e. each bears the same genes, but in some cases the genes at corresponding points on the two chromosomes may be similar but not identical *(allelic genes or alleles)*. The amount of DNA in eucaryotic cells is much greater than in procaryotic cells: the genome of the fruit fly, for instance, contains about 40 times as much DNA as does *E. coli*, and the genome of humans almost 1000 times as much.

Fig. 6.11 Chromosome pattern of a human male: 46 pairs of chromatids in a tissue cell.

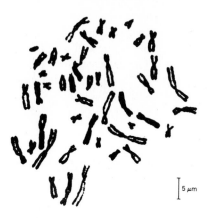

Reproduction in eucaryotes may be asexual (by simple division, *mitosis*) or sexual (Figs 6.12 and 6.13). In sexual reproduction, germ cells arise by a special type of division *(meiosis)* of the diploid cells, in which the progeny cells acquire only one of each chromosome and are termed *haploid*. One haploid cell from each parent fuses to form a diploid zygote, which then divides and differentiates to generate a new individual. (On a sociological note: in the higher animals the male contributes only nuclear DNA; mitochondria, which do much of the cell's work, come solely from the female.)

Fig. 6.12 Eucaryotic cell dividing — *mitosis*. Each chromosome consists of a single double-stranded DNA molecule. In most cells the chromosomes are present as identical pairs (*diploid* state). Before cell division starts, the chromosomes are not visible in the nucleus; during this phase they replicate. At the beginning of cell division the chromosomes become visible as threads and then condense into distinct rods, the *chromatids*, joined at the centromere. The pairs of chromatids are drawn apart by the contractile fibres of the *spindle*, and a nuclear membrane forms around each set. The cytoplasm of the cell divides and two identical cells are formed.

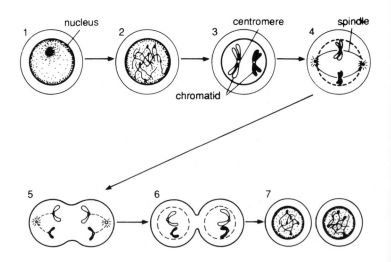

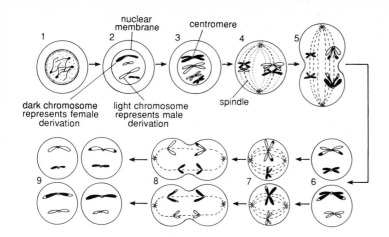

Fig. 6.13 Eucaryotic cell dividing — *meiosis*. The first phase of meiosis resembles mitosis and results in the formation of two cells, each of which is diploid (containing identical pairs of chromosomes). Each of these cells now divides again with no duplication of the chromosomes, so that the four resulting cells each contain a single representative of each chromosome.

REPRODUCTION OF VIRUSES

Viruses can only multiply inside living cells. Let us take herpes simplex virus as an example. The virion consists of DNA enclosed in a capsid of protein encoded by viral genes, outside which is an envelope consisting of both viral and host proteins. The virion attaches to the susceptible cell (in a mucous membrane, for example) by the glycoproteins in the envelope and is taken into the cell. The capsid enters the cytoplasm and releases the viral nucleic acid into the nucleus, where it takes over the metabolism of the cell and directs the production of viral nucleic acid and viral proteins. The nucleic acid acquires its coat of viral protein, picks up its envelope at the nuclear membrane and passes through the cytoplasm to be released from the cell surface (Fig. 6.14).

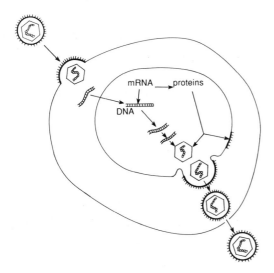

Fig. 6.14 Reproduction of herpes virus. The envelope of the virus fuses with the cell membrane, and the capsid enters the cell. The capsid releases its DNA into the nucleus where it is transcribed into mRNA, which is translated into proteins necessary for the synthesis of viral components and into the components themselves. The DNA is also replicated. The DNA is enclosed in capsid proteins while in the nucleus, and the capsid acquires its envelope on passing through the nuclear membrane.

CHAPTER REVIEW

1   Define:
     (a)   a gene
     (b)   an enzyme
2   What is necessary to synthesise a protein?
3   What is the function of DNA?
4   How does the replication of DNA occur?
5   What does an enzyme do?
6   What is an inducible enzyme?
7   Explain mutation and its significance.
8   What is a plasmid?
9   Outline the process of cloning a gene.

MICROBES IN THE ENVIRONMENT

MICROBES AS NORMAL FLORA

We have seen in chapter 2 that the surface of the throat is colonised by large numbers of bacteria. In fact, every body surface of
every animal is more or less densely populated by bacteria. A
human body, for example, is made up of about 10 million million
human cells accompanied by 100 million million bacterial cells.

MICROBES OF THE HUMAN BODY

Table 7.1 indicates the types of microbes found at different sites of
the human body. These microbes are referred to as *normal flora* or
as *commensals*. As can be seen, the flora of the nose, mouth and
throat is made up largely of Gram-positive cocci and Gram-positive rods. Because of the gastric acid, the stomach contains few
microbes or none. In the small intestine there are small numbers of
streptococci, lactobacilli, diphtheroids and yeasts *(Candida albicans)*.
Towards the lower part *Enterobacteriaceae* and anaerobes appear, and
in the colon (which has the densest bacterial flora of the body) there
is an impressive variety of species: about 400 have been detected so
far. More than 99% of these are strict anaerobes, Gram-negative
nonsporulating species such as *Bacteroides* or *Fusobacterium*, Gram-positive cocci (e.g. *Peptococcus*) and Gram-positive rods (e.g. *Eubacterium*).
Facultative anaerobes such as *Escherichia coli*, *Klebsiella pneumoniae* or
Proteus mirabilis and strict aerobes such as *Pseudomonas aeruginosa* make
up only 1% or less of the organisms in faeces. Those few anaerobic
species with strong pathogenic potential, mainly *Bacteroides* and
Fusobacterium, are present only in small numbers.

73

TABLE 7.1 BACTERIAL FLORA OF THE BODY SURFACES

*Surface**	*Main types of bacteria found*
Nose	Staphylococci, corynebacteria
Mouth, throat	Staphylococci, streptococci and enterococci, *Neisseria* species, corynebacteria, *Haemophilus,* lactobacilli, enterobacteria such as *E. coli* and *Klebsiella,* many types of anaerobes
Lower small bowel, large bowel	*Enterobacteriaceae,* enterococci, staphylococci, streptococci, lactobacilli, *Bacteroides, Fusobacterium, Clostridium* and other anaerobes
External genitals	Staphylococci, streptococci, enterococci, corynebacteria, *Enterobacteriaceae,* yeasts
Vagina	Lactobacilli, streptococci, enterococci, staphylococci, many types of anaerobes, *Enterobacteriaceae*
Skin	Staphylococci, corynebacteria, yeasts

(*Organs such as the nose and the gut are referred to as 'surfaces' here because they are in direct contact with the environment.)

The numbers of bacteria involved are very large: faeces or vaginal secretions may contain 10^{11} bacteria per gram and scrapings from the surface of the teeth are almost as rich. Smaller numbers, but still very large, are present on the skin. These populations are not simply 'passers-by'; they are apparently specialised for the human environment and even for the particular body site. Many adhere to receptors in the gut wall or throat and remain intimately associated with the epithelial cells.

BENEFITS OF NORMAL FLORA

All animals likewise have huge populations of *commensals*. Herbivorous animals largely depend on microbes to digest cellulose and other plant materials (Under normal circumstances gut bacteria make little contribution to *human* nutrition). The importance of the normal flora in humans lies in preventing colonisation of the throat, gut and other sites by bacteria not normally present and possibly pathogenic. They do this by occupying the sites of attachment on surface cells, by monopolising the available nutrients, and by secreting substances that are actively toxic to many other bacteria. These microbes are adapted to the environment that we provide, and under normal circumstances do not invade our tissues (how they avoid the surface defences is not known).

When the normal flora of the throat is eliminated by antibiotics, *Escherichia coli, Klebsiella* and other enterobacteria establish themselves (and are then more likely to infect the lungs). Any severe illness appears to disturb the normal flora; for this reason it is very common to isolate enterobacteria from the respiratory tract of patients in the Intensive Care Unit. On the skin, bacteria are present in micro-colonies on the surface and in hair follicles and sweat glands — because they are largely inaccessible in the latter sites, it is impossible to destroy all bacteria on the skin by disinfectants, and there is always the possibility that a needle (inserted to administer a drug or collect blood) will encounter one of these bacterial deposits.

MICROBES AND THE BIOSPHERE

The biosphere is the thin rind of this planet which can be colonised by living creatures (Fig. 7.1). It extends about a hundred metres into the earth, 30 or so kilometres into the atmosphere and some 10 kilometres into the ocean's depths. Wherever in the biosphere there is 'life', there is microbial life. Microbes are the hardiest living creatures, existing in the Arctic oceans at temperatures close to 0^0C, in hot springs where the water is close to boiling, on bare rocks and in the presence or absence of oxygen. In all these places they survive and even multiply, in soil and water, on dust particles in the air, on all the objects with which we come into contact and in the food we eat. It is also important to note that *the vast majority of environmental microbes have no ability to cause disease in animals or humans.*

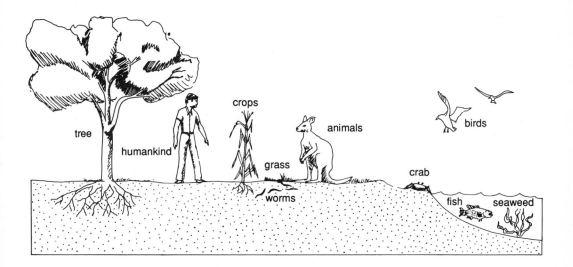

Fig. 7.1 The biosphere, the zone around the planet where life is possible — in the air, on land and in the sea.

Environmental bacteria may be grouped into *autotrophic* 'self-sufficient' organisms, which can use solar or chemical energy to synthesise their requirements, and *heterotrophic* ones, which use the chemicals built up by the autotrophs or the green plant — either directly, or after they have nourished animals. Algae such as *Chlorella* and the cyanobacteria contain the machinery for photosynthesis (Fig. 7.2). Given sunlight, carbon dioxide and inorganic ions (including nitrates) they will grow and multiply. Almost all the others derive their food, just as we do — from the green plant. Plants use the energy of sunlight to convert carbon dioxide to carbohydrates. They take up nitrogen from the soil in the form of nitrates and ammonia and synthesise proteins, carbohydrates, lipids and other organic compounds.

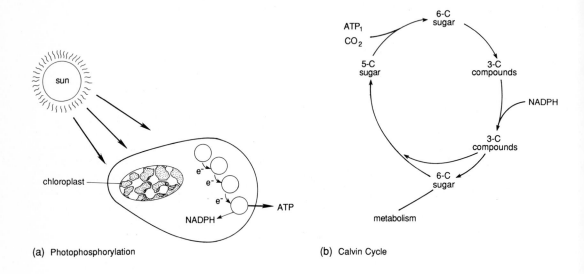

(a) Photophosphorylation

(b) Calvin Cycle

Fig. 7.2 Photosynthesis: **(a)** photophosphorylation and **(b)** the Calvin cycle. Solar energy is captured by the chloroplast and used to generate ATP and NADPH. These two molecules drive the Calvin cycle, in which atmospheric carbon dioxide is converted into carbohydrates.

CYCLES OF MATTER

The total microbial mass on the planet is about 25 times the animal mass, terrestrial and aquatic. Rich soil contains millions of microbes per gram: bacteria, fungi, algae, protozoa and nematodes; this amounts to 200-500 kilograms of microbes per hectare (or about 200-500 pounds per acre). In the oceans microbes occur more sparsely, but the volume of sea water is so great that they represent a significant fraction of the total. When plants or animals die, the chemical compounds which make up their bodies must be broken down and re-utilised, otherwise very soon the earth would become covered in their remains and all the raw materials needed for life would be locked up. It is the microbes which play the main part in ensuring that the constituents of dead plants and animals are made available again; these processes constitute cycles, in which carbon, nitrogen, phosphorus, sulphur and other elements alternate between organic and inorganic compounds.

THE NITROGEN CYCLE

One of the most important cycles is the *nitrogen cycle* (Fig. 7.3). The reservoir of nitrogen is the atmosphere, of which it makes up four fifths. In its gaseous form nitrogen is rather inert and does not readily take part in chemical reactions. Only certain bacteria — the *Rhizobium* species in the root nodules of clover, peas and other legumes, and free-living species, chiefly blue-green algae and *Azotobacter* — can use solar or chemical energy to 'fix' nitrogen, i.e. cause it to combine with hydrogen to form ammonium ions, which are then incorporated into the amino acids and proteins of plant tissues. The plants may then be eaten by animals. When the plant or animal dies, the protein is broken down to amino acids, then to ammonia and nitrates. These may be re-used by plants and microbes, or converted to gaseous nitrogen by other bacteria and re-enter the atmosphere.

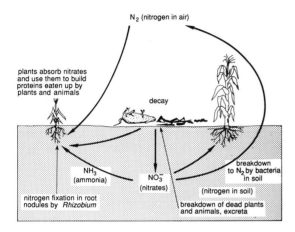

Fig. 7.3 The nitrogen cycle. Atmospheric nitrogen is 'fixed' (converted into ammonia) by bacteria, mostly in root nodules of plants. The ammonia is incorporated into proteins by plants, which may be eaten by animals. When plants and animals die, their proteins are broken down. The amino acids may be reused, or their amino groups may be converted to nitrate and then to nitrogen gas.

THE CARBON CYCLE

Another important cycle is the *carbon cycle*. By the processes of photosynthesis green plants and bacteria convert the carbon dioxide of the atmosphere into organic carbon compounds such as glucose; these serve as food to animals and microbes and are 'burned' to carbon dioxide and water in the processes of respiration. When plants, animals and microbes die, their bodies are attacked by other microbes, the complex organic compounds of which they are made are broken down, and carbon dioxide is released. This cycle is outlined in Figure 7.4.

THE PHOSPHORUS CYCLE

In the carbon and nitrogen cycles, these elements appear in different chemical forms at various points in the cycle. In the phosphorus cycle (Fig. 7.5.) this is not so. Throughout the cycle, phosphorus remains in the form of phosphates, PO_4^{3-} or HPO_4^{2-}. On land, phosphates are taken up from the soil and incorporated into

Fig. 7.4 The carbon cycle. Carbon dioxide in the atmosphere is converted to carbohydrates by plants, which may serve as food for animals. Animals burn the carbohydrates for energy, producing carbon dioxide again. The carbohydrates in dead plants and animals are broken down in the soil by saprophytes, and CO_2 is produced.

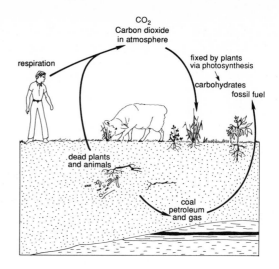

plant tissues, which then are eaten by animals and are then included in the proteins, lipids and nucleic acids of tissues and the framework of bones. When the animal dies, phosphates are liberated into the soil by microbial decomposition and re-enter the cycle. In the ocean similar events take place. There are losses of phosphates as dead creatures sink into the ocean depths, where there is little biological activity. Losses from the land cycle are accentuated if sewage is disposed of in the ocean and phosphate is often a limiting factor in the growth of crops.

Fig. 7.5 The phosphate cycle. Phosphates in the soil are taken up by plants and then used by animals which eat them. The phosphates return to the soil when plants and animals die. There is continual loss to the sea, since phosphates are leached out of the soil by water and carried away by rivers — this loss sometimes being accentuated by the quaint custom of depositing sewage in the ocean (or on Bondi beach).

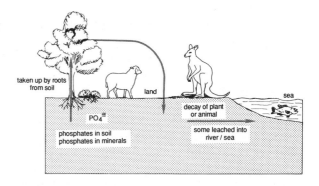

CHAPTER REVIEW

1   (a)   Define normal flora.
       (b)   What areas of the body have a normal flora?
       (c)   What parts of the body are normally sterile?

2   Where on/in the body would you expect to find Gram-positive organisms?

3   What is the importance of the normal flora?

4   (a)   How may the normal flora be modified or eliminated?
       (b)   What effect does this have?

5   Outline the carbon cycle.

6   Outline the nitrogen cycle.

CLASSIFYING AND IDENTIFYING MICROBES

In biological science, it is necessary for us to identify the creature we wish to study, to attach a label to it (if only to know that it is the same creature we studied last week).

In medical microbiology there are other good reasons for identifying the organism that one isolates from a patient. A particular set of symptoms (a *syndrome*) may be caused by different microbes. For example, an infection of the lungs — pneumonia — may be due to *Streptococcus pneumoniae* (the pneumococcus), to *Haemophilus influenzae*, to *Staphylococcus aureus*, or to *Mycoplasma pneumoniae*, to name only a few of the possible causes. The illness each causes will differ somewhat in its course, the likely complications, and the response to antibiotic treatment, so it is desirable to ascertain the microbe to blame. To identify the causative organism may advance medical knowledge (in recent years, for example, these investigations have led to the recognition of *Chlamydia trachomatis* as a cause of pneumonia). In a hospital, precise identification may reveal unsuspected spread of infection from patient to patient within the hospital (see chapter 13). Hence, identifying the microbes that are isolated from patients is a most important task of the medical microbiology laboratory.

CLASSIFICATION

Investigations which enable us to identify a microbe can also be employed to *classify* them. In a classification, the relationships between different creatures are set forth. Classification is based on the premise that organisms which are nearly related will share more characteristics than distant relatives (Fig. 8.1).

Fig. 8.1 Family tree of man and apes, and relationship to other mammals. This classification is based on anatomical and biochemical features. Our closest relatives are the gorilla and the chimpanzee; all three species are equally close to the orangutan, and then more distantly related to the other apes and monkeys. The other mammals are further away still.

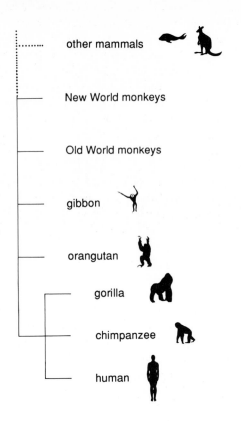

IDENTIFYING MICROBES

The identity, the uniqueness, of a microbe or any other creature is primarily embodied in the structure of the DNA — in the sequences of the nucleic acids themselves. At the second level, it finds expression in the proteins, carbohydrates and other constituents of which the cell is composed, and in the enzymes which carry out its essential reactions. At the third level we must consider the cell's products and the biochemical reactions it can carry out, and lastly we should think of the morphology and the behaviour of cells. Techniques for identification have evolved in the reverse order. Microscopy and biochemical reactions are the 'classical' tests, investigations of cellular constituents and of DNA sequences have come later. We shall approach this topic largely from the point of view of the medical microbiologist.

1 MICROSCOPY

Bacteria have not much variety in their shape and only in certain situations can one be reasonably confident of an identification based on microscopy alone. Gram-positive cocci in clumps seen in pus are probably staphylococci, species uncertain (Plate 2); Gram-

positive cocci in chains from a similar source would be streptococci, of any one of a good number of species (Plate 3); small
Gram-negative rods seen in the cerebrospinal fluid of a child with
fever and a stiff neck would almost certainly be *Haemophilus influenzae* (Plate 4); acid-fast bacilli in sputum are probably *Mycobacterium
tuberculosis* (Plate 15). But in most cases microscopy gives only
hints. Note, however, that in all of the examples cited, microscopy
yields sufficient information to guide initial chemotherapy, while
fuller investigations continue (see p.91 'A case of pneumonia').
Immunofluorescence (see p.127) is often capable of giving a rapid
and accurate answer.

In general eucaryotes have a much greater variety of shape and
microscopic characteristics may be adequate for identification. For
instance, an encapsulated yeast seen in cerebrospinal fluid or
sputum is almost certainly *Cryptococcus neoformans* (see p.235 and
Plate 5). A motile, pear-shaped protozoon observed in vaginal secretions is *Trichomonas vaginalis* (see p.253). Parasites are normally
identified by the appearance of their eggs or trophozoites. Motility,
the ability to swim or to crawl over a surface, can be detected
microscopically and often contributes to the identification of a
microbe. In secretions from the large gut, for example, *Entamoeba
histolytica* (p.240 and Plate 60) is detected by its motility (and by
the presence of red cells in its food vacuoles).

2 BIOCHEMICAL REACTIONS

Biochemical reactions include analysis of factors required for
growth or biochemical capabilities such as utilising a particular
organic compound or producing a distinctive substance.

GROWTH REQUIREMENTS

Some bacteria have characteristic growth requirements that help
us to identify them. An example is *Haemophilus influenzae*, a small
Gram-negative rod which causes lung disease and meningitis. We
distinguish it from similar organisms by the fact that it needs two
factors for growth (known as 'X' and 'V' factors). Suppose we isolate a small Gram-negative rod. We spread it on a nutrient agar
plate and place on the surface 3 paper disks impregnated with X,
V and X + V; then *H. influenzae* will grow only around the X + V
disk (Fig. 8.2).

BIOCHEMICAL CAPABILITIES

Another characteristic used in the identification of many species is
the sugars, amino acids and the like which they can metabolise.
The sugar under test is added to a dilute broth containing an acid-
base indicator dye such as bromthymol blue. This dye changes colour when the pH of the solution is altered, being blue at pH 7.0
and yellow at pH 6.0. The initial pH of the medium is close to 7.0,

Fig. 8.2 Identification of *Haemophilus influenzae*. An agar plate is inoculated with the organism to be tested (a small Gram-negative rod) and disks containing X, V and X+V substances are placed on it. If the bacterium requires both substances, it will grow only around the X+V disk (and is *H. influenzae*). If it grows around both X+V and V disks, it is *H. parainfluenzae*, which does not usually cause disease.

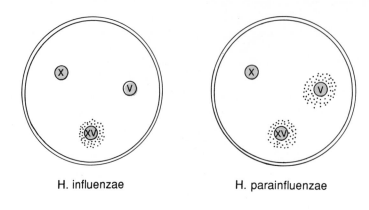

H. influenzae   H. parainfluenzae

so the dye is blue. If the sugar is metabolised, acid is produced and the dye changes colour to yellow. Such a medium can detect organisms capable of using lactose and thus distinguishes *Escherichia coli* (a member of the normal gut flora) from *Salmonella* and *Shigella*, organisms which cause infectious diarrhoea. The ability to break down amino acids can be detected in a similar manner — arginine, lysine and ornithine are commonly used.

Another identification test looks at the capacity to produce indole from the amino acid tryptophane. Indole is detected by a chemical reaction — after the medium has been inoculated and incubated, reagents are added and production of indole is indicated by a change in colour. Many bacterial cells contain the enzyme catalase, which breaks down hydrogen peroxide, an extremely toxic substance which can be formed in bacterial cells. Production of catalase can be detected by mixing the bacterial colony with hydrogen peroxide and watching for the evolution of gas bubbles. Streptococci and anaerobic bacteria do not possess catalase.

Other bacteria liberate into the medium proteins with various properties. *Staphylococcus aureus*, for instance, secretes coagulase, an enzyme which causes plasma to clot, and this fact is used to identify it (p.196). Likewise some bacteria secrete an enzyme that breaks down proteins: to detect this, fine particles of charcoal are embedded in gelatin and added to the broth; if a proteinase is produced, the charcoal is released and the medium becomes uniformly black (Fig. 8.3). Other secreted enzymes break down starch, DNA, urea and many other substances; tests are available to detect these reactions. Many of these tests are included in the API 20E gallery (Plate 7), a disposable plastic set of 20 wells each containing a different test material. Such kits are now widely used, since they save the laboratory the trouble of maintaining stocks of many different test media. New biochemical tests and new ways of applying old tests are constantly being developed.

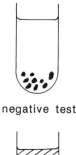

negative test

positive test

Fig. 8.3 Gelatin breakdown, −ve and +ve tests. Particles of charcoal are embedded in gelatin and added to the medium. If the microbe can digest gelatin, the particles are released and the medium is uniformly black when shaken. Otherwise the black pieces of gelatin remain intact.

3 SEROLOGICAL TESTS/DETECTION OF ANTIGENS

Many bacteria produce distinctive substances unique to the species. Streptococci, for instance, contain group antigens and are classified as group A, group B, C and so on. These groupings correlate with other biochemical features and with clinical characteristics (chapter 14). The group antigens (A, B, C etc) are polysaccharides. The *Enterobacteriaceae, Escherichia coli, Salmonella typhi, Shigella* and others, carry on their surfaces O antigens in great variety. *Streptococcus pneumoniae, Haemophilus influenzae, Cryptococcus neoformans* and other microbes produce characteristic capsules. Toxins are an important group of microbial products. The diphtheria bacillus causes illness by releasing a toxin which is absorbed and acts on the heart. *Clostridium tetani* and *Clostridium difficile* are two other organisms which cause disease in this way.

Any of these substance may be identified by *serological* methods. If a suitable preparation of the bacterium, the polysaccharide or the toxin is injected into an animal, the resulting *antiserum* (chapter 10) can be used to detect the substance injected and hence to diagnose the corresponding infection or identify the microbe once isolated. It is now the normal practice in the diagnosis of meningitis, for example, to test the cerebrospinal fluid for the antigens of *H. influenzae, N. meningitidis, S. pneumoniae* and *C. neoformans*. It is also possible to demonstrate microbial antigens in the urine. A positive result in such a test provides a diagnosis much more rapidly than cultural techniques. (See following, 'Stephanie has a stiff neck'.)

DNA PROBES

It is now possible to 'clone' a segment of DNA from the genome of a microbe (see chapter 6). If one selects a segment that is unique for that microbe, this can be used to identify it. Such probes are now available for the detection or identification of *Mycobacterium tuberculosis*, *Legionella*, *Mycoplasma pneumoniae*, herpes simplex virus and cytomegalovirus.

IN THE WARD
Stephanie has a stiff neck

Apart from a 'cold' some 10 days before, Stephanie Jacobs had been quite well, until she awoke one morning looking rather 'strange'. Her mother noticed that she did not seem 'quite to know where she was', she was irritable and cried and she felt very hot.

Her local doctor found that her temperature was 39.3°C and her neck was stiff, and arranged her immediate admission to hospital as a 'probable meningitis' case (neck stiffness probably results from irritation of the nerves because of inflammation in the covering membranes, and is the hallmark of meningitis).

On arrival in the hospital a lumbar puncture was immediately carried out. The cerebrospinal fluid was turbid, its glucose content was low and the white-cell count was 2400×10^6 /L, made up of 2100 neutropils and 300 mononuclear cells (lymphocytes and monocytes); a normal cell count would be 0 and <5 respectively.

The laboratory technologists searched the Gram-stained film of the cerebrospinal fluid very carefully without finding any bacteria. Tests were carried out to detect the antigens of the common causes of meningitis; antigens of *Neisseria meningitidis* were present (Fig. A).

Stephanie was given penicillin intravenously and made a good recovery over the next few weeks.

The cerebrospinal fluid was inoculated into several different media; a few colonies of *Neisseria meningitidis* grew from one of these cultures. Failure to see the organism in the Gram stain is explained by the fact that not many bacteria were present and that *Neisseria meningitidis* is a small Gram-negative coccus, hard to see amid all the white cells, which also stain Gram-negative.

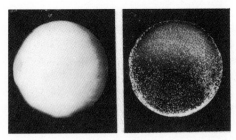

Fig. A Antigen detection by slide agglutination. The test reagent was made by attaching antibodies against the capsular antigens of *Neisseria meningitidis* to the surface of fine particles of latex. When the reagent is mixed with cerebrospinal fluid containing the antigen, the particles are clumped. If no antigen is present, the suspension remains uniform.

CHAPTER REVIEW

1 Why is it necessary to identify an organism?
2 Give examples of bacteria which can be provisionally identified by microscopy.
3 Give examples of biochemical tests used in the identification
   and classification of microorganisms.
4 What biochemical test is used in the identification of
   (a) *Haemophilus influenzae?*
   (b) *Staphylococcus aureus?*
5 (a) Define a *toxin.*
   (b) How are toxins detected?
6 (a) What is serological identification?
   (b) How is it performed?

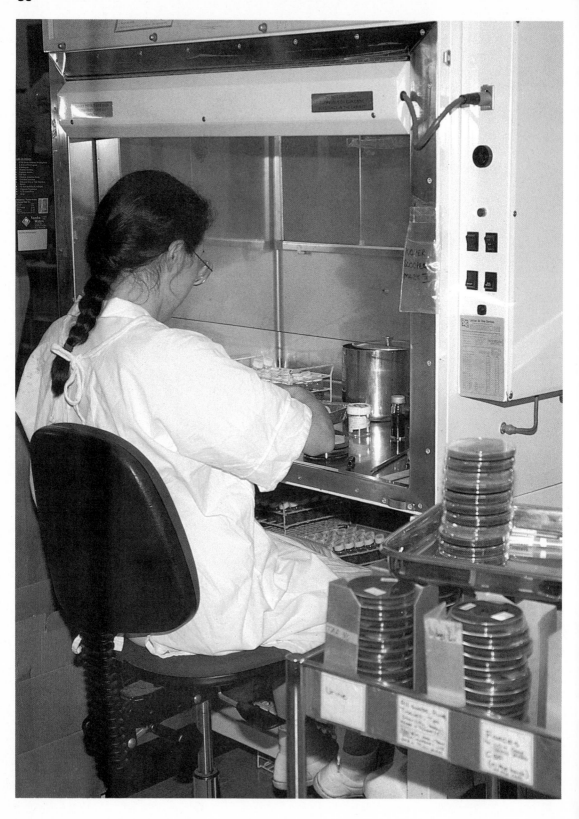

9

IN THE HOSPITAL MICROBIOLOGY LABORATORY

Most hospitals of any size, and all teaching hospitals or referral hospitals, have a *microbiology laboratory*, staffed by scientists (some of whom may have training in medicine also). In a large hospital laboratory, services will be available day and evening, and at weekends, with staff on call at other times. The laboratory examines by-products and bits of people, secretions and fluids sampled with swabsticks, even pieces of tissue (biopsies) — and attempts to identify in them microbes likely to cause disease. The laboratory also tests the antibiotic susceptibilities of any pathogens, looks for antibodies to bacteria, viruses and parasites as evidence of infection, and estimates the levels of antibiotics in blood in order to guide treatment.

PERSONNEL

Microbiologists carry out a wide range of tests and must have a good deal of knowledge and experience, since they advise on the interpretation of laboratory results, the diagnosis of infections, and on antibiotic therapy. Microbiology relies less on automated equipment than do other divisions of pathology. Infection control nurses form an important unit within the microbiology department; they must work in close liaison with the microbiologists. Their role is hospital epidemiology. This involves monitoring the occurrence of infections in the hospital, tracing routes of spread, advising on problems of sterilisation and cleaning, and taking part in the education of nursing and other staff.

87

SPECIMENS: TYPES, QUALITY, PROCESSING, TIME-SCALES

The microbiology department receives many sorts of specimens. Initially, we must distinguish between specimens from sites that are normally sterile, and from sites that are not (see Table 9.1). If an organism grows from blood or cerebrospinal fluid or another site where the body's defences normally prevent the access of bacteria, this fact is strong evidence that the organism is producing disease, and it will be fully investigated. On the other hand, secretions in contact with body surfaces normally teem with bacteria (chapter 7): the microbiologist must decide, by choosing suitable methods for examining the specimen, and by assessing the results, whether a potential pathogen is present amongst the normal flora.

TABLE 9.1 MICROBIOLOGY SPECIMENS AND THEIR ORIGINS

From normally sterile sites	*From normally unsterile sites*
Blood	Sputum
Cerebrospinal fluid	Faeces
Body fluids (from pleural, peritoneal or joint cavity, deep abscess)	Swabs (from throat, nose, eye, ear, skin, vagina, urethra)
Tissue biopsies (Urine)*	

(*Urine is bracketed, because it is passed through a tube, the urethra, which is unsterile in its lower part.)

The *quality* of the specimen is all-important. The quality depends on the care of collection and the patient may need to be given instructions. For example, the ward staff should ensure that, before providing a specimen of sputum, the patient washes out his or her mouth and gives a deep cough. Or a specimen of pus to be examined for anaerobes must be protected from air (it is best collected into a syringe and left there).

The specimen must also be conveyed to the laboratory promptly. Some bacteria (e.g. gonococci) die rapidly when removed from the affected tissues. If a number of different bacteria are present in the specimen, holding it at room temperature for some hours may lead to confusion, since some species will grow faster than others, and the relative numbers in the sample will change. For the same reason, the laboratory must process the specimen as soon as possible after receipt — normally in less than an hour — and, in order to ensure that all bacteria present in the specimen can grow, the media used must be of high quality, be suitable and be *fresh*.

The *time-scales* of microbiological investigations are determined primarily by the nature of microbes. Once the specimen has been received, the minimum time for completing typical investigations would be about 10 minutes for microscopy of a Gram stain (preliminary report), 15-18 hours for a culture, and an additional 5-24 hours for antibiotic susceptibilities. However, it is increasingly true that rapid methods of detecting and identifying microbes are coming into use. (It is occasionally necessary to point out that these laboratory delays arise from the rates of bacterial growth and cannot be influenced by the seniority of the inquirer — or by profanity!). In some cases much longer times are involved, e.g. a blood culture should be incubated for three weeks when brucellosis is suspected.

THREE MAIN CLINICAL QUESTIONS

The three main clinical questions which the clinician asks the laboratory are:

1   Is this patient suffering from a microbial infection?
2   If so, which microbe causes it?
3   How can it be treated?

They can be answered in different degrees and circumstances. When the specimen comes from a *normally sterile site*, it is often possible to answer all three questions. The blood, the cerebrospinal fluid, fluids from the pericardial, pleural or peritoneal cavities or from joint cavities would normally be sterile, since in these sites there is no normal flora. Likewise, pus withdrawn from an abscess in the deep tissues of the body would usually contain only the microbes responsible for the infection. In all of these cases, if a bacterium is seen or grown, it is likely that the patient has an infection due to it. The presence of any organism in the Gram stain of the fluid will give an immediate clue. However, if the specimen comes in contact with a body surface before collection then the results are much more difficult to interpret.

TYPICAL MICROBIOLOGICAL INVESTIGATIONS
1 BLOOD CULTURE

A *blood culture* is frequently carried out in the investigation of fever. Blood is drawn with precautions to avoid contamination by the skin flora, and inoculated into two flasks of medium, — one suitable for the growth of aerobes and one for anaerobes. As less than one bacterium may be present per mL of blood, even in serious illness, it is important to collect at least 10 mL of blood for culture, and preferably 20. Blood cultures are inspected daily for at least one week, and preferably two. Any organism appearing in the blood culture needs to be identified, since bacteria are not normally present in the blood.

2 CEREBROSPINAL FLUID (CSF)

If *meningitis* is suspected, it is essential to investigate the *cerebrospinal fluid*. This is an emergency, the procedure for collecting the fluid ('lumbar puncture'), must be carried out immediately, and the cerebrospinal fluid be taken directly to the laboratory. As several different tests need to be carried out it is important that enough fluid is obtained (5 mL at least).

The first step is to carry out a cell count on the csf, for which a microscope and a special counting chamber are used. One records the numbers of red cells, polymorphonuclear and mononuclear cells and any other objects seen. Then some of the csf is centrifuged, the deposit is re-suspended in 1-2 drops and a film is made, Gram-stained and examined for microbes. Even the presence of two or three bacterial cells is considered significant (it is usually difficult to be certain that the object is a bacterial cell if you only see one). The fluid is also examined for antigens derived from the organisms commonly causing meningitis: *Haemophilus influenzae, Streptococcus pneumoniae, Neisseria meningitidis,* and *Cryptococcus neoformans.* A positive result indicates the corresponding infection (see box 'Stephanie has a stiff neck', chapter 8, p.84). The deposit is cultured on rich media such as blood agar and chocolate agar and in cooked meat broth, and the cultures are kept for at least three days. If any colonies appear on the plates after culturing this specimen, they *need to be identified*, since their presence in a sterile site is strong evidence that they are the cause of disease.

3 SPUTUM

The specimen most often presented to the laboratory in cases of *respiratory infection* is *sputum*. The lung is normally sterile beyond the main air-passages (bronchi), but specimens cannot be easily and safely collected from them. The healthy person does not produce secretions from the lungs by coughing, so to persuade such a person to provide 'sputum' will actually result only in saliva, the examination of which is unhelpful.

When lower respiratory tract secretions are present and sputum can be coughed up, it will pass through the throat and mouth. Here there is a dense normal flora, which may include most of the bacteria that cause infections in the lung. In fact infection of the lung normally arises because of some failure of the normal defences to prevent the flora of the upper respiratory tract descending into the lungs. Hence, except in the case of tuberculosis, it is impossible to say with certainty from the examination of sputum that the patient has a microbial infection; that is, it is impossible to answer question 1: 'Is this patient suffering from a microbial infection?'. Only the clinician can decide that. If the patient has clinical and X-ray evidence of infection, and the clinician concludes that pneumonia is likely, then the laboratory may be able to help by providing an answer to question 2, 'Which microbe is causing the infection?'.

The normal examination of sputum includes a Gram stain and culture. On the Gram stain the technologist will note the numbers of epithelial cells and may reject the specimen if too many are present, since epithelial cells come from the surface of the mouth and their presence is evidence that the specimen is heavily contaminated with saliva. The report should also comment on the numbers of 'polymorphs' or 'pus cells' (polymorphonuclear leucocytes), on the presence of normal upper respiratory tract flora and indicate the predominant organism(s). Sometimes the microscopic examination is diagnostic, or virtually so (see following, 'A case of pneumonia').

IN THE WARD
A case of pneumonia

Allan Brown, age 45, was feeling well until 24 hours ago, when he developed a cough with 'rusty' sputum, chills and fever. His temperature is now 39⁰C, his breathing is rapid and he looks ill.

Examination of the chest suggests pneumonia. A sample of his sputum is sent to the laboratory (while he himself is taken to the X-ray department). The clinical notes accompanying the specimen read: 'Cough, temp 39, chest - probable pneumonia. Urgent.'

A film is made from the sputum and stained by Gram's method. As well as the normal flora, numerous Gram-positive cocci are seen, in pairs and surrounded by a capsule (Plate 8). These are likely to be pneumococci — *Streptococcus pneumoniae* — the commonest cause of pneumonia acquired outside hospital.

This report is telephoned to the ward immediately.

The chest X-ray shows 'consolidation' of the lungs, the typical appearance of pneumococcal pneumonia. Thus both the Gram-stained film and the X-ray confirm the clinical diagnosis.

The appropriate treatment is penicillin by injection and this is started without delay.

Sputum is cultured on blood agar, and preferably on a selective medium which will reveal *Haemophilus influenzae* as well as other Gram-negative rods; *H. influenzae* grows relatively slowly and forms small transparent colonies, which may not be seen amid the hundreds of others representing the flora of the upper respiratory tract. There will inevitably be fairly large numbers of colonies from the flora of the upper respiratory tract: alpha-haemolytic streptococci, diphtheroids and others. The technologist must decide if any of the hundreds of colonies on the plate(s) are likely to cause respiratory tract infection. Fortunately these colonies belong to relatively few types. Organisms likely to be the cause of pneumonia are *Streptococcus pneumoniae, Haemophilus influenzae, Staphylococcus aureus, Branhamella catarrhalis* and various Gram-negative rods, and any colonies suggesting these organisms would be considered more closely. *H. influenzae, B. catarrhalis* and *S. aureus* would be thought significant only if present in relatively large numbers, +++ or ++++, and a Gram-negative rod only if it was predominant and replacing the normal flora almost completely. Culture results are often reported on a scale of + to ++++: 'scattered colonies' to 'predominant growth'. If any unusual cause of pneumonia is suspected, this should be mentioned in the request, so that additional media can be inoculated. For example, *Legionella,* the cause of Legionnaires' disease, would not usually be detected by the routine sputum cultures.

4 URINE

Urine is the premier microbiology specimen: constituting about 25% of the laboratory's workload. Primarily it is examined for evidence of infection, and also to detect *haematuria* (blood in the urine). The number and types of cells present are determined by means of a phase-contrast microscope; with this instrument one can visualise cells without staining them.

As an example, a microscopy report might read:
>100×10^6 white cells /L (per litre)
<10×10^6 red cells /L
<10×10^6 epithelial cells /L

In this case the number of white cells is abnormally high and usually indicates infection; the numbers of other cells are within normal limits. Large numbers of epithelial cells, >100×10^6 /L, usually mean contamination of the urine with vaginal secretions; this often makes interpretation of the culture results impossible.

In examining urine the microbiologist makes use of another method of assessing the significance of microbes in the specimen; the number of bacteria in the urine are counted. There are several ways of doing this. We may plate out a measured quantity using a special loop that delivers, say, 1 microlitre; we may dip a slide covered with medium in the urine, drain it and incubate it, counting colonies the next day and comparing them with standards. The bladder urine is normally sterile and the urethra (the passage leading from the bladder to the exterior) contains only small numbers of bacteria. Hence, if large numbers of bacteria are detected, it is likely that the urine is infected. In urinary infection there are usually 10^8 organisms per litre of urine or close to it and a single organism is present or clearly predominates. Such an organism will be identified. Because the lower urethra has a microbial flora, most urine specimens contain small numbers of Gram-positive cocci and diphtheroids ($< = 10^4$/ mL); their presence, however, does not mean urinary infection.

5 SWABS

Investigations of other specimens from sites possessing a normal flora follow similar lines; skin swabs for example are examined for *Staphylococcus aureus,* and also for beta-haemolytic streptococci if impetigo is suspected. When sent up by the Sexually Transmitted Disease (STD) clinic, vaginal and urethral swabs are examined for specific pathogens: *Neisseria gonorrhoeae*, *Trichomonas vaginalis*, *Candida albicans*, *Gardnerella vaginalis*, while throat and rectal swabs from this clinic would be cultured for *N. gonorrhoeae* only. Because *N. gonorrhoeae* is easily outgrown by the flora of these sites, special selective media containing antibiotics are used to detect it. In all these cases the normal flora would be disregarded.

FURTHER INVESTIGATIONS

IDENTIFICATION

How does the technologist decide which of the colonies she or he sees on the plate can be neglected, and which merit further investigation? This task demands considerable training and only the most experienced staff are rostered to 'read' cultures. They look at:

- size
- shape
- colour
- texture
- other features of the colony

Is it smooth or rough, shiny or dull, opaque or translucent, pigmented or colourless?

Has the organism spread over the surrounding medium?

Has it attacked the red cells? *Beta-haemolysis*, for instance, is seen as a clear red zone around the colony; in this zone the red cells are lysed (have disintegrated). In *alpha-haemolysis*, the blood pigments are changed to green, but the cells are not lysed, so that there is a turbid green zone around the colony.

On the basis of what appears on the plate, the type of specimen and the history of the illness (see following, 'Clinical notes help the laboratory'), one or more colony types are selected for identification and testing of their susceptibility to antibiotics. Plates 31–34 illustrate the work of the microbiology laboratory.

IN THE LAB
Clinical notes help the laboratory

The request form which is filled out for a microbiological test includes a space for 'clinical notes'. This should indicate what illness is suspected (the *provisional diagnosis*) and explain why the test is thought necessary. The clinical notes are important, since they help the laboratory staff:

- select the proper media for cultures
- decide on any necessary additional tests
- interpret the results

Sputum specimen — 'cavity in R lung': mycobacteria will also be looked for.

Urine specimen — '? chronic renal failure': a special, more accurate cell count and microscopy will be performed, since in this case a small increase in white cells in the urine may be important.

Eye swab — 'probable conjunctivitis': the technologist will know to test any organism that is isolated for susceptibility to chloramphenicol, which is often used in eye infections.

Unfortunately, clinical notes are often omitted. And at other times the notes that are supplied are unhelpful — even mysterious, such as the following examples:

'? abscess, right lung'
'swelling, right side of neck' } accompanying vaginal swabs
'fever, ? urinary infection' accompanying an eye swab
'? fracture skull'
'dementia, ? stroke' } with 50 mL urine in each case

Start your own collection!

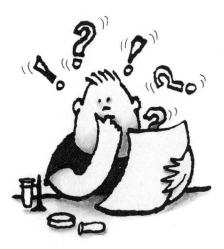

LABORATORY REPORTS

It is the laboratory's responsibility to *issue reports* promptly. If investigations are not complete within 48 hours, a preliminary report should be issued (we are assuming that the laboratory's records are not part of a computerised hospital information system which allows medical and nursing staff to look at progress results of laboratory work by means of ward terminals).

The report should be *comprehensible*. If, for instance, we report that 'the sputum grew ++++ of *Enterobacter agglomerans* and it is sensitive to gentamicin and trimethoprim and resistant to ampicillin', we should not be surprised that the patient receives unnecessary antibiotics, since most of the clinicians will never have heard of this organism, and reporting susceptibilities is often taken to indicate that the isolate is significant and should be treated. In reality, however, this reading usually means that the patient has already *received* too many antibiotics and it should therefore be accompanied by the note '*Enterobacter agglomerans* is an inhabitant of the gut; it appears in sputum usually as a result of antibiotic therapy. Treatment is unnecessary unless the patient has clinical signs of respiratory tract infection'.

The results of microbiological tests must be interpreted in the clinical context. There are relatively few results capable of only one interpretation. Examples of these would be: the culture of *Haemophilus influenzae* from the cerebrospinal fluid of a 3-year child; the appearance of *Streptococcus pneumoniae* in a blood culture; growth of *Neisseria gonorrhoeae* from the urethral discharge of a young man recently returned from an Asian holiday.

But, as stated, only a small proportion of the laboratory reports are so unequivocal. For instance, a urine specimen yielding 10^8 *Escherichia coli* per litre would mean urinary infection requiring treatment in a healthy woman of 30, but may simply represent colonisation and the need for further observation in a catheterised man of 60. Likewise, in about 75% of cases, *Staphylococcus aureus* in a blood culture is significant; in the remaining cases, however, it is probably derived from the skin. Organisms such as *Escherichia coli*, *Klebsiella pneumoniae*, *Pseudomonas aeruginosa* and *Haemophilus influenzae*, however, which are rarely present in the skin flora, are almost *always* important when isolated from the blood.

And always the *patient* must be evaluated clinically: *one must not treat a laboratory report.* For example, infection is normally accompanied by fever, and numerous inflammatory cells appear in the infected site — but some patients do not observe the rules: after a surgical operation an old person may develop a major infection without any rise in temperature. Similarly, a patient with neutropenia (a common consequence of the drugs used to treat leukaemia) may have almost no white cells for any purpose; in such a patient an infection, for example, of the lung, urine or cerebrospinal fluid may take place without the appearance of the numerous inflammatory cells we would expect to see in such circumstances.

We must remember that laboratory testing makes a relatively small contribution to diagnosis — although often a vital one. A doctor will have made a correct diagnosis in close to 90% of patients by the time he has finished taking the history of the patient's illness and carrying out a physical examination. *And the laboratory is most likely to make a useful contribution when there is good communication between the laboratory staff and the clinicians.*

CHAPTER REVIEW

1   Which body sites are normally bacteriologically sterile?
2   (a)   What is the best method of collecting pus for anaerobic culture?
     (b)   Why is it important?
3   List the specimens commonly processed by the microbiology laboratory.
4   Outline how a urine specimen is examined in the microbiology laboratory.

5   How long does it normally take to complete the culture and sensitivity tests on a specimen?

6   Why should the specimen arrive promptly at the laboratory following collection?

7   What precautions should one take in collecting a specimen of
(a)   sputum?
(b)   urine?

Part Two
Bacteria and Humankind

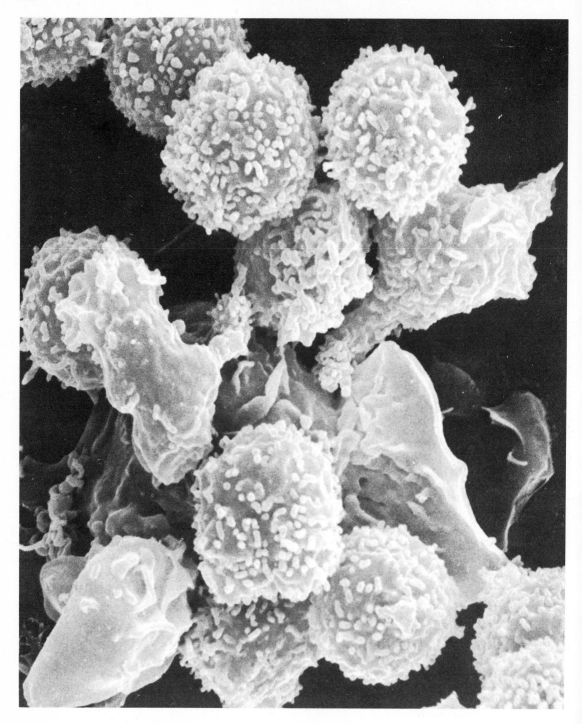

T-cells (the small, spherical objects) recognise antigen on the surface of
a macrophage (the larger flat object). The macrophage ingests the bacterial
protein, breaks it down and displays the pieces together with certain of the cell's
surface proteins, aiding the programmed T-cells to recognise the bacterial
antigens.

10

THE BODY'S DEFENCES

As we have seen, bacteria and other microbes (thousands of different species) swarm on our bodies and in the general environment. Most of these are harmless and even beneficial (see p4), but there nevertheless remains a large number of microbes which can invade the body in one fashion or another and cause *disease*. Such microbes are called *pathogens*. The mechanisms by which they cause disease will be studied later — firstly we shall consider *immunity*, the body's defences against infectious disease.

1 INNATE (OR NON-SPECIFIC) IMMUNITY

Some of these defences are innate and non-specific, i.e. they are normally present in healthy humans and do not depend upon a response to an invading microbe.

The first line of defence against pathogens is the barrier formed by the body surfaces: covered by the *skin* and *mucous membranes* (Table 10.1). The intact skin cannot be penetrated by most microbes, and its effectiveness is reinforced by antibacterial substances in sweat and secretions of skin glands: *lactic acid* and *fatty acids*. The *mucus* secreted by mucous membranes traps microbes and hinders their adherence to the surface. In the stomach the low pH of the gastric juice kills most bacteria.

If microbes do manage to pass these barriers, they encounter further mechanisms of defence — collectively referred to as the *acute inflammatory response*, the signs of which are *heat, redness, swelling* and *pain*. The components of the *acute inflammatory response* are set out in Figure 10.1.

TABLE 10.1 INNATE DEFENCES — NON-SPECIFIC IMMUNITY

Barriers	skin, mucous membranes of gut, respiratory tract and genito-urinary tract
	fluids on skin and mucous membranes
	acid in stomach
	cleaning action of cilia, saliva, urine
	antagonism of normal flora
Phagocytes	neutrophils
	macrophages
Dissolved substances	lysozyme, acute phase proteins, interferons

Fig. 10.1 The acute
inflammatory response.
Staphylococci multiplying
in a hair follicle liberate
chemotactic factors, and the
reaction of staphylococci
with antibodies and
complement has the same
effect. In response to these
stimuli, polymorphonuclear
leucocytes pass out from the
blood vessels and gather at
the site of infection. These
reactions also enhance the
permeability of the
capillaries and facilitate the
accumulation of cells and
antibodies around the site
of infection.

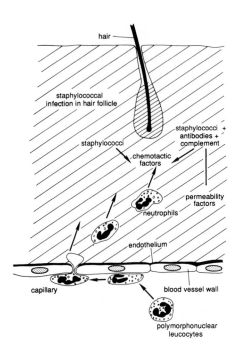

PHAGOCYTES: NEUTROPHILS AND MACROPHAGES

Phagocytes are cells which eat foreign substances (even animals as
primitive as the earthworm can destroy invading bacteria by means
of phagocytes, so they are an ancient weapon). In higher animals
there are two types of phagocytes, the *neutrophil* and the *macrophage*.
Polymorphonuclear neutrophil leucocytes, or 'neutrophils' for short,
are the commonest white cells in the blood, easily recognised by
their multi-lobed nuclei (Plate 10) ('polymorphonuclear' means
'nucleus of many shapes'). Their cytoplasm contains granules of
various substances, by means of which they kill the microbes they
engulf. Macrophages are produced in the bone marrow (as are all
the blood cells) and travel in the blood to the tissues, settling especially in the lungs, liver, spleen and lymph nodes, where they constitute the *mononuclear phagocytic system*.

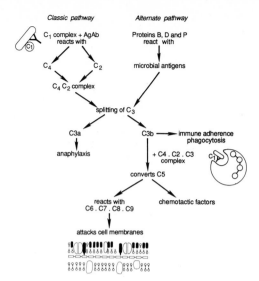

Composition of the blood

Blood consists of cells and a liquid, plasma.

1 Blood cells:
- red — carrry oxygen to the tissues
- white — polymorphonuclear leucocytes
  - neutrophils
  - eosinophils
  - basophils
  - monocytes → macrophages
  - lymphocytes, large and small
  - platelets, involved in the clotting of blood

2 Plasma — contains ions, Na^+, K^+, Cl^- and others
- many proteins, including antibodies
- amino acids, and vitamins
- coagulation factors

3 Serum — the fluid left after plasma has clotted

DESTRUCTION OF MICROBES: INFLAMMATION, COMPLEMENT

To destroy microbes, phagocytes must first *locate* them and then *engulf* them. Both neutrophils and macrophages are motile, and move towards microbes, attracted by chemicals the microbes release: this is termed *chemotaxis*. Some of these attracting molecules are produced by bacteria and others are generated by the activation of *complement*, a system of proteins found in plasma (Fig. 10.2). Many microbes react with complement and activate it, a complicated sequence of chemical events causing the production of molecules which:

1 attach to the microbe and make it stick to the surface of phagocytes
2 attract phagocytes and stimulate them to produce microbicidal agents
3 modify capillary blood vessels so that they become more permeable, and phagocytes and plasma constituents gather where the microbes are located
4 punch holes in the membranes of certain cells (e.g Gram-negative bacteria)

As a result of complement activation, phagocytes move towards the invading microbes, which adhere to their surface and are then (usually) engulfed (Fig. 10.3). The cytoplasm extends around the microbe and fuses to contain it in a phagocytic vacuole. Next, the cytoplasmic granules merge with the membrane of the vacuole and discharge their contents into it. The vacuole has available a number of microbicidal systems, some of which convert oxygen to active toxic forms (superoxide anion and hydrogen peroxide), while others damage the cell wall of the microbes *(lysozyme)* or deprive them of the iron needed for growth *(lactoferrin)*. Once killed, the microbes are digested by enzymes.

Some pathogens, however, such as helminth worms, are much too large to be engulfed by a phagocyte. In these instances, eosinophils (a type of neutrophil which shows reddish granules

Fig. 10.3 (a) and **(b)**
Phagocytosis. When a bacterium reacts with an antibody, complement is 'fixed', i.e. part of the C_3 component binds to the bacterial surface. The surface of the leucocyte carries receptors for the Fc part of the antibody molecule and for C_3. The bacterium binds to these receptors, the cytoplasm of the leucocyte extends around it, and it is enclosed in a phagocytic vacuole. Lysosomes (packages of enzymes) release their contents into this vacuole and the bacterium is digested.

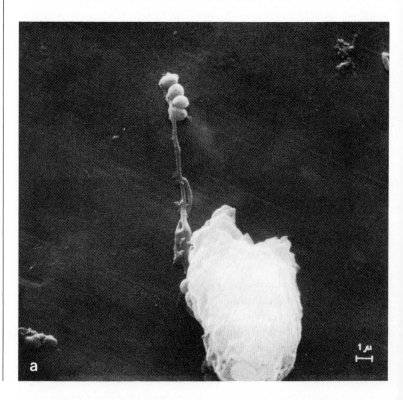

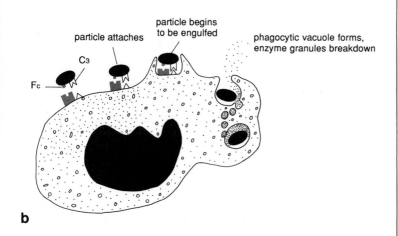

particle begins
particle attaches to be engulfed
phagocytic vacuole forms,
enzyme granules breakdown

C₃

Fc

b

when stained by the usual technique for blood films) can attack parasites by sticking to them and releasing toxic substances (Plate 10d).

Among the soluble factors active in defence we can include lysozyme, present in most body fluids as well as in phagocytes, the acute phase proteins and the interferons. Lysozyme is an enzyme which breaks down the peptidoglycan cell wall and kills the bacterium — unfortunately, in most bacteria the peptidoglycan meshwork is covered by other layers (protein, lipoprotein or capsule) and is thus protected.

The acute phase proteins increase rapidly in concentration in blood and tissue fluids during the 'acute phase', i.e. the early stages, of the response to infection or injury. Some assist in the formation of a *fibrin clot* to wall off the injury and prevent spread of microbes; others attach to invading organisms and trigger the complement system. One of these proteins, *C-reactive protein*, has been part of body defences for quite a while — a very similar protein is present in the horseshoe crab, which first appeared on earth about 300 million years ago! C-reactive protein can bind to some microbes, and then activates complement. This leads to the linkage of a complement component to the surface of the microbe and promotes its phagocytosis.

Interferons are anti-viral substances produced by lymphocytes and other cells. They are secreted by a virus-infected cell and bind to neighbouring cells, preventing viral replication within them and creating a zone of uninfectable cells around the infected cell, thus restricting the spread of the virus. *Natural killer cells*, a type of large lymphocyte, achieve the same end by attacking and lysing the virally infected cells.

2 SPECIFIC IMMUNITY: THE ACQUIRED IMMUNE RESPONSE

ANTIBODIES

In higher animals innate immunity is supplemented by a second, *specific immunity* generated by the *acquired immune response*. We know, for instance, that a child who has had measles or mumps is not at risk of catching that disease again, and that immunisation in early childhood protects against diphtheria, tetanus, whooping cough and poliomyelitis. In some way the body 'remembers' the previous experience with the infection or immunising injection.

Furthermore this second type *immunity* is specific, e.g. immunisation against diphtheria does not protect one against tetanus or 'polio'. We can therefore see that the important features of the adaptive immune response are *specificity* and *memory*. If we were to investigate a young girl who had had measles, we would find that her blood and tissue fluids contained antibodies that reacted with the virus (antibody-mediated immunity) and that specifically sensitised cells were present that also recognised the virus (cell-mediated immunity).

Antibody molecules are *proteins*, and they have three functional regions: one recognises and binds to the antigen (constituent of a microbe, a toxin, a viral coat protein or whatever); one activates complement by a pathway somewhat different to the one we have already discussed, and one links to receptors on the surface of the phagocyte and triggers engulfment. Some microbes are not readily ingested by phagocytes and do not initiate the cascade of complement reactions. Once antibody molecules are bound to the surface of such organisms, complement is fixed and phagocytosis is made easier. The specifically sensitised cells are called *lymphocytes*. Some recognise antigen by means of antibody molecules on their surfaces, others have another type of receptor molecule for this purpose. After contact with antigen, some develop into antibody-producing cells, while others activate macrophages.

We can learn a great deal about the immune response by injecting a rabbit on two occasions with tetanus toxoid and measuring the amount of antibody (tetanus antitoxin) in the blood. This experiment is described following ('In the lab'). We see that after the first injection the animal takes some time to produce antibodies and these reach only a relatively low level ('primary response'). A second injection some weeks later stimulates a brisker response and a much higher final level of antibody ('secondary response'). In this experiment, what exactly has happened?

IN THE LAB
Immune response to tetanus toxoid

On day 1 three rabbits were injected with tetanus toxoid. On day 80 the rabbits were given a second injection of toxoid.

Blood samples were collected at intervals of five days. The levels of anti-toxoid antibody, both IgG and IgM, were determined.

Figure A records the mean antibody response of the three animals.

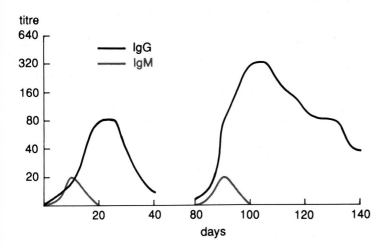

titre

Fig. A Antibody to tetanus toxoid. After the first injection a small amount of IgG and IgM is formed. Both disappear fairly rapidly. After the second injection IgM again disappears rapidly. IgG appears more promptly after the second injection, the titre reaches a higher level and antibody persists in the serum for much longer, even for years.

The foreign molecule, tetanus toxoid, enters the body and sets up a response in which antibodies are formed (an antigen is any molecule which is treated as 'foreign' by the body and which therefore provokes an immune response). The ability to make each antibody is genetically determined and *not* acquired after encounter with the antigen. Just as growth and development lead to specialised cells in liver, lung and brain, so does a similar process generate a large number of lymphocytes, each of which has a different antibody on the surface: antibody to the type 3 pneumococcal polysaccharide, to tetanus toxin, to the coat protein of influenza A virus, to grass pollen. When a lymphocyte encounters 'its' antigen, it is stimulated to divide again and again, generating a large set or *clone* of antibody-forming cells, termed *plasma* cells. Thus the antigen 'selects' the corresponding cell — this theory of antibody formation is termed the *clonal selection* theory. Although the animal is born with antibody-producing lymphocytes, we talk of an *acquired* immune response, because antibodies appear in the serum only as a result of contact with the antigen (Fig. 10.4).

As well as plasma cells, a number of memory cells are formed. These are retained after the initial burst of antibody formation and persist for years — even for life. Hence, after contact with antigen, there are more cells available with the potential for producing the

Fig. 10.4 Clonal selection.
Reaction of the antigen
with 'its' antibody on the
surface of the lymphocyte
triggers cell division and
maturation of the daughter
cells into antibody-
producing cells (plasma
cells) and memory cells.

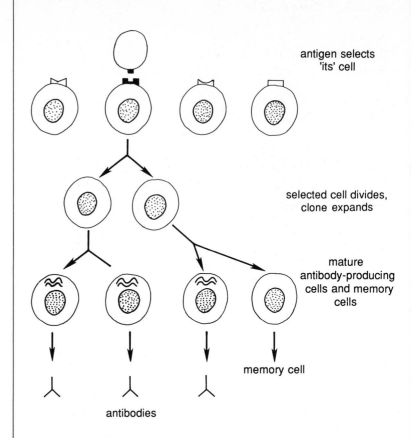

antigen selects
'its' cell

selected cell divides,
clone expands

mature
antibody-producing
cells and memory
cells

memory cell

antibodies

particular antibody, and these cells come into action more rapidly,
so that the secondary response to the same antigen is more rapid
and of greater magnitude.

'SELF' AND 'NOT-SELF'

If we are born with the ability to make antibodies to any antigen
we encounter, then we may ask why do we not react in this way to
our *own* proteins and carbohydrates? The answer is that they are
recognised as 'self' because the cells that could have made antibodies against them have been rendered 'tolerant'. Round about
the time of birth the immune system is immature; antigens that the
lymphoid cells encounter at this period somehow inhibit them from
responding to the same antigens in later life, when the immune system reaches maturity. Obviously, among the substances that the
lymphoid cells encounter at this time are all the components of the
body. The immune system thus develops 'tolerance' towards these
components — a tolerance that persists in most cases throughout
life. It is possible to render animals tolerant to foreign antigens by
injecting them into the immature animal — normally this does not
occur and the animal retains the capacity to respond to molecules
that it does not make itself (i.e. that are 'not-self').

THE SMALL LYMPHOCYTE

One particular cell, the *small lymphocyte*, plays a central role in both forms of the immune response. Lymphocytes are produced in the bone marrow and develop further either in the bone marrow or the thymus (Fig. 10.5).

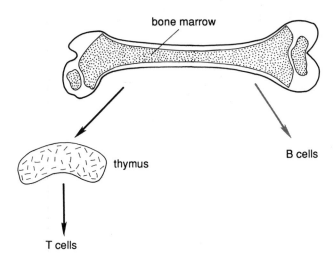

Fig. 10.5 Production of T- and B-cells. Both types of cells are formed in the bone marrow. T-cells mature and differentiate in the thymus; B-cells acquire their final competence while still in the bone marrow.

T-CELLS AND B-CELLS

The T-lymphocytes are dependent in some way on the thymus gland, a structure at the root of the neck, most prominent in children and gradually atrophying with age. T-lymphocytes are responsible for cell-mediated immunity. The B-lymphocytes (so called because in birds their development is controlled by the 'bursa of Fabricius') are responsible for the production of immunoglobulins. In many animals, including man, the final maturation of the B-cells occurs in the bone marrow. T- and B-cells look the same under the light microscope, but can be distinguished by the proteins on their surfaces.

MILESTONES
Thanks for the 'memory': The role of the lymphocyte
In the 1950s the English scientist J.L. Gowans inserted a cannula into the thoracic duct (the main lymph channel) of a rat and drained away the lymph containing the lymphocytes.
    After a time he found that such rats:

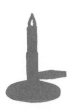

1 made little antibody to tetanus toxoid;
2 could not reject a skin graft — a manifestation of cellular immunity.

The rat's ability to do these things could be restored by injections of small lymphocytes. This experiment proved the central role of the small lymphocyte in the immune response.

This was confirmed by later experiments. If we inject tetanus toxoid into a rat, the rat mounts a primary response, i.e. it produces relatively small amounts of antibody fairly slowly. And if we inject lymphocytes from this rat into a second rat that has not previously been given tetanus toxoid, and then give the second rat toxoid, the second rat produces antibodies in high concentration, and rapidly: i.e. in the fashion characteristic of the secondary response.

So the 'memory' of the first experience of toxoid has been transferred from the first rat to the second rat by the small lymphocytes. Gowans received the Nobel Prize for his work.

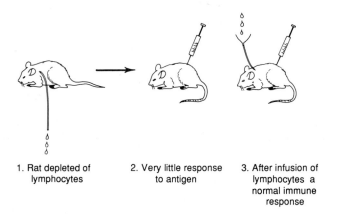

1. Rat depleted of lymphocytes

2. Very little response to antigen

3. After infusion of lymphocytes a normal immune response

Fig. A Role of the lymphocyte.

LYMPHOID ORGANS AND THE LYMPHATIC SYSTEM

The organs of the immune response (Fig. 10.6) are the lymphoid tissues. Like other organs they are made up of cells, located in lymph glands around the body, in the spleen and the mucous membranes. All the lymphoid cells arise in the bone marrow. The B-cells mature there, while the T-cells pass to the thymus and 'learn their trade' in this organ. From the thymus and the bone marrow the cells travel all over the body, settling in well-defined organs, the lymph nodes and the spleen, or scattered through the mucous membranes.

The spleen is an important lymphoid organ, containing both T- and B-cell areas. It filters foreign particles from the blood and bacteria entering the bloodstream are mainly removed here and in the liver. There are many other collections of lymphoid cells in other tissues (e.g. in the tonsils, in the wall of the gut — the appendix is

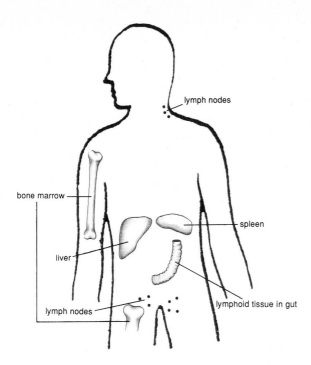

Fig. 10.6 The organs of the immune response: the bone marrow (where all the cells of the immune response originate), the liver and spleen, the lymph nodes (scattered throughout the body) and the lymphoid tissue in the gut.

a lymphoid organ — the respiratory tract, the genito-urinary tract and the bone marrow). The macrophages of the mononuclear phagocytic system in liver, spleen, lung and elsewhere take up antigens from the blood, but do not initiate an immune response, although they play an important role in the process.

Lymph nodes are linked by the *lymphatics*, a network of fine channels running all through the tissues and rivalling the blood vessels in complexity. The blood capillaries permit the outflow of water and small molecules which convey nutrition to the tissues. This fluid rejoins the circulating blood via the lymphatic system. Lymphoid cells also circulate in these channels. From the blood they enter the tissues, eventually reach the lymphatics, are carried to lymph nodes and end up in the bloodstream again. This traffic makes it easier for the antibody-forming cells to encounter 'their' particular antigens, and thus to initiate the appropriate defence reaction.

Once antigen has made contact with the immune system, what, we can ask, happens to it? An antigen that enters the body through a break in the skin will usually end up in the regional lymph nodes (thus an infection of the hand may cause swollen glands in the armpit); an antigen that is inhaled or swallowed is trapped by the lymphoid tissue in the upper respiratory tract or the gut; while an antigen that reaches the blood induces an immune response in the spleen.

ANTIBODY SYNTHESIS: SEQUENCE OF EVENTS

As we have seen, the manufacture of antibody takes place in the lymph nodes, spleen or bone marrow. The antigen is trapped by antigen-processing cells — a type of macrophage — and concentrated on their surface for presentation to lymphocytes (Fig. 10.7). Antigens may be 'soluble' or 'particulate' (particulate antigens are first taken up by macrophages in lymphoid tissue or spleen and partly digested before presentation). The antibody-forming cells are B-cells. Some antigens, such as pneumococcal polysaccharides, which are made up of repeated units, can stimulate the B-cells directly, without the aid of T-cells, but in most cases the antigen is received from the antigen-processing cells by other lymphocytes, the T-helper cells, which somehow reinforce the stimulus of the antigen for the B-cells. In each case the response of the B-cells is to divide, expanding the clone of antibody-producing cells, and then to differentiate into plasma cells secreting immunoglobulin, or memory cells. Division and maturation are controlled by soluble growth factors produced by T-cells. IgM is produced first, then another growth factor switches production to IgG. The IgM and the IgG produced by the same cell have identical specificities.

STRUCTURE OF ANTIBODIES

Antibodies are proteins of a type known to biochemists as globulins and are therefore called immunoglobulins. Antibodies occur in the gammaglobulin fraction of serum and this fraction is used as a source of antibodies if they are needed for medical treatment. They combine with the corresponding antigen by means of various chemical forces such as hydrogen bonds and attractions between positively and negatively charged ions. Under the right conditions of pH and salt concentration, the combination between antigen and antibody is reversible. What the antibody molecule 'recognises' is the shape of the antigen molecule, not the presence of individual atoms in it. The better the two molecules fit together, the stronger and more numerous will be the bonds holding them. Such an antibody is said to have a high affinity for its antigen (Fig. 10.8).

Because there is more than one antibody-forming cell per antigen before the primary response and because mutations occur as the clone expands, the immune response to any antigen includes many different antibodies, which have the same general specificity, but which differ in their affinity for the antigen (i.e. some fit more closely and therefore combine more firmly than others).

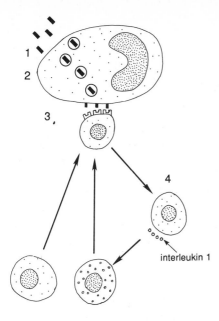

Fig. 10.7 Antigen presentation and antibody formation.
1. The antigen is taken in by the macrophage.
2. Macrophage processes the antigen.
3. Macrophage 'presents' the antigen on its surface for recognition by the T-cell. Macrophage also secretes interleukin-1.
4. T-cell is stimulated (by antigen and interleukin-1) to divide.

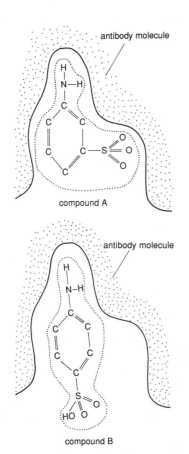

Fig. 10.8 Antibody affinity. The tightness with which the antigen and antibody combine depends on the quality of fit between the two. Thus compound B fits much more 'loosely' than compound A into the recognition site of the antibody to compound A. The antibody is said to have a lower *affinity* for compound B. The antibody 'recognises' the overall shape of the molecule, and not particular atoms or chemical groups.

When the dose of antigen is small, only those cells with high-affinity antibodies on the surface can hold sufficient antigen to be stimulated, while with large doses cells with lower-affinity receptors will also be stimulated. Antibody produced in a secondary response tends to have a high affinity.

There are many different proteins in serum. These include various immunoglobulins, which differ in size and electrophoretic mobility (the distance they migrate under the influence of an electric field). The main immunoglobulin is immunoglobulin G, abbreviated IgG. The IgG molecule consists of four peptide chains, two light and two heavy, which are held together by disulphide bridges (bonds between two sulphur atoms, each in a different chain). Near the point of attachment of the light chains there is a 'hinge', a region where the molecule is flexible, so that its usual configuration is that of a Y.

There are many different immunoglobulin molecules in serum, so many that to purify one in order to analyse it was an impossible task (until recently). To study the structure of immunoglobulins, scientists profited by an experiment of nature: there is a cancer called myeloma, a cancer of antibody-forming cells. The malignant change takes place in a single cell originally and all the others are its descendents, so that all produce exactly the same immunoglobu-

Fig. 10.9 Structure of IgG. Immunoglobulin G consists of two heavy and two light polypeptide chains held together by disulphide bridges. The variable regions (V_L and V_H) are responsible for antibody specificity. The Fc portion is recognised by phagocytes, and binds complement.

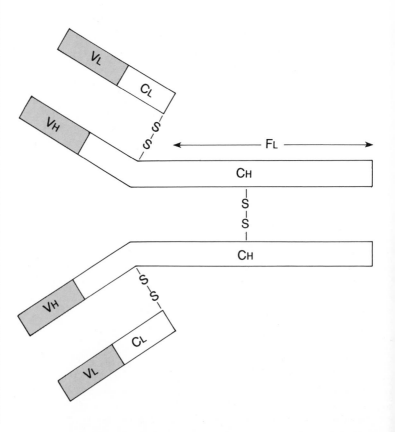

lin. Thus the patient has a very large amount of this immunoglobulin in their serum and it can be purified with relative ease.

When purified immunoglobulins are analysed it is found that certain regions are very similar, while others differ considerably. Thus the region of IgG shaded in Fig. 10.9 is found to differ from molecule to molecule (i.e. it is composed of different sequences of amino acids), whereas the unshaded regions have an (almost) identical structure. The shaded region of each chain is called the variable or 'V' region and the unshaded region the constant or 'C' region. In fact this diagram gives a very poor idea of what the molecule actually looks like. Each pair of light and heavy chains is folded upon itself so that six loops grip the antigen; hold an orange in the middle three fingers of each hand and you will see an IgG molecule embracing an antigen (Pl 11). Differences in the amino acids forming the tips of the loops account for the differing specificities of antibodies.

FIVE IMMUNOGLOBULIN CLASSES

The constant regions of human antibody molecules show two different sorts of light chains and five different sorts of heavy chains. Each of the heavy chains distinguishes a distinct immunoglobulin class (see Table 10.2). *IgG* (Fig. 10.9) is the main immunoglobulin synthesised during the secondary response. It consists of two light and two heavy chains. It is present in serum in the largest quantity (8-16 mg/mL); serum contains about 75 mg protein/mL. IgG can pass through the walls of blood vessels and so is found in areas of inflammation, promoting the phagocytosis of microbes and neutralising their toxins. It can also pass through the placenta and is present in the blood of newborn babies (vaccinating a mother against tetanus, for instance, protects her child for some months). IgG has two antigen-combining sites. Four different types of IgG molecules can be distinguished, by variations in the makeup of the heavy chains.

TABLE 10.2 IMMUNOGLOBIN CLASSES

Class	IgG	IgM	IgA	IgD	IgE
MW	150,000	900,000	160,000	185,000	200,000
Light chains	Kλ	Kλ	Kλ	Kλ	Kλ
Heavy chains	γ	μ	α	δ	ε

IgM is the biggest immunoglobulin molecule. It consists of five sets of pairs of light and heavy chains (Fig. 10.10(a)) and thus has 10 antigen-combining sites. Its large size means that it cannot readily pass through the walls of blood vessels and so is largely confined to the bloodstream and of importance in the defence against bacteraemia.

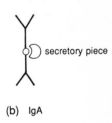

(a) IgM

(b) IgA

Fig. 10.10 Structure of **(a)** IgM and **(b)** IgA. The IgM molecule consists of 5 IgG-like molecules linked together. The IgA molecule in secretions consists of two IgG-like units plus a secretory piece.

The blood-group antibodies anti-A and anti-B are IgM.

IgA is a secretory immunoglobulin (Fig. 10.10(b)), appearing in the secretions coating the respiratory tract, the gut, the genital tract, in tears and in sweat. Here it has a role in protecting these surfaces against microbial attack. It consists of two pairs of light and heavy chains with an additional component which protects it against digestion by proteolytic enzymes, for example in the digestive tract.

IgE has a specialised role in body defences. It is present in very low concentration in the blood and is mostly found attached to mast cells. When an antigen (e.g. a bacterium or other pathogen), comes in contact with the specific IgE, the reaction causes the mast cell to release substances that promote the inflammatory response by increasing the permeability of blood capillaries and facilitating the accumulation of cells, antibodies and other serum factors at the site. When a person has IgE antibodies to the wrong antigen (such as grass pollen) the result is hayfever or asthma.

IgD, the remaining immunoglobulin, is found on the surface of some lymphocytes; its role is unclear.

CELL-MEDIATED IMMUNITY

It is easy to understand how antibody can react with microbes living free in tissue fluids *outside* the cells of the host (extracellularly), but what if the organisms can *enter cells* and survive there? Viruses must enter cells to replicate. A number of bacteria and other pathogens — *Mycobacterium, Salmonella typhi, Listeria, Chlamydia, Rickettsia, Leishmania* and more — can survive and multiply *inside* the phagocytes that engulf them. Antibody does not offer an effective defence against these parasites. To cope with this problem, another form of immunity evolved, *cell-mediated immunity*, (Fig. 10.11) in which the weapon is a cell specialised to detect antigen on the surface of another cell.

Just as B-cells do, T-cells possess on their surfaces antibody-like receptors specific for antigen. The receptors on these T-cells recognise an antigen only when it is accompanied by another marker molecule which indicates that the antigen is located on the surface of a cell. These marker molecules are part of the major histocompatibility complex (MHC), and are the antigens responsible for rejection of grafts.

When an intracellular parasite establishes itself inside a macrophage, the macrophage manages to display antigens of the parasite on its surface. When such a macrophage encounters a helper T-cell that recognises that antigen, the T-cell binds to the antigen + MHC marker and is activated. T-cells are stimulated by contact with antigen to divide and undergo clonal expansion, just as B-cells do. Some of these T-cells release soluble factors (lymphokines) which modify the behaviour of other T-lymphocytes and of macrophages. Lymphokines have several activities (see Table 10.3).

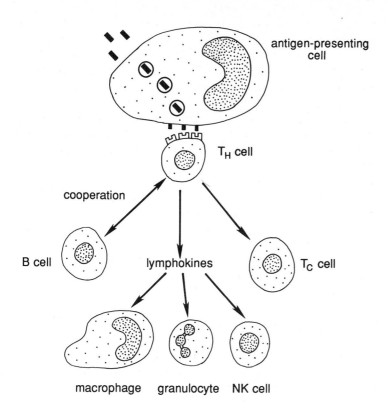

TABLE 10.3 RESULT OF INTERACTION BETWEEN MACROPHAGE AND T-CELL

Production of Memory cells
Production of Lymphokines which:
- stimulate macrophages to kill intracellular parasites
- attract macrophages
- induce proliferation of T-cells
- induce production of cytotoxic T-cells
- act as interferons

Cytotoxic T-cells, which recognise antigen only in association with MHC markers of a different class, destroy cells parasitised by viruses and are also responsible for rejection of skin and other tissue and organ grafts. Other T-cells become memory cells capable of delivering an accelerated response to further contact with the antigen. This type of immunity can be transferred, not by antibodies in serum, not by macrophages — but by T-cells (lymphocytes). Once macrophages are activated by lymphokines, they can kill other intracellular bacteria, not just the organism that provoked the original immunity.

TRANSPLANTATION IMMUNITY

If a surgeon tries to cover a burn by placing on it skin from another person, the grafted skin survives and looks healthy for some days, but then starts to break down and in two weeks or so has sloughed off completely. Only skin from the burn victims themselves or their identical twin will survive. In the same way a graft of a kidney or heart will be rejected unless special treatment is given to prevent this. This *graft rejection* is due to cell-mediated immunity. Lymphoid cells infiltrate the graft and attack the foreign cells. The role of lymphocytes can be shown experimentally. An animal that is depleted of lymphocytes will reject a skin graft very slowly (p.107). An animal that has rejected one skin graft will reject another from the source more rapidly and this *accelerated* rejection can be transferred with cells. The antigens that are recognised in the rejection of a graft, the *transplantation* or *histocompatibility antigens*, MHC antigens, are quite numerous; in humans over 100 are recognised so far. All nucleated cells bear MHC antigens. In the rejection of organ grafts such as kidneys, antibody also plays a role.

Today transplantation of organs — kidney, bone marrow, liver and heart — is commonly performed. These transplants, however, are only possible if rejection of the grafted tissue can be prevented. This can often be achieved:

1 by selecting a donor whose HLA antigens match closely those of the recipient (HLA is the abbreviation for the system of human MHC antigens most relevant in transplantation) and/or

2 by treating the recipient with drugs that suppress the immune response to the graft (unfortunately these also suppress most other immune responses, not just those aroused by the grafted tissue, and transplant patients are therefore more susceptible to infections: see p.262).

Organ transplantation is an expensive and complex procedure. The resources available for health care are limited; decisions may have to be made as to the justification for organ transplantation (see following, 'Two transplant cases: consider your verdict').

IN THE WARD
Two transplant cases: consider your verdict

Now that it is technically possible to transplant a major organ, heart, liver or bone marrow with a good chance that the graft will survive, complex ethical problems arise.

Transplantation is extremely costly, both for the surgical and hospital expenses and for the drugs needed to prevent rejection of the organ; these drugs need to be taken for years. It is unlikely that the cost will fall appreciably as the operations become more common.

To an increasing extent these operations are being paid for by the community. In the USA, health care accounts for about 12% of the gross national product, in Australia the figure is 8%. Can we afford high-technology medicine for everyone? One state in the USA has already decided that it cannot: Oregon now refuses to pay for transplants other than of kidney and cornea, unless three quarters of the cost is raised privately. The state authorities estimated that one transplant cost as much as one year's basic medical care for over 80 people.

If we can afford such operations, *who* should benefit from them?

Consider the following candidates for transplantation (paid for by Medicare, not the patient).

Case 1

Peter M, a bank manager aged 46 , married with two children aged 12 and 9, has a six-year history of coronary artery disease. He had a coronary-artery-bypass graft four years ago. Now he has severe pain again and the coronary arteriogram shows that his grafted vessels have almost blocked. Six years ago he was 20 kg overweight; he has managed to lose only half of this. He has given up smoking several times, but admits that he now smokes 20 cigarettes a day (cigarette-smoking is clearly associated with heart disease).

Case 2

Alfred S, aged 60, is a widower with one grown-up daughter. He is a pharmacist and an alderman of his local council active in community affairs. He has cirrhosis of the liver due to chronic alcoholism. He gave up drinking a year ago, but his liver disease has progressed and complete liver failure is only months away.

In making your decisions on the above cases, consider the following. It is essential for the success of the operation that the patient take anti-rejection drugs regularly.

Both patients have diseases at least in part self-inflicted. It would obviously be important that they should avoid prejudicing their new organs by smoking or excessive drinking. Do you think they will?*

Setting aside the question whether these 'addicts' will reform, is organ transplantation the most effective use of health resources.

Are there other forms of health-care that should have priority?

* Rather surprisingly recipients of liver transplants usually abstain from drinking. But it is perhaps less certain that smoking can be given up so easily.

BLOOD GROUPS

We have seen that Gram-negative bacteria have polysaccharide molecules on their surfaces, the O antigens. The cells of eucaryotes carry similar markers. On the surface of red cells are oligosaccharide molecules, by which the cells can be 'grouped'. There are numerous sets of related blood-group antigens, but the most important from a practical standpoint are the ABO and Rh groups, which largely define the compatibility of blood transfusions. All red cells possess on the surface an H substance, a disaccharide linked to a lipid in the cell membrane. Cells which bear the simple H substance are group O, while group A and B-cells have additional sugars linked to the H substance. The blood groups are under genetic control by the A and B genes.

TABLE 10.4 ABO BLOOD GROUPS

Blood Group	Antigens	Antibodies
O	H	anti-A, anti-B
A	A	anti-B
B	B	anti-A
AB	A, B	none

If one has group A red cells, one has anti-B antibodies in the blood also, apparently because some antigens of the gut flora resemble A and B substances so closely that the antibodies they give rise to react with A and B. Conversely anti-A agglutinins are found in the blood of a group B individual. Anti-A and anti-B are IgM antibodies. Table 10. 4 sets out the pattern of antigens and antibodies in different individuals. Blood group O is the commonest and AB the rarest. The practical importance of blood groups is in transfusion. If a transfusion is *mismatched*, e.g. A red cells are given to a group B individual, his anti-A agglutinins cause the A red cells to clump and undergo destruction; the blood is said to be incompatible and the resulting *transfusion reaction* may be fatal.

RH BLOOD GROUPS

The Rh blood group system has considerable importance because of possible effects on the fetus. If a woman is RhD-negative (D is the most important antigen in this context) and her husband is RhD-positive, she may conceive an RhD-positive child. At its birth bleeding from the placenta may allow some of the baby's blood to enter the mother's circulation; these RhD+ red cells will sensitise her to produce anti-RhD. As these antibodies are mainly IgG, they can cross the placenta and react with the red cells of a second RhD+ child, leading to *haemolytic disease of the newborn*.

Anti-RhD antibodies are more difficult to detect than say anti-A or anti-B. Red cells carry very few D antigen sites on the surface and so few antibody links can be set up between cells, too few to draw the negatively charged cells together. This difficulty can be overcome by adding an anti-human-IgG antibody — the Coombs test (Fig. 10.12).

UNDESIRABLE EFFECTS OF IMMUNITY

HYPERSENSITIVITY: FOUR TYPES

Sometimes immune reactions are exaggerated, causing damage and even death. Such hypersensitivity reactions are of four types.

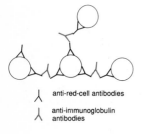

λ anti-red-cell antibodies

λ anti-immunoglobulin antibodies

Fig. 10.12 The Coombs test. In some antigen-antibody reactions involving cells, the antibody molecules bind to the cell surface but do not link up to bring the cells together and cause clumping — so that the reaction is not detected. If an antibody to the immunoglobulin is added, the cells are clumped.

In type I (or *anaphylactic* hypersensitivity reactions, Fig. 10.13) the antigen reacts with IgE bound to the surface of mast cells. This causes the breakdown of granules in the mast cell and the release of messenger molecules including histamine, leukotrienes and chemotactic factors. The commonest examples of this hypersensitivity are *hay fever* and *asthma*. A bee sting may cause fatal anaphylaxis in a person who has been stung before; in rare cases the injection of penicillin may do likewise. Type I hypersensitivity is often detected by skin tests.

In *type II (antibody-dependent cytotoxic* hypersensitivity, Fig. 10.14) antibodies to surface antigens of a cell will cause the destruction of that cell, either by phagocytosis or complement-mediated lysis (breakdown). This form of hypersensitivity is responsible for transfusion reactions and the problems of Rh-negative babies (see p.118).

Type III reactions are due to *immune complexes* (Fig. 10.15). If a lot of a 'foreign' antigen is present, as may happen with a chronic infection (e.g. in a HBV carrier who has large amounts of surface antigen in the blood), antibody may combine with it and lead to deposition of antigen-antibody complexes in the kidneys, joints, skin or elsewhere, and consequent disease: glomerulonephritis, rheumatoid arthritis, or serum sickness.

Type IV, or *delayed-type* hypersensitivity (Fig. 10.16), unlike Types I, II and III, is a manifestation of cell-mediated immunity. If, for instance, we inject tuberculin (a preparation of antigens of *M. tuberculosis*) into the skin of a person who is infected by this organism, redness and swelling develop, but only after several hours. The reaction takes 48 hours or so to reach its peak and then subsides. Most of the swelling is due to immigration of lymphocytes and macrophages into the area. T-cells recognise the antigen and secrete lymphokines which summon macrophages and other lymphocytes. The tuberculin reaction is used in the diagnosis of tuberculosis (see 'In the wards', The tuberculin reaction p.205). Cell-mediated hypersensitivity occurs with many intracellular infections: measles, herpes simplex and other viruses, and fungi, as well as some bacteria.

AUTOIMMUNITY

If our cells carry certain HLA antigens we are more likely to suffer from some forms of arthritis and other diseases. Most have an *autoimmune* basis. Sometimes the mechanisms which ensure that immune responses are not provoked by self antigens break down, and autoantibodies are produced — antibodies to the body's own proteins and other antigens. There is quite a long list of diseases which are thought to be caused by antibodies specific for one or another organ or of a more general reactivity: diseases of the thyroid gland, pernicious anaemia, one form of diabetes, myasthenia gravis, ulcerative colitis, systemic lupus erythematosus and more. Autoimmune diseases often tend to be commoner in persons who carry a particular histocompatibility (HLA) gene. Table 10.5 lists some of these diseases and the HLA genes associated with them; if the relative risk is 6, a person who has the HLA antigen DR4 is six times more likely to suffer from rheumatoid arthritis than the population at large.

Fig. 10.13 Type I hypersensitivity reaction. Allergen links two IgE molecules on the surface of the mast cell. This reaction causes release of granules from the mast cell and liberation of histamine and other mediators of anaphylaxis, leading to hayfever, asthma and other allergic diseases.

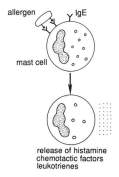

Fig. 10.14 Type II hypersensitivity reaction. Antibodies against antigens on the surface of the target cell lead to its destruction either by (a) phagocytosis and/or lysis by the complement system, or by (b) cytotoxic 'killer' cells.

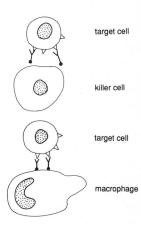

Fig. 10.15 Type III hypersensitivity reaction. Antigen-antibody complexes form deposits in tissues and lead to various reactions, all of which result in inflammation.

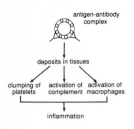

Fig. 10.16 Type IV hypersensitivity reaction. A sensitised T-cell is activated by a second contact with antigen, either directly or via an antigen-presenting cell, and produces lymphokines, which activate macrophages and killer T-cells and cause migration of lymphocytes.

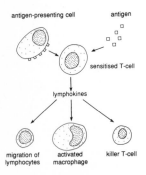

TABLE 10.5 DISEASES ASSOCIATED WITH HLA GENES

Disease	HLA gene	Relative risk[1]
Rheumatoid arthritis	DR4	6
Multiple sclerosis	DR4	5
Ankylosing spondylitis	B27	87
Post-Salmonella arthritis	B27	30

[1] Expressed as multiple compared to the risk of people who do not have the gene, e.g. the person with the DR4 gene is 6 times more likely to acquire rheumatoid arthritis.

IMMUNITY IN THE NEWBORN

A baby does not begin to synthesise its own antibodies until the age of 4-12 weeks, and adult levels are not achieved until several months later. In a newborn baby the lymph nodes are poorly developed and groups of antibody-forming cells are not much in evidence. So a newborn baby does not respond as well to vaccination as one who is say 2-3 months old, at which age immunisation with DPT (diphtheria, pertussis and tetanus) is begun. Some antigens will elicit a response when given soon after birth.

Unlike IgM and IgA, IgG can pass through the placenta into the fetal circulation. The human infant acquires maternal IgG across the placenta and also receives maternal IgA in the colostrum (first milk). Thus any antibodies that the mother possesses will also be present in the baby's blood and will offer passive immunity for the first few months of life. In this way the baby gains protection for some months against tetanus or bacterial and viral infections of the gut — *if* his mother has antibodies to the relevant microbes.

PREVENTION OF INFECTION

In the last hundred years most of the infectious diseases which 'carried off' our ancestors have become much rarer. Antibiotics have played a major role, but we must remember that other factors have been important.

For much of the world's population standards of living have risen, and well-fed people resist infection better. One of the most effective ways of protecting people against infection is to *keep the infection away*. Improvements in hygiene, purer water supplies, efficient sewerage systems and better housing have in fact contributed more than antibiotics. Transmission of infection by the faecal-oral route is interrupted when people wash their hands after defaecation and when an efficient sewerage system is available to remove the faeces. Transmission of infection by inhalation is less likely when housing conditions improve and people sleep under less crowded conditions. Additionally, a number of important pathogens of both humans and animals (e.g. rabies, foot-and-mouth disease) do not occur in islands (Australia is an island) and can be prevented in such places by controlling the entry of animals. Educating people, and especially foodhandlers, in the need for handwashing and other aspects of personal hygiene also helps. Table 10.6 summarises the prevention of infection.

TABLE 10.6 PREVENTION OF INFECTION

Specific   Acquired immunity

Non-specific   Various immune defences
                  Enhancement of 'natural' resistance by better
                      nourishment
                  Preventing contact with infection by:
                  • better living conditions
                  • personal hygiene
                  • adequate services — water, sewerage
                  • quarantine measures

We can also tackle the problem of prevention by *enhancing the immunity* of the individual. This is an appropriate place to review the forms of immunity (Table 10.7). Acquired specific immunity may be divided into *active* and *passive* forms.

TABLE 10.7 THE FORMS OF IMMUNITY

• innate, acquired
• specific, non-specific

Forms of acquired specific immunity:
Method of acquisition   *Examples*
Active: natural infection   Measles, hepatitis A,
                                 rubella, poliomyelitis

           vaccination   Measles, hepatitis B,
                                 rubella, tetanus,
                                 diphtheria, poliomyelitis

Passive: placental transfer
           injection of immune serum, immunoglobulins

1 ACTIVE IMMUNITY: VACCINES

Recovery from infection usually leads to *active immunity*. Moreover, we can invoke a similar state artificially; we can induce the body to form the antibodies and sensitised cells found in immunity by the use of *vaccines*. At the end of the eighteenth century Edward Jenner (1749-1832) showed that cowpox, now known to be a viral infection of cows analogous to smallpox, produced only a mild local infection in humans, but protected against smallpox (the practice of inoculating persons with cowpox was called vaccination from the Latin *vacca*: a cow). Cowpox was the first vaccine, and an extremely effective one.

LIVING AND NON-LIVING VACCINES

Vaccines may be live and attenuated, or non-living. It has been found that vaccines consisting of live organisms usually produce a stronger immunity than non-living vaccines. Live vaccines are prepared either by selecting a strain of the pathogen that produces only mild disease in humans, or by inducing some change in the microbe so that it loses most of its virulence. In either case the immune response is similar to that evoked by the pathogen. Cowpox was the first example of such a vaccine. Attenuated vaccines are also available against tuberculosis (the BCG strain of *M. tuberculosis*), poliomyelitis, measles, mumps and rubella. The vaccine strain of poliomyelitis virus multiplies in the gut and induces local production of IgA as well as IgG; IgG alone results from injecting killed polio vaccine. The live vaccine is both more effective (producing protection with fewer doses) and more convenient (since it can be taken by mouth).

Killed vaccines are used against diphtheria, tetanus and pertussis, cholera, meningococcal meningitis and pneumococcal infection. They have the disadvantage that the preparations must be injected. Against diptheria and tetanus, the vaccine consists of the toxin chemically inactivated, so that it is harmless, but capable of eliciting the same antibody response. These preparations are extremely effective. Against cholera and pertussis the vaccine consists of killed bacteria. The vaccines against *Neisseria meningitidis* and *Streptococcus pneumoniae* are made from capsular polysaccharides, a dozen or more in the case of the pneumococcus. Typically, three injections of killed vaccines are needed to initiate an adequate immune response and regular booster injections are also required.

If attempts to make an attenuated vaccine by conventional bacteriological methods fail, the techniques of genetic engineering can now be called upon. For example, genes coding for antigens of *Vibrio cholerae* can be cloned and inserted into *Escherichia coli*, yielding a non-pathogenic strain that expresses antigens of *Vibrio cholerae* on its surface and so induces immunity to cholera. It is now possible to include genes coding for several antigens into the one strain of vaccinia virus. (See following, 'Teaching an old cow new tricks'.) Vaccines prepared by these or similar methods are now coming into use. The hepatitis B vaccine now available is a cloned vaccine (see following, 'Molecular biology and hepatitis B vaccine').

IN THE LAB
'Teaching an old cow new tricks': multivalent vaccinia

The gene for HBsAg is cloned and inserted it into a vector, a plasmid.

The vector is transformed into a cell culture and the culture is infected with vaccinia.

During growth inside the cell DNA from the vector recombines with vaccinia DNA.

Some of the progeny vaccinia particles will contain the

HBsAg gene as part of their DNA.

Infection with these virus particles will lead to immunity against HBV, as the HBsAg protein is produced when the vaccinia multiplies.

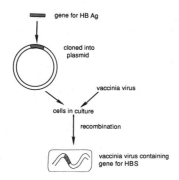

IN THE LAB
Molecular biology and hepatitis B vaccine.
The first HBV vaccine contained the surface antigen (HBsAg) prepared from the serum of carriers. It was expensive to prepare and was potentially dangerous, since it could theoretically carry other viruses (though in practice there is no evidence that this ever occurred). More recently, a vaccine has been prepared with the techniques of molecular biology.

HBV cannot yet be grown in cell culture. HBV DNA was purified from the blood of carriers, was cut up and the fragments then incorporated into an *Escherichia coli* plasmid and grown up in *E. coli.*

The result was an *E. coli* culture containing plasmids with various fragments of HBV DNA in them. The *E. coli* strain containing the gene encoding the HBV surface antigen was identified. This strain was then grown up and the plasmid isolated and cloned into a yeast. (It was necessary to transfer the gene to yeast because in *E. coli* very little HBsAg was produced.)

To produce the vaccine the yeast strain was grown up in a fermenter — a culture vessel containing several thousand litres, in which all growth conditions can be carefully controlled — and the HBsAg purified.

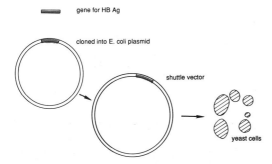

Fig. A Molecular biology and hepatitis B.

Some pathogens can infect animals as well as humans or can survive in the environment *(Clostridium tetani, Pseudomonas aeruginosa)*. If the only host of the pathogen is humans and infection does not set up a carrier state and there is an effective vaccine, immunisation can not only protect the individual, but may even eliminate the infectious agent from the community. Once sufficient individuals are immunised the microbe may not be able to find a susceptible host, the chain of transmission is broken and the infection rate in the community falls sharply. Once about three quarters of the children in England had been immunised against diphtheria, the disease almost disappeared (Fig. 10.17). Smallpox virus has recently been completely eliminated from the world: the first infection for which this has been achieved.

Fig. 10.17 The decline of diphtheria. As can be seen, the introduction of immunization produced a precipitative fall in the number of cases of diphtheria in England and Wales.

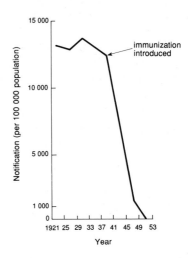

2 PASSIVE IMMUNITY

To confer immunity by means of a vaccine requires weeks or months and there are occasions when this process is too slow. For instance, a man who has been in contact with a case of hepatitis A, or a pregnant woman who meets a rubella-infected child needs more rapid protection. Injection of *human serum* will 'lend' such persons antibodies for long enough to prevent infection (see p.120, immunity in the newborn). More effective still are preparations of *gamma globulins* derived from human serum. 'Hyperimmune' immunoglobulins can be collected from persons recently infected or who have high levels of antibody (to e.g. tetanus) because of immunisation. In the near future it is likely that monoclonal antibodies (see p.128) produced by human cells will be available to protect against common viral and other infections. Antibody molecules, like other serum proteins and many body components, are eliminated from the body at a constant rate and so the protection that can be afforded in this way is temporary. Immunoglobulins from horses immunised against tetanus and diphtheria were much used in the past, but less commonly nowadays because of the greater risks associated with injecting foreign proteins (see *anaphylaxis* p.119).

IMMUNODEFICIENCY

We have seen that the 'machinery' of immunity is complex — it is not surprising therefore that diseases due to failure of a component in the machinery have been recognised; a good number of these are hereditary, due to *genetic* defects in the immune response (Table 10.8). For instance, a deficiency of the 3rd component of complement makes the patient unduly susceptible to certain bacterial infections; a defect in B-cells leads to failure to produce immunoglobulins, and susceptibility to bacterial infections. These diseases can be recognised by measuring the amount of immunoglobulins or complement in the blood, by testing the patient's ability either to react to antigens injected into the skin or to form antibodies in response to e.g. diphtheria toxoid. There are ways to test the ability of phagocytes to engulf and destroy bacteria and to enumerate the number and the different types of T-cells.

TABLE 10.8 DISEASES DUE TO IMMUNOLOGICAL DEFECTS

Disease	Defect	Characteristic infections
Agammaglobulinaemia	B-cell	Staphylococci, streptococci
Thymic hypoplasia	T-cell	Some viruses *Candida*
Chronic granulomatous disease	Phagocytes	Catalase+ve bacteria
C3 deficiency	Complement	Staphylococci, streptococci

Many other factors can also depress the reactivity of the immune system. One such factor is *malnutrition* (even the malnutrition of the very poor in Western society). Leukaemia of some types and myeloma may affect the production of antibodies, and patients with Hodgkin's disease often have impaired cellular immunity. Leprosy, malaria and viral infections such as measles depress the immune system temporarily, while HIV does so permanently, destroying the helper T-cells.

Many drugs also affect the immune system. Cytotoxic drugs are toxic for rapidly growing cells, such as cancer cells, but also kill bone marrow cells: (the bone marrow produces many cells important for the immune defence, especially the neutrophils). Corticosteroids and other drugs, and X-rays are also used in medical treatment; these agents also often gravely depress the immune response.

USING IMMUNOLOGICAL REACTIONS

In the clinical laboratory we often wish to detect or estimate antibodies, and to detect microbial or other antigens. Many methods are now available for doing so, from the simple to the highly sophisticated.

Fig. 10.18 Mechanism of precipitin reaction. Antigen molecules react with antibodies forming a network which precipitates from solution when large enough.

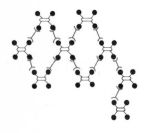

Fig. 10.19 Precipitin reaction in tubes. When a solution of the antigen is carefully layered onto the surface of the antibody solution in a test-tube, a precipitate forms at the interface between the two solutions.

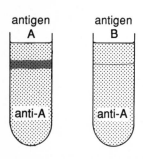

PRECIPITIN REACTION

A rabbit is injected several times with ovalbumin, a soluble protein of eggs. The rabbit is bled, the blood is allowed to clot and is then centrifuged (in a centrifuge with a sealed head, to avoid dangerous aerosols if a tube breaks). The serum is removed and mixed with a solution of ovalbumin. After a time a white precipitate forms in the tube. This is a *precipitin reaction* (Fig. 10.18), the first immunological reaction to be demonstrated in the test-tube . The simplest way of estimating the amount of antibody is to titrate it, i.e. to dilute it in two-fold steps and then add antigen to each tube (Fig 10.19). The mixture is then kept for some hours and examined. The dilution in the last tube showing a reaction is the *titre*. We can also detect the precipitin in an agar medium (Fig 10.20).

If the antigen is an insoluble particle, a bacterium or a red cell, antibodies to it will cause clumping of the particle suspension. Group A red cells are agglutinated by anti-A antiserum. *Salmonella typhi* is clumped by antiserum to the O antigens of *S. typhi*. This is a convenient technique and it has been adapted to soluble antigens. The antigen is linked to tiny latex particles or 'pickled' red cells and the antibody clumps the suspension. The tests used to detect antigens in clinical specimens (p.83) are often based on this technique.

IgM is the first immunoglobulin to appear in the primary response and it tends to disappear rapidly, so that the presence of IgM is evidence of a current or recent infection. IgG is also produced in the primary response, but takes longer to reach its peak (see p.104). In a secondary response IgM again arises early and falls away quickly, but IgG reaches a much higher titre and persists for much longer. A test which detects IgM is often more helpful than one which does not distinguish between IgG and IgM.

ELISA

Several sophisticated chemical techniques are now used in the measurement of antibodies or in the detection of microbes. For instance, in the ELISA technique (Fig. 10.21) for estimation of antibodies to *Toxoplasma gondii*, the *Toxoplasma* antigen is fixed to wells in a plastic tray and the serum to be tested is added. If it contains antibodies to *Toxoplasma*, these will bind to the antigen molecules and will remain in the wells after the plate is washed. Then another antibody is added — an antibody to human immunoglobulin. To these anti-human antibodies are coupled an enzyme, phosphatase. The antibody-phosphatase complex links itself to any human immunoglobulin adhering to the *Toxoplasma* antigen. The antibody-phosphatase complex can be detected by adding a colourless chemical which the phosphatase transforms to a coloured product.

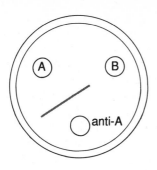

Fig. 10.20 Precipitin reaction in agar. Anti-A antibody is placed in one well cut in the agar plate, and different antigens A and B in two other wells. The antigens and antibody diffuse out from the wells. Where the antigen meets the corresponding antibody a line of precipitate forms.

IMMUNOFLUORESCENCE

The technique of immunofluorescence (Fig. 10.22 and Plate 12) utilises antibodies linked to a dye. When illuminated by ultraviolet light, the dye fluoresces and the antibody can then be seen. For instance, if *Legionella* organisms are present in a specimen taken from a patient, a fluorescent antibody to *Legionella* will combine with them and the bacteria will then be visible when viewed with a suitable microscope and light source. (They appear as bright yellow or green rods.) Fluorescence methods can also be adapted to estimate the concentration of an antibody in a serum.

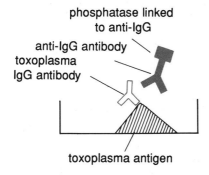

Fig. 10.21 In the ELISA technique for detection of antibody (*enzyme-linked immunosorbent assay*), the antigen, (e.g. of *Toxoplasma*) is bound to a well in a plastic tray. Antibody in the test serum combines with the antigen. This antibody is detected by adding another antibody, an anti-immunoglobulin antibody to which has been coupled an enzyme. Next, a chemical is added which the enzyme transforms into a coloured compound and the amount of this compound is measured. This method is a very sensitive one for detecting and measuring antibodies.

MONOCLONAL ANTIBODIES

When we immunise an animal in the ordinary way and collect the serum, more than 90% of the antibodies present will not be directed against the antigen we are interested in, and those that do have the appropriate specificity will vary greatly in affinity. A method is now available for producing antibodies all of the same specificity and affinity. By chemical treatment it is possible to cause two cells to fuse into one and for the resulting hybrid cell to survive. If we fuse a cell producing a particular antibody with a cell from a B-cell tumour, we can obtain a line of cells which multiplies indefinitely — a property acquired from the tumour parent — and which synthesises the antibody of interest (Fig. 10.23). All the cells in a monoclonal culture represent a single clone, derived from one parent cell and produce exactly the same immunoglobulin. It is thus possible to produce very large quantities of a very pure antibody. Such monoclonal antibodies have numerous uses, in research, in diagnosis and in therapy (Table 10.9).

Fig. 10.22 Immunofluorescence. To detect *Legionella* in lung tissue, a thin slice of the tissue is washed with an anti-*Legionella* antibody. If *Legionella* is present, the antibody is bound to the tissue. Next, the tissue is washed with an anti-immunoglobulin antibody labelled with a dye such as fluorescein. If antibody is bound to the tissue, the anti-immunoglobulin antibody will react with it. When the specimen is illuminated with ultraviolet light and examined under the microscope, the labelled antibody shines a bright green. Single bacteria or virus particles can be seen with this technique.

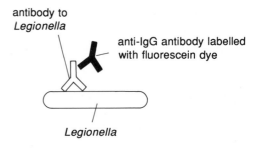

Fig. 10.23 Production of monoclonal antibodies. The mouse is immunised with antigen A. Spleen cells from the mouse are fused with myeloma cells; myeloma cells survive and multiply indefinitely in culture. The cell suspension is diluted in a medium which selects for the hybrid cells and is placed in the wells of plastic trays. After some time in culture the wells are assayed for the desired antibody.

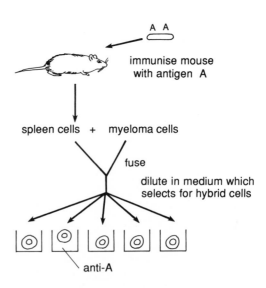

TABLE 10.9 USES OF MONOCLONAL ANTIBODIES

Research:
- Identify T4 or T8 lymphocytes
- Locate immunoglobulin-producing cells in tissues
- Detect viruses inside cells and study where they multiply

Diagnosis:
- Identification of *Legionella*
- Detection of *Chlamydia* in genital specimens
- Identification of viruses after isolation

Treatment:
- Several uses under development

CHAPTER REVIEW

1   List the body's innate, non-specific defence mechanisms.
2   (a)   What are *phagocytes*?
      (b)   What roles do they play in immune defence?
3   (a)   Describe the *acute inflammatory response*.
      (b)   Why is it important?
4   (a)   What is *specific immunity*?
      (b)   Define *antibody*.
      (c)   What are the major types, and what do they do?
5   (a)   What is *passive immunity*?
      (b)   Give examples.
6   Describe the various types of vaccines.
7   (a)   Describe the different types of hypersensitivity.
      (b)   Give examples of diseases due to this mechanism.
8   Define *B-cells and T-cells* and briefly describe their functions.
9   How can rejection be prevented?

11

HOW MICROBES CAUSE DISEASE: INFECTION MECHANISMS

In order to understand microbial disease we need to locate the reservoirs of infection (where the disease-producing microbes are found), establish the routes of infection (how they reach and enter the human body), and analyse the mechanisms of invasion (how they overcome the body's defences).

RESERVOIRS OF INFECTION

For humans the main infection reservoir is other humans (Table 11.1). Usually our permanent resident flora causes trouble only when our defences are weakened by injury, illness or drug treatment. But as well as our permanent flora there are transients. Organisms such as *Corynebacterium diphtheriae, Neisseria gonorrhoeae, Treponema pallidum, Bordetella pertussis, Streptococcus pyogenes* and *Streptococcus pneumoniae* have no host other than humans and survive because they are constantly passed from individual to individual. Rhinoviruses (common cold viruses), measles, mumps, herpes simplex, rubella and numerous other viruses are maintained by the same mechanism. The same is true of some parasites: *Plasmodium, Trichomonas vaginalis*.

TRANSMISSION OF INFECTION

The environment (soil, air, dust, water *and* our food) teems with microbes, the vast majority of which are harmless to us, but a few of which can cause harm. In soil there are toxin-producing clostridia such as *Cl. tetani* and *Cl. botulinum*, and also *Listeria monocytogenes*

130

TABLE 11.1 RESERVOIRS OF HUMAN INFECTIONS

Humans	*Haemophilus influenzae, Streptococcus pneumoniae, Neisseria meningitidis,* hepatitis B virus, herpes simplex, rubella, *Plasmodium* spp, *Trichomonas vaginalis.*
Animals	*Brucella abortus, Rickettsia* spp, *Chlamydia psittaci,* rabies virus, yellow fever virus
Environment	*Clostridium tetani, Clostridium botulinum, Listeria monocytogenes, Legionella* spp., *Vibrio* spp.

and the anthrax bacillus. In air microbes are usually on dust particles or droplet nuclei. A cough or sneeze liberates several thousand droplets of secretions containing microbes. When the droplets dry they constitute droplet nuclei and are so light that they remain airborne indefinitely. In water, fresh, brackish or salt, we may encounter *Vibrio cholerae* and other vibrios, *Aeromonas hydrophila*, *Legionella* and numerous parasites.

Animals of all types — rodents, birds, snails — may carry infections to which humans are subject. Infections carried by animals and transmissible to humans are termed *zoonoses.* Many of these infections are endemic in the animal host and are well tolerated. The human infection is outside the normal life-cycle of the pathogen, the parasite is rarely transmitted to another human and the infection does not contribute to the propagation of the microbe. Some of these infections are transmitted by animal bite (rabies), by contact with animals or their excreta *(Brucella, Chlamydia psittaci, Echinococcus)* or through the efforts of biting insects *(Borrelia,* plague bacillus, *Rickettsia;* see Fig. 11.1).

Some microbes are maintained in a host-vector cycle consisting of an animal or bird and a biting insect or other arthropod. Thus yellow fever and dengue circulate through monkeys and mosquitoes, Murray Valley encephalitis virus through water-birds and

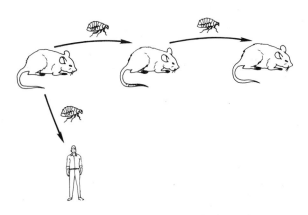

Fig. 11.1 Transmission of plague. The normal cycle is: rodent → flea → rodent → flea ... A human does not usually transmit the disease.

mosquitoes (Fig. 11.2), murine typhus through rodents and fleas. Some infections transmitted by insect vectors, such as malaria, have no other host than humans. The infection is spread from human to human by the bite of an infected mosquito (Fig. 11.3). The ways in which infections spread are summarised in Table 11.2.

TABLE 11.2 HOW MICROBES SPREAD

1 Direct physical contact   Organism
Sexual   Treponema pallidum, Neisseria gonorrhoeae, Human immunodeficiency virus, Herpes simplex, Hepatitis B
Non-sexual   *Salmonella typhi,* Rhinoviruses
Congenital   Rubella virus, Cytomegalovirus, Hepatitis B, *Toxoplasma gondii, Listeria monocytogenes,* HIV, *Streptococcus agalactiae*

2 Indirect transfer
Aerial   *Streptococcus pneumoniae, Corynebacterium diphtheriae, Mycobacterium tuberculosis,* influenza viruses, *Legionella*
Food/water   *Salmonella,* hepatitis A, *Giardia lamblia, Entamoeba histolytica, Taenia saginata*
Via fomites   *Ps. aeruginosa, S. aureus,* hepatitis B,
(environment)   *Schistosoma*
Via bite   malaria, plague, rabies
Via wound   *Staphylococcus aureus, Clostridium perfringens*

[Note: this list is incomplete, also one microbe may be spread by two or more routes.]

Once the potential pathogen reaches a possible host, the major problem arises: how to establish itself in the tissues of that host. Its ability to do so is referred to as its *pathogenicity* or *virulence;* the two

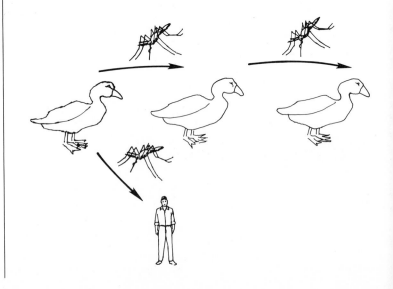

Fig. 11.2 Transmission of Murray Valley encephalitis. The normal cycle is: bird → mosquito → bird → mosquito → ..Again, the human does not usually transmit the disease.

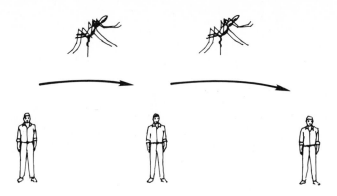

terms mean roughly the same thing. Microbial disease is the outcome of an interaction between the microbe with its virulence factors and the host with his/her defences. Virulence is difficult to quantitate and is not an absolute characteristic of a microbe, but may vary with the number of infecting organisms, the route by which they gain entry, the state of health of the host, the level of immunity, specific and non-specific, and the condition of other defences. Immunological factors in the host's defences are discussed in chapter 10. However, disorders of anatomy and physiology can also undermine resistance (Table 11.3).

TABLE 11.3 IMPAIRED RESISTANCE TO INFECTION

May occur in:

- malnutrition,
- alcoholism,
- diabetes mellitus,
- cancer,
- chronic disease of liver or kidneys,
- disease of the heart and circulation,
- chronic respiratory disease.

SYMBIOSIS AND PARASITISM

Close association between living creatures can be *symbiotic*, where both benefit, or *parasitic*, where one profits at the expense of the other. We live in something close to symbiosis with our flora, since they confer some advantages on us (p.74), whereas for example *Neisseria gonorrhoeae*, *Vibrio cholerae* or hepatitis B have a purely parasitic relationship to us. From the standpoint of the microbe, what is the ideal outcome of an encounter with a potential host? 'Successful' microbes — like any other successful life form — must survive, must find an environment in which they can reproduce. Peaceful cohabitation is the rule for relationships between microbes and the higher animals. Microbes which are specialised for life in and on humans will do best if they do not interfere with the survival of their hosts, so that those hosts can continue to provide food and lodging. The anaerobes which swarm in the gut are well adapted to a gut habitat; every human provides food and shelter for a few hundred grams of them. Only infrequently does one of these organisms pass beyond the gut wall and cause an infection. *E. coli, Klebsiella, Proteus mirabilis* and the other facultative anaerobes of the gut are also very successful. The coagulase-negative staphylococci, the streptococci and diphtheroids which are so common on the skin and other body surfaces also live in peace with humans. From their point of view the onset of a fatal infection, whatever the cause, is a disaster.

If an infection produces a high mortality in healthy humans, then either this is a relatively new disease in humans and the host-parasite relationship is evolving, or human infection is 'accidental' and the true host is another creature. Rabies is lethal in humans, but in a natural host, the vampire bat, it gives rise to a trivial illness and the virus is shed in the saliva for a long time. A number of other serious infections (plague, scrub typhus, psittacosis, and Lassa fever) only incidentally cause infection in humans; normally they are maintained by a host-vector cycle in which the host is another animal.

INVASION

When entry to the body is considered, microbes can be classified into 3 groups:
1 those that can adhere to the healthy body surface (and often penetrate it), usually a mucosal surface — gut, respiratory tract, or genito-urinary tract
2 those that need the services of a biting arthropod (an insect, mite or tick) to pass through the skin
3 those that can enter only when the normal defences are damaged, either locally (by a wound, or insertion of a catheter) or generally (by illness, drugs).

Table 11.4 lists the portals of entry of some common infectious agents. Obviously portal of entry correlates with route of dissemination; an organism that spreads by the aerial route is likely to enter the body via the respiratory tract and so on.

TABLE 11.4 PORTALS OF ENTRY OF SOME COMMON PATHOGENS

	Organism	Disease
Respiratory tract	Neisseria meningitidis	meningitis
	Streptococcus pneumoniae	
	Mycobacterium tuberculosis	pneumonia
	influenza virus	
	Epstein-Barr virus	glandular fever
Gut	Salmonella typhi	typhoid fever
	Salmonella typhimurium	enteritis (food poisoning)
	hepatitis A virus	hepatitis
	human immunodeficiency virus	AIDS
Genito-urinary tract	Neisseria gonorrhoeae	gonorrhoea
	Treponema pallidum	syphilis
	HIV	AIDS
Skin or wound	Clostridium tetani	tetanus
	hepatitis B virus	hepatitis
	human immunodeficiency virus	AIDS
	Plasmodium vivax	malaria

ADHERENCE

Adherence is the first stage of infection via a mucous membrane. Microbes must attach to host cells before they can cause infection (unless the disease is due to the absorption of preformed toxin). The surface of many microbes includes molecules, *adhesins*, which link to receptors on host cells. The bacterial structures involved are often pili or outer membrane proteins. Attachment of gonococci to epithelial cells or of *Escherichia coli* to cells of the urinary tract is mediated by these reactions. Many bacteria have similar mechanisms: *Bordetella pertussis, Mycoplasma pneumoniae, Streptococcus pyogenes*. The coats of viruses include proteins which link with molecules on the surfaces of host cells. In general the presence or absence of the corresponding receptor on the host-cell surface determines whether the virus is infective for that particular cell and host. Poliovirus attaches to lipid-glycoprotein receptors on gut cells. The coat of influenza virions includes molecules termed haemagglutinin, because they cause red cells to agglutinate (clump). These bind to specific mucoprotein receptors on the epithelial cells of the respiratory tract. Attachment to the mucosal surface may be hindered in various ways. The mucosal secretions themselves have a 'washing' effect and contain sticky substances (mucin), which may interfere with the motility of bacteria. Molecules resembling the cell receptors may be present in the secretions; microbes that combine with them will be prevented from attaching to the mucosal cells. IgA directed against the microbial adhesins will have the same effect (Table 11.5).

TABLE 11.5 ANTI-MICROBIAL DEFENCES OF MUCOUS MEMBRANES

Against adhesion	IgA
	washing by secretions
	'receptor-like' molecules
	mucin
	normal flora
Against multiplication	IgA
	normal flora
	antibacterial substances
	• lactoferrin
	• lysozyme
	interferon

Some microbes do not need to enter the body to cause disease. *Corynebacterium diphtheriae*, the organism responsible for diphtheria, adheres to the mucosa of the throat and multiplies there, but does not invade the tissues. Its toxin is absorbed and attacks the heart. *Vibrio cholerae* and *Shigella* liberate toxins that produce an outpouring of fluid from the intestinal cells and hence diarrhoea. *Streptococcus mutans* colonises the surfaces of teeth in dental plaque and the result is dental caries. The effects of toxins can often be prevented by vaccination.

LOCAL PROLIFERATION

After attachment, the microbe must be able to survive and multiply despite the host's local defences. At different sites there are a variety of defences, both immunological and non-specific. The resident flora can prevent colonisation of a mucosal surface by foreign bacteria. Thus the gut surfaces of newborn calves or piglets are readily occupied by enterotoxigenic strains of *Escherichia coli*, which produce severe diarrhoea. Within a few days of birth the gut is colonised by the typical flora, and susceptibility to enterotoxigenic *E. coli* is sharply reduced. Antibiotic treatment often alters the flora of the mouth and throat in humans. Gram-negative rods such as *Klebsiella*, *Enterobacter* or *Proteus* replace the Gram-positive cocci and rods that normally live there and are more sensitive to antibiotics. Soon after the antibiotic therapy stops the Gram-positive flora usually re-establishes itself and the Gram-negative rods disappear.

Mucosal secretions contain antibacterial substances and antibodies. *Lactoferrin* is a protein which binds free iron and competes with microbes for iron in the environment. Iron is essential for bacterial growth and bacteria which cannot scavenge iron from lactoferrin may not survive. IgA is normally present in secretions and specific IgA regularly results from local infection. Microbes may also possess defences against these antibodies. A number of organisms, e.g. *Haemophilus influenzae*, *Neisseria meningitidis* and *N. gonorrhoeae*, possess enzymes that break down IgA. At frequent intervals variations occur in the surface proteins of some bacteria, with the result that antibody formed in a previous infection does not recognise the new protein and does not offer protection against a fresh infection. The pili and outer-membrane proteins which attach gonococci to epithelial cells undergo rapid spontaneous variation. Trypanosomes use the same strategy. At any one time the coat consists of one major protein; coat proteins are encoded by numerous different genes, which appear to be switched on at random, so that antibody is always being synthesised to a protein no longer present. The numerous different capsular polysaccharides of *Streptococcus pneumoniae* have presumably evolved for the same purpose. In the absence of the specific antibody the possession of a capsule is an effective means of evading phagocytosis.

Once they have adhered to the mucosal surface and multiplied, many organisms can invade the cells of the mucosa, and even destroy them and spread throughout the body. The mechanisms by which they do this are largely unknown. Even when ingested by phagocytes, many bacteria can resist destruction by mechanisms that are not understood. Clinical illness probably involves either release of toxins or invasion of host cells, leading to tissue damage and inflammation. Plasmids are in control of invasive mechanisms in *Shigella sonnei* and in *Yersinia enterocolitica*.

DEFINITION OF 'PATHOGEN'

Having penetrated into the tissues, microbes are exposed to the specific and non-specific defences we have already discussed (chapter 10). Because infection is the outcome of interaction between the microbe's weapons and the host's defences, it is not possible to label each microbial species as either 'pathogenic' or 'non-pathogenic'. Most microbes that cause disease in humans are capable of producing infections that range in severity from 'inapparent' to fatal. If the victim's defences are undermined by severe injury or drug treatment, a normally harmless organism may overwhelm them. If the patient is healthy and well-nourished, a virulent organism may set up only a trivial infection.

The classical rules formulated by Robert Koch (1843-1910) a century ago required that, to be considered the cause of an infection (i.e. to be 'pathogenic') the organism must: be regularly found in the lesions of the disease, be grown in pure culture from the sufferers, and be capable of producing a similar illness in experimental animals. Thus the task of the laboratory was simpler; the isolation of any such pathogen was 'significant'. Organisms which were not pathogens were not significant and need not be reported. These rules make it possible to label *Mycobacterium tuberculosis*, *Clostridium tetani* or *Staphylococcus aureus* as pathogens. They fail in the case of *Mycobacterium leprae*, *Treponema pallidum* or hepatitis A virus, which cannot be cultured, or *Neisseria meningitidis*, which affects no experimental animal. Many of the infections we deal with today are caused by members of our normal flora; only under unusual circumstances do they cause disease at all.

We cannot here discuss all the possible manifestations of infectious disease, which are very varied. Infection may lead to *overt disease* or to *sub-clinical infection*, in which the organism multiplies in the host and elicits an immune response without obvious symptoms or signs, and is then eliminated from the body of the host. *Colonisation* is the presence and multiplication of an organism in or on the host without any of the manifestations of infection, other than (possibly) an immune response. Such an individual is often termed a carrier. A carrier may be colonised as a result of previous infection, but show no reaction to the organism at the time it is isolated from him, or overt signs of infection may never have been present. Carriage may be transient, intermittent or chronic. Thus one finds that roughly 30% of people carry *Staphylococcus aureus* in the nose most of the time, another 50% intermittently and the rest rarely or never. Up to 70% of people associated with hospitals (staff or patients) carry it in the nose. Its presence has no particular significance except that the bearer may infect himself elsewhere or transfer it to others. Dissemination may occur from carriers, but usually only from a proportion of them, and sometimes because of other disease (e.g. a baby may shed *S. aureus* when it has a viral upper respiratory infection, or a physician may do so, when re-activation of his chronic dermatitis leads to scaling of skin). At any given time, *Streptococcus pneumoniae*, *Haemophilus influenzae* or *Neisseria meningitidis* may be isolated from the nose or throat of a few healthy, symptomless individuals. Infection with *Salmonella typhi* leads to carriage of the organism in a small number of cases.

In general, infection results in a defence reaction on the part of the host, the cells of which are predominantly polymorphonuclear if the invader is bacterial and predominantly mononuclear when a virus is to blame. The site of infection and its intensity will differ with the causative agent, the route of infection, and the general health of the individual. Bacteria are more versatile than viruses and tend to cause a wider range of infections. We shall illustrate the various possibilities with examples.

SYMPTOMS AND SIGNS OF INFECTION

Any infection of moderate severity will be accompanied by fever, malaise and prostration. If it is localised there may be pain, redness, heat and swelling of the affected part. Involvement of the respiratory tract may lead to a running nose, cough +/− sputum; infection of the gut may lead to abdominal pain, vomiting and/or diarrhoea; a stiff neck, confusion or coma may indicate infection of the central nervous system.

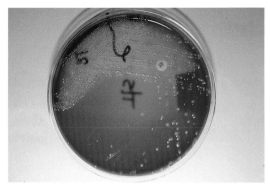

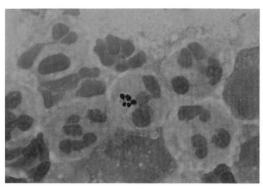

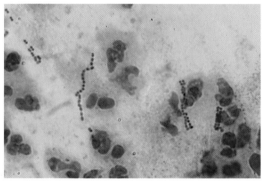

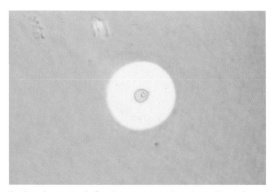

1 Culture of throat swab on blood agar. Note that the colonies differ in size and appearance and that some are surrounded by haemolysis. Actual diameter of plate 9 cm.

2 Gram stain of pus. A clump of Gram-positive cocci in or on a neutrophil is surrounded by other neutrophils, 'pus cells'. The cocci appear to be staphylococci (they were in fact demonstrated to be so by culture).

3 Gram stain of pus. Gram-positive cocci in chains and pairs lie among 'pus cells'. On the basis of this film, a streptococcal infection would be diagnosed.

4 Cerebrospinal fluid from a case of meningitis. Neutrophils and large mononuclear cells are seen and a number of small Gram-negative rods and coccobacilli. Provisional diagnosis: *Haemophilus influenzae* meningitis.

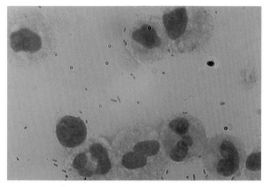

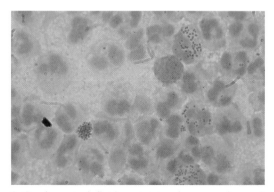

5 Cerebrospinal fluid was mixed with India ink to reveal the large transparent capsule surrounding the yeast cell. Provisional diagnosis: *Cryptococcus neoformans* meningitis.

6 Cerebrospinal fluid containing large numbers of 'pus cells'. Some neutrophils contain large numbers of small Gram-negative diplococci. Provisional diagnosis: *Neisseria meningitidis* meningitis.

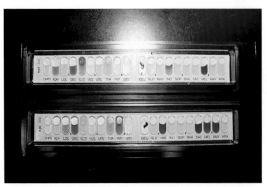

7 Two API galleries. Each small plastic cup contains a growth medium plus a different test chemical. Most media change colour if the test is positive, e.g. in the sugar media on the right, yellow = 'positive'.

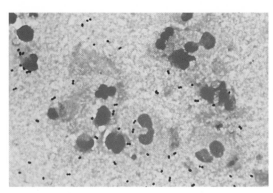

8 Sputum from a case of suspected pneumonia. Numerous 'pus cells' (which often look rather 'battered' — their life-span is less than a day) and Gram-positive cocci mostly in pairs. Provisional diagnosis: pneumococcal pneumonia.

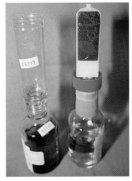

9 Roche blood-culture device. Bacteria from the blood grow in the liquid medium. When the device is inverted bacteria are deposited on the media on the plastic paddle inside the cylinder. These form colonies on further incubation.

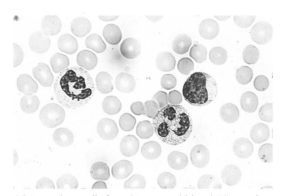

10a-e White cells found in normal blood. These play important roles in the immune defences. Neutrophil polymorphonuclear leucocytes ('neutrophils') are the commonest white cells in the blood, followed by lymphocytes and monocytes. Eosinophils and

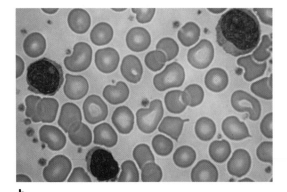

b

basophils are seen fairly infrequently. The neutrophils, eosinophils and basophils have multilobed nuclei and granules in the cytoplasm. Lymphocytes have round or oval nuclei and no granules in the cytoplasm. The monocyte is a large cell with an indented kidney-

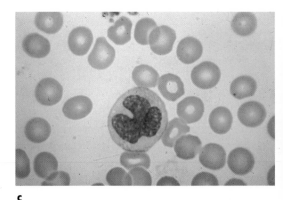

c

shaped nucleus. It becomes a macrophage in the tissues. (**a**) Two neutrophils and one large lymphocyte, (**b**) 2 small and 1 large lymphocyte, (**c**) a monocyte, (**d**) an eosinophil, (**e**) a basophil (precursor of a tissue mast cell) and a neutrophil.

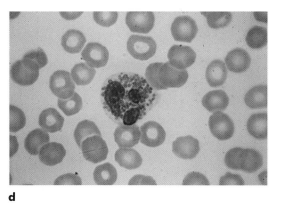

d

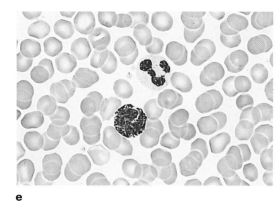

e

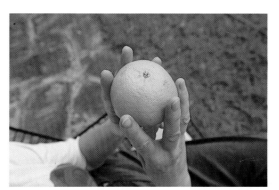

11 Representation of the antibody molecule. The three fingers of each hand represent the three loops formed by the light and heavy chains of the antibody molecule. These make up the antigen-binding site into which the antigen (orange) fits.

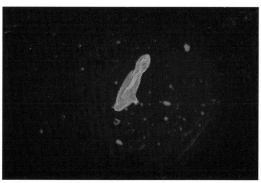

12 Immunofluorescence. Fluorescent antiserum is used to detect and identify a schistosome larva (cercaria), outlining it in green.

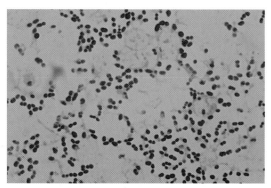

13 Gram stain showing *Streptococcus pneumoniae*, pneumococci singly and in pairs (diplococci).

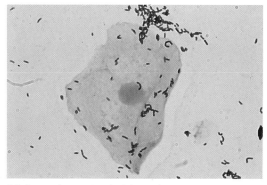

14 Corynebacteria, 'diphtheroids', on and around an epithelial cell from the mouth. These Gram-positive rods characteristically occur as V-shaped pairs and in clumps like 'Chinese letters'.

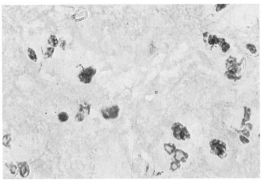

15 In this Ziehl-Neelsen stain of sputum the tubercle bacilli, 'acid-fast bacilli', stain pink, while pus cells and other material stain blue. The tubercle bacilli are seen as fine, beaded rods, mainly in clumps.

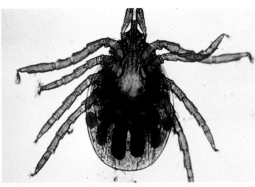

16 A tick. Note the eight legs, and the mouth by which the arachnid sucks blood. The photograph is taken with transillumination, so that internal organs are visible.

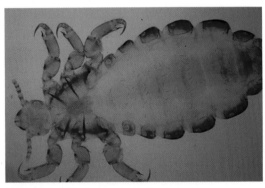

17 Adult female louse, *Pediculus humanus*.

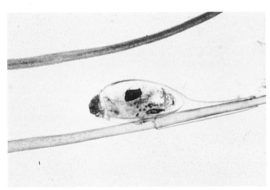

18 A 'nit', i.e. an egg of a louse, attached to a hair.

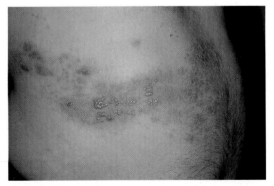

19 Shingles (due to the recurrence of *Herpes zoster*). The fluid-filled vesicles occur in the area of distribution of a nerve, since the virus lies latent in the nerve ganglia. Hence, on the trunk, the vesicles appear in a band.

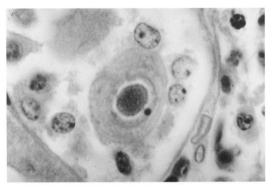

20 Inclusion body in cytomegalovirus-infected epithelial cell in urine. Note the greatly enlarged cell with a central nuclear inclusion.

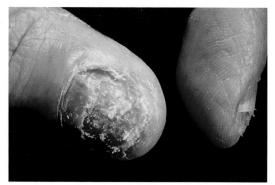

21 Chronic *Candida* infection of the finger-nails showing destruction of nail tissue.

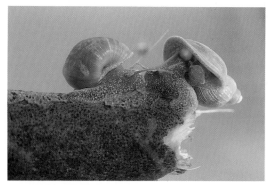

22a Snails, *Bulinus* species — intermediate host of *Schistosoma*.

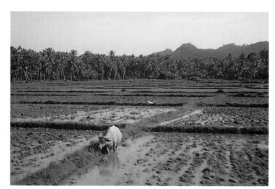

22b A paddy field is a typical environment in which the *Schistosoma* finds its intermediate host — a snail. Workers in such fields are infected by the cercariae subsequently liberated from the snails. (Ko Samui, Thailand.)

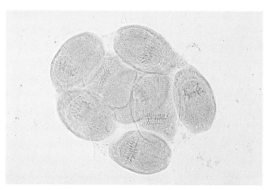

23a 'Hydatid sand', unattached protoscolices of *Echinococcus*, from a cyst.

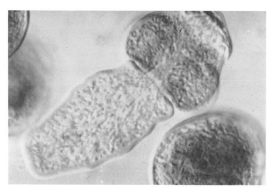

23b Scolex of *Echinococcus granulosus* in urine. Note the 'crown' of hooklets (top right). Hooklets are also visible in Pl 23a.

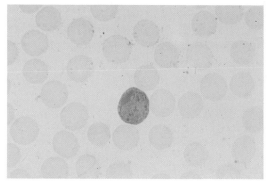

24a *Plasmodium vivax* — female gametocyte. The parasite completely fills the red cell.

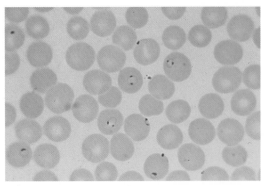

24b *Plasmodium falciparum* — ring forms. The rings are small and some red cells are multiply infected.

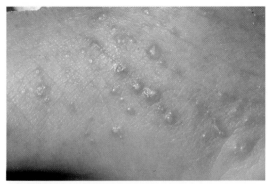

25 Scabies on a baby's foot. In infants, the rash often becomes vesicular (i.e. forms blisters).

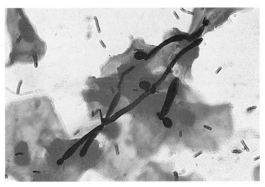

26 *Candida vaginitis*. Vaginal swab showing Gram-positive rods (lactobacilli — normal vaginal flora) and yeast cells and hyphae.

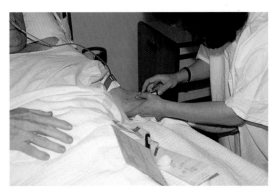

27 A nurse collecting blood for culture.

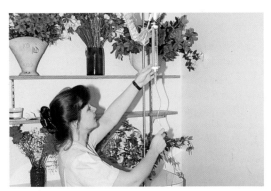

28 A nursing sister adjusting the flow of an intravenous infusion.

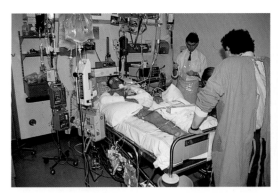

29 A severely ill patient in intensive care, festooned with tubing and surrounded by equipment: a 'compromised' patient.

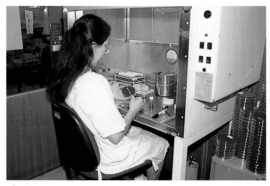

30 A technologist inoculates a blood-agar plate with a swab from an infected wound. She is working in a safety cabinet, which prevents spread of infectious material to her or others.

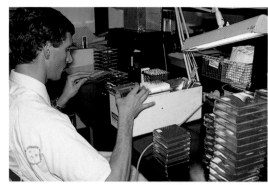

31 A technologist uses a replicator to inoculate a large number of different cultures onto the one plate. This allows antibiotic susceptibility tests to be performed economically.

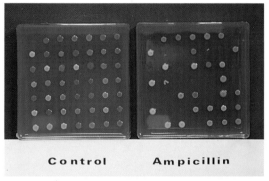

Control   Ampicillin

32 Agar dilution susceptibility plates inoculated with the replicator illustrated in Plate 31. The control plate contains no antibiotic. Bacteria susceptible to ampicillin grow on the control, but not on the ampicillin plate.

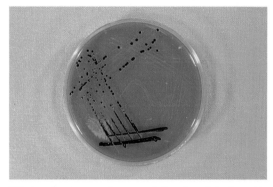

33 A selective medium used for the detection of intestinal pathogens. The black colonies are *Salmonella typhi*, the cause of typhoid fever.

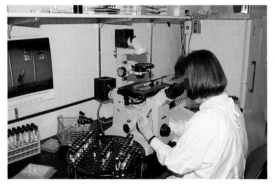

34 A technologist uses an inverted microscope to check cell cultures for evidence of viral growth. With this instrument the cells are viewed 'from underneath' and remain in the medium while being examined.

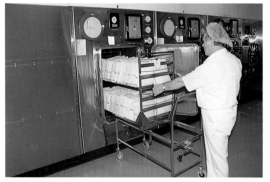

35 Unloading drapes from an autoclave after sterilisation. (Sterilising Services Dept, RNS Hospital).

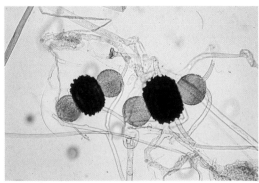

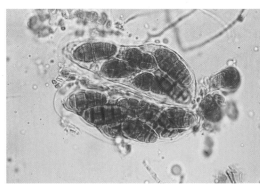

36 Reproduction in fungi. The black rough-walled structures are zygospores, sexual spores produced by the fusion of two cells, one from each parent.

37-44 Fungal spores. These plates illustrate the great variety of types: small, large, thin-walled, thick-walled, in long chains or in groups of 2, 4 or 8. These differences are important in the identification of fungi. Pl 37 — 41 are environmental saprophytes and do not usually cause disease.

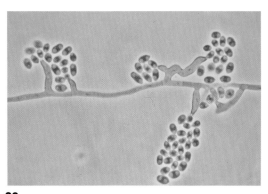

38

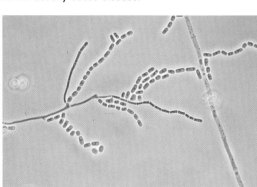

39

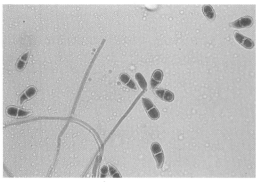

40

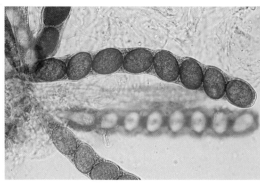

41

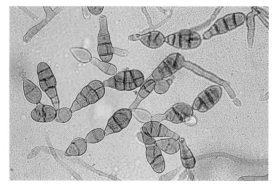

42 This organism, a species of *Alternaria*, was isolated from a corneal ulcer.

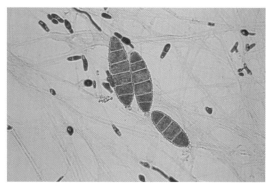

43 The fungus *Microsporum gypseum* is a cause of infections of the skin.

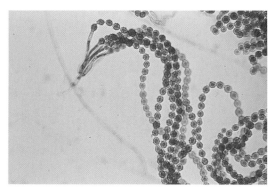

44 The long chains of small, rough-walled spores are produced by a *Penicillium* species (some strains of the mould *Penicillium* produce penicillin).

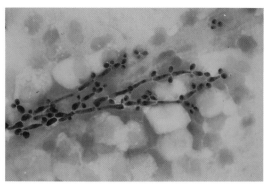

45 Mycelia of the yeast *Candida albicans* in urine; the patient's kidneys were infected with this yeast.

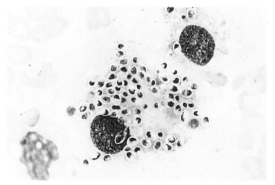

46 Macrophages containing numerous cells of the fungus *Histoplasma capsulatum*. Infection with this organism is usually inapparent, but occasionally serious.

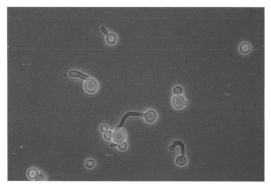

47 When *Candida albicans* is incubated in serum, it forms a characteristic outgrowth within 2-3 hours — the 'germ tube'. This feature serves to distinguish it from other yeasts.

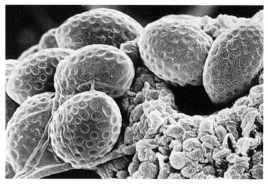

48 Fungal spores being discharged from the structure in which they were formed (scanning electronmicrograph).

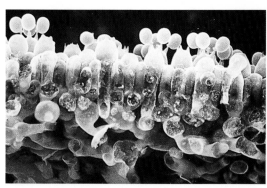

49 The gill of a mushroom showing spores in groups of four and the structures which bear them (scanning electronmicrograph).

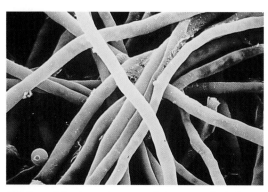

50 Fungal hyphae, the normal form in which fungi grow (scanning electronmicrograph).

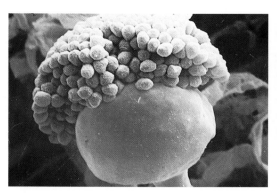

51 A fungal sporangium bearing a dense mass of spores (scanning electronmicrograph).

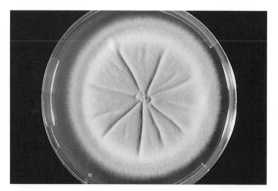

52-55 Cultures of various fungi: a *Microsporum* (**52**) and a *Trichophyton* (**53**), both common causes of skin disease; an *Aspergillus* (**54**) and a *Fusarium* (**55**), environmental organisms which very occasionally cause infections in compromised patients. Such

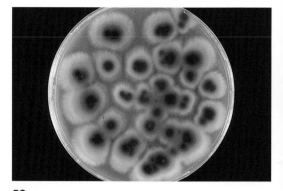

53
colonies take days or weeks to develop to the extent seen here. Colonial appearance is of importance in the identification of fungi.

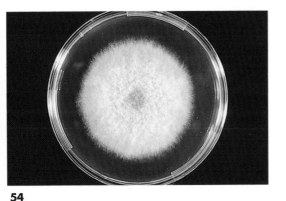

54

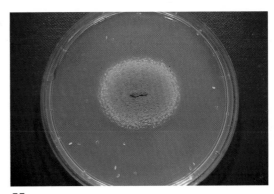

55

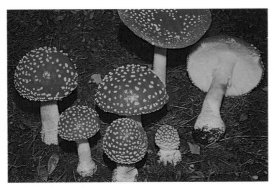

56 This spectacular mushroom, *Amanita muscaria,* produces dangerous hallucinogenic drugs.

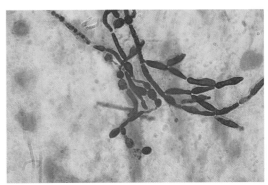

57 A Gram stain of sputum showing *Candida*: yeast cells and pseudohyphae. Such a picture may indicate *Candida* infection of the mouth or even the lung; such an infection is most likely in a compromised patient.

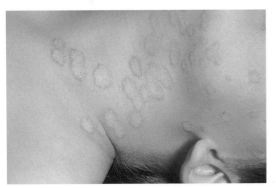

58 The circular, scaling lesions of ringworm (actually a fungus, not a worm). The cause in this case was *Microsporum canis.*

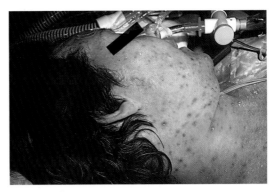

59 *Varicella pneumonia.*

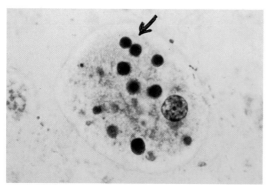

60 A stained film showing a trophozoite of *Entamoeba histolytica*. At the lower right of the cell can be seen the nucleus. The black dots are red cells which have been engulfed, a feature diagnostic of this parasite.

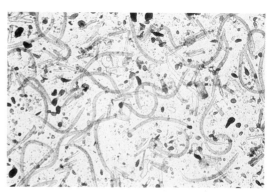

61 Large numbers of the nematode worm *Strongyloides stercoralis* in faeces create the effect of a Jackson Pollock painting.

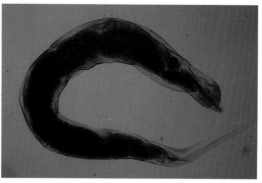

62 Adult female of *Enterobius vermicularis*. Note the typical long pointed tail and the plentiful stock of eggs.

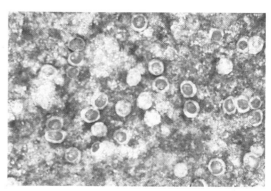

63 This delicate pastel-toned slide represents the protozoon *Cryptosporidium* in faeces. Diarrhoea due to this parasite is being recognised more often, both in immunocompetent and immunocompromised persons.

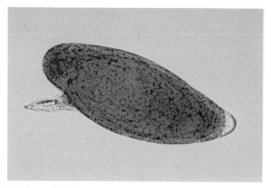

64 Egg of *Schistosoma mansoni*. The large size and the lateral spine are characteristic.

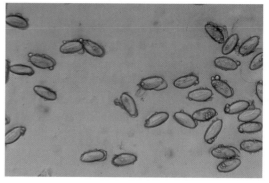

65 'Sticky-tape' preparation showing large numbers of *Enterobius vermicularis* eggs.

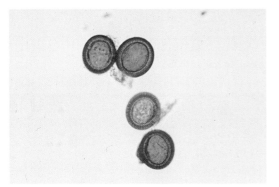

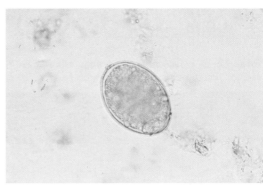

66-71 The eggs of many tapeworms are distinctive. Since they are the life-form of the parasite most likely to be seen in faeces (the usual diagnostic material), a good deal of attention is devoted to their identification. The eggs shown here are of *Taenia* sp,

67
Diphyllobothrium latum, Ascaris lumbricoides (with and without its outer coat), *Fasciola hepatica, Trichostrongylus* and *Trichuris trichiura*. As can be seen, the eggs vary a great deal in appearance.

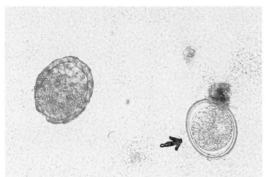

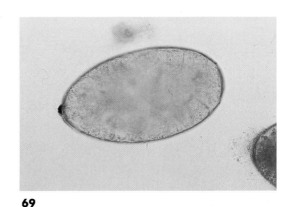

68

69

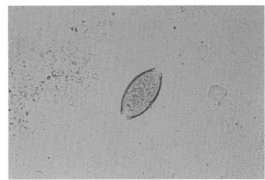

70

71

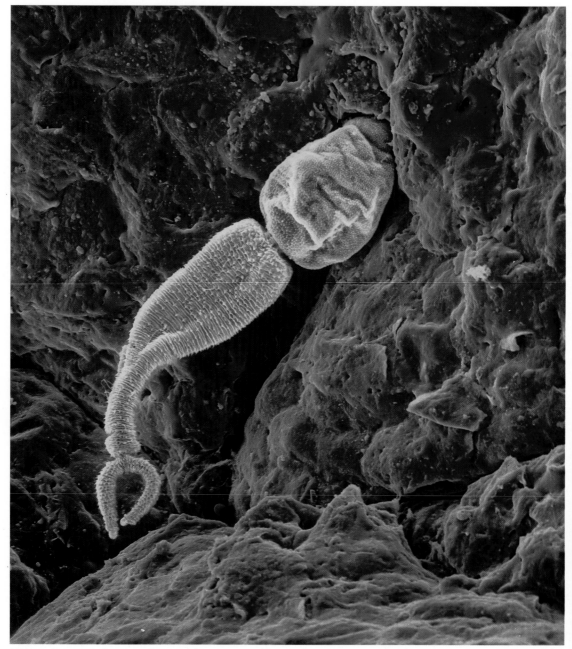

72 A schistosome larva in the act of penetrating human skin. The motile larva (cercaria) emerges from its intermediate host (a water snail) to swim off to find its definitive host (a human being). It requires only 30 seconds or so to vanish below the surface of the skin, shedding its tail in the process.

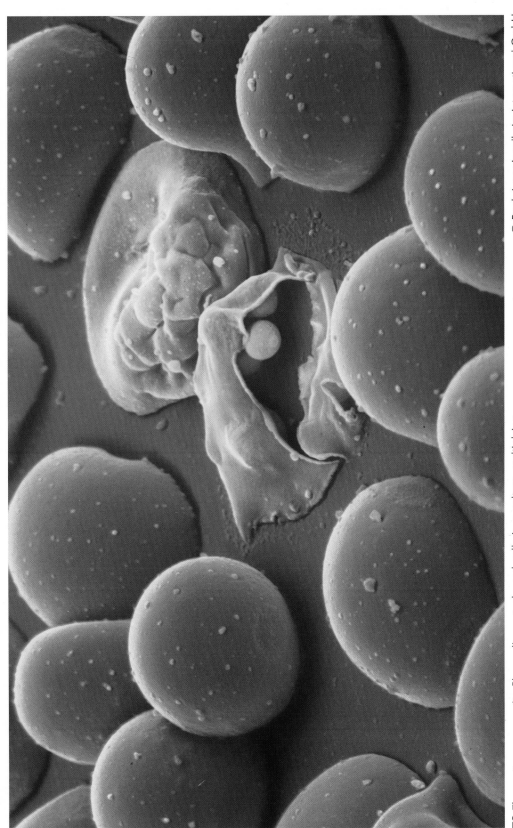

73 The protozoan parasite Plasmodium attacks red cells in a culture, multiplying inside two of them. One red cell has already been lysed, releasing parasites to attack other red cells. The parasite adheres to the cell by specific receptors and enters to multiply inside a vacuole.

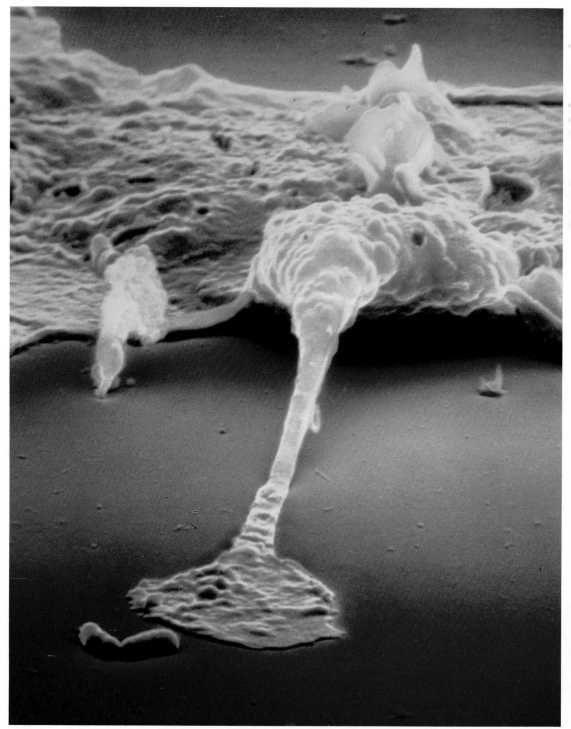

74 A macrophage extends a pseudopod to ingest a bacterium. Substances liberated by the bacterium and by its reaction with antibody and complement attract the phagocyte, a process called *chemotaxis*.

TYPES OF INFECTIONS

Infections may be *local* or *systemic* (generalised).

1 *Local infections* may be relatively trivial (e.g. a pimple or boil) or more serious, but still involving mainly a single organ (urinary tract infection, appendicitis, gastroenteritis, pneumonia).

2 *Systemic infections* involve several organs; examples are bacteraemia, infective endocarditis, brucellosis and typhoid.

THE BOIL

Let us look first at a boil or furuncle, in which *Staphylococcus aureus* sets up infection in a hair follicle. The early events in the development of a boil have been described above (pp.99–101) as an example of the acute inflammatory response. This defence reaction may be rapidly successful in overcoming the invasion; the signs of inflammation will then promptly subside. If not, tissues surrounding the multiplying bacteria will break down, the infection spreads and the inflammation intensifies, causing an enlarging abscess that eventually penetrate the overlying skin and 'points' (discharges pus). The infection may break through the deeper tissues, forming a carbuncle, and even enter lymph channels and blood vessels to result in bacteraemia (see below).

URINARY INFECTIONS

The bladder urine is normally sterile. It has some antibacterial properties and ascent of bacteria from the external genitals is prevented by the washing of the urethra when urine is passed. Urinary infection (urinary tract infection, often abbreviated UTI) is much commoner in women than men, presumably because of the relative shortness of the female urethra. Urinary infection is usually due to a faecal bacterium (most often *Escherichia coli*), which ascends to the bladder from the exterior. Infection which reaches no further than the bladder is often termed 'cystitis'. Multiplication of bacteria in urine leads to an outpouring of inflammatory cells, and symptoms of 'burning and scalding' on passing urine. Microscopy of the urine shows large numbers of white cells and culture typically yields a bacterial count of 10^7-10^9/L. Antibiotic treatment is rapidly effective in most cases, although increasingly the causative bacteria are resistant to the older antibiotics. Much less often the infection extends further up the urinary tract and sets up *pyelonephritis*, infection of the kidney itself, a more serious disorder accompanied by fever and pain in the loin.

THE URINARY CATHETER

In many hospital patients an 'indwelling' catheter (i.e. a catheter that is left in the bladder for days or weeks) is necessary because the patient is unconscious; in the case of incontinent or demented patients also, this arrangement is convenient for nursing purposes. Bacteriuria is very common in such patients. Antibiotics should only be given when the patient develops signs of infection (e.g. local discomfort, fever and malaise).

RESPIRATORY TRACT INFECTION

The respiratory tract must remain in contact with the environment, because its function is to be constantly flushed with air. There is the risk that microbes will be inhaled along with air, since that air contains microbes in droplet nuclei and on dust particles. Yet the defences of the respiratory tract (Fig. 11.4) are so effective that below the level of the main bronchi the healthy respiratory tract is sterile. How is this accomplished? The nasal passages present a large surface covered with mucous secretions, so that inhaled particles are trapped and eventually swallowed. This filter system probably removes over 90% of inhaled particles. Small particles, however, may manage to pass further down. Many of these will be deposited on the mucous membranes of the trachea, bronchi and bronchioles: this material is removed by the cilia on the respiratory membranes, which carry a constant stream of particle-laden mucus up the bronchi and trachea into the pharynx, where it is swallowed. Consequently, only *very* small particles will reach the alveoli — where they will be phagocytosed and destroyed by macrophages. As well as these 'mechanical' defences, the nasal secretions contain various antibacterial substances, such as lysozyme and secretory IgA; immunoglobulins and complement are present in the lung secretions.

Additionally, the epiglottis closes off the trachea and prevents upper respiratory tract secretions from trickling down into the lungs and carrying bacteria and viruses with them. Any depression of consciousness (anaesthesia, stroke, abuse of alcohol or drugs — even sleep) can interfere with the function of the epiglottis and contribute to lower respiratory tract infection. Inhaling vomitus while in such a state may lead to pneumonia caused by mixed anaerobic bacteria from the gut. Coughing helps to remove foreign material from the lungs and prevents accumulation of secretions. A weakened or absent cough reflex greatly increases the risk of lower respiratory tract infection.

Pneumonia is an inflammation of the lungs, usually due to a bacterium or a virus (viral infections of the respiratory tract are discussed in more detail on pp.225-227). A very large number of microbes can cause pneumonia and Table 11.6 shows only the commonest. The organism passes down the trachea from the mouth or throat and sets up an acute inflammation in lung tissue. Fluid exudes and fills up the air-spaces, so that the lung becomes 'consolidated' and air cannot enter; the amount of functioning lung tissue is reduced and the respiratory rate rises. X-ray of the lung shows consolidation; lung tissues filled with fluid rather than air are more opaque to X-rays . It is important to establish the

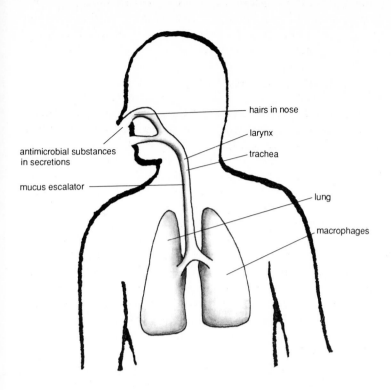

hairs in nose

larynx

antimicrobial substances
in secretions

trachea

mucus escalator

lung

macrophages

Fig. 11.4 Defences of the respiratory tract. All surfaces are covered with mucus, leading to the trapping of inhaled particles. Hairs in the nose cause eddies in the air stream, also helping to trap particles. The epiglottis at the inlet to the larynx stops upper respiratory tract secretions (and food or vomitus) from entering the lungs. Coughing removes foreign materials and secretions from the lungs. The cilia on the respiratory membranes drive the 'mucus escalator' — a stream of mucus that carries foreign particles up and out through the larynx to be swallowed. Macrophages and other phagocytes in the lungs engulf foreign particles.

causative organism, since most are susceptible to some antibiotic. Microscopy and culture of a *properly collected* specimen of sputum will be of great help in this.

TABLE 11.6 COMMON MICROBIAL CAUSES OF ACUTE PNEUMONIA

Bacteria and similar agents:

Streptococcus pneumoniae	Mycoplasma pneumoniae
Staphylococcus aureus	Chlamydia
Haemophilus influenzae	Coxiella burnetii
Escherichia coli	
Klebsiella pneumoniae	Viruses:
Pseudomonas aeruginosa	Influenza viruses
Legionella	Respiratory syncytial virus (children)

Mixed anaerobic bacteria
Mycobacterium tuberculosis

INFECTIONS OF THE GUT: DIARRHOEA

Like the respiratory tract, the gut is constantly exposed to microbes from the environment. Much of the food we eat contains bacteria, though usually not pathogenic ones. We swallow numerous bacteria which make up the flora of the upper respiratory tract. The gut has powerful defence mechanisms (Fig. 11.5). Most of the microbes swallowed will be destroyed by the *gastric acid:* the pH of the stomach, close to 1, keeps it sterile or almost so. Further down in the upper small intestine there are few bacteria, but numbers increase in the terminal ileum, and the colon contains vast quantities of bacteria, which make up about half the weight of faeces. The integrity of the gut wall and its mucous secretions, which contain antibodies, help to protect the gut and there is also the mechanical effect of secretions 'washing' the walls and of peristalsis (gut contractions) moving the gut contents along to the exterior.

Fig. 11.5 Defences of the gut. The gastric acid kills many microbes. Mucus and other secretions together with the contractions of the gut 'wash' the surfaces. Mucus and antibodies interfere with adherence of pathogens. Microbes which pass through the mucosa encounter phagocytes in the gut wall, the bloodstream and the liver. Plasma cells are found in the lymphoid tissue of the gut wall.

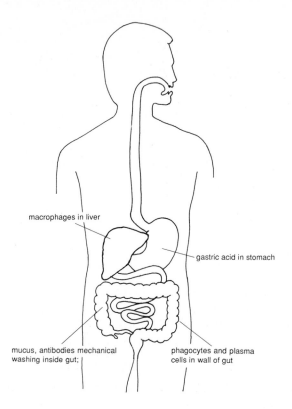

Within the gut wall are found phagocytic cells (whose role is presumably to destroy microbes that succeed in passing any tiny breach in the mucosa), and plasma cells synthesising immunoglobulins (especially IgA). The veins draining the small and large intestine go directly to the liver, which has a great phagocytic capacity (p.109), and bacteria that pass through the gut wall are removed here before they reach the general circulation.

Most of the faecal bacteria live in comfortable symbiosis with the human host. Of the several hundred different species of bacteria that occur in the faeces, only a comparative few cause infections in normal persons, and then only when they elude the defences of the gut and reach another part of the body: the urinary bladder, lung, meninges. Infectious diarrhoea is almost always due to an agent recently acquired from outside (Table 11.7). Known variously as gastroenteritis, 'food poisoning', 'travellers' diarrhoea', 'Montezuma's revenge', 'Greek gallop', 'Bali (or Delhi) belly' and by many other colourful terms, infectious diarrhoea is actually responsible for an enormous death toll in the developing countries; in rural India 5% of infants aged 7-12 months die of this cause. In the developed countries such infections are also among the commonest, but are rarely fatal.

TABLE 11.7 MAIN INFECTIVE CAUSES OF DIARRHOEA

Organism: *Mechanism of disease*

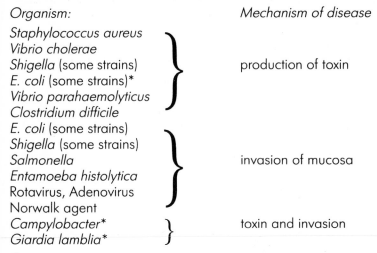

Organism	Mechanism of disease
Staphylococcus aureus *Vibrio cholerae* *Shigella* (some strains) *E. coli* (some strains)* *Vibrio parahaemolyticus* *Clostridium difficile*	production of toxin
E. coli (some strains) *Shigella* (some strains) *Salmonella* *Entamoeba histolytica* Rotavirus, Adenovirus Norwalk agent	invasion of mucosa
*Campylobacter** *Giardia lamblia**	toxin and invasion

[*a major cause of travellers' diarrhoea].

We are protected against these infections by the factors discussed above, by personal hygiene and by immunity acquired in previous attacks. Almost all the agents involved are acquired by the faecal-oral route, by consuming food or drink that is contaminated by the faeces of humans or animals. For most of the bacterial causes of diarrhoea the infecting dose is large: 10^8 for enteropathogenic *Escherichia coli* or *Vibrio cholerae*; 10^5 for *Salmonella*. At the other extreme, *Shigella*, which can survive the gastric acid, may set up infection with only 10-100 bacteria.

The ability to adhere to and colonise the gut mucosa appears to be necessary for many enteric pathogens, which may go on to produce disease in at least two ways: by *secreting toxins* or by *invading the mucosa*.

SECRETION OF TOXIN

Staphylococcal food poisoning and botulism are due to toxins acting on the nervous system (the botulism toxin actually causes paralysis, not diarrhoea). The organisms multiply outside the body, in the food before consumption. Enterotoxins active on the intestinal mucosa and causing excessive fluid secretion are produced in the gut by *Vibrio cholerae*, by enterotoxigenic *E. coli* and by several other species. *Clostridium difficile* elaborates a cytotoxin that destroys mucosal cells and leads to inflammation and diarrhoea.

INVASION OF MUCOSA

Shigella and some *E. coli* strains actually invade and multiply in the the mucosal cells, destroying them and leading to diarrhoea. *Salmonella typhi* and *Yersinia* penetrate the mucosa and multiply in the lymphoid and reticuloendothelial cells, then enter the bloodstream, producing a systemic infection with fever, but often without diarrhoea. The mechanisms by which some enteric pathogens e.g. *Giardia lamblia* cause disease are unknown.

The presence of one of these infections is usually clinically obvious. Laboratory investigations should be capable of revealing at least *Salmonella, Shigella, Vibrio, Campylobacter* and *E. coli*. The specimen should also be examined for *Giardia lamblia* if the diarrhoea has lasted more than 1 week. Antibiotics are needed for typhoid (a systemic infection) but hitherto have been of little avail for infective diarrhoeas. However, it appears that the quinolones (especially ciprofloxacin) are quite effective in the treatment of these disorders. Nevertheless, *in most infective diarrhoeas it is more important to re-hydrate the patient adequately than to give antibiotics*. In any severe diarrhoea fluid loss may rapidly lead to *fatal* dehydration.

MENINGITIS

Meningitis is an inflammation of the membranes covering the brain and spinal cord (Fig. 11.6). Acute bacterial meningitis is a medical emergency requiring the most skilful diagnosis and treatment. The death rate remains about 30%. The main causes of this condition, *Haemophilus influenzae, Neisseria meningitidis* and *Streptococcus pneumoniae*, have their normal reservoir in the nose and throat. From here they apparently enter the bloodstream and, evading destruction because they possess capsules, reach the cerebrospinal fluid and multiply there. Meningitis due to group B streptococci most often appears in the newborn. Meningitis caused by *Listeria monocytogenes* occurs in this age-group, but also in older persons, especially in the immunocompromised. Viral meningitis is usually a mild infection, rarely fatal (Table 11.8).

TABLE 11.8 CAUSES OF MENINGITIS

Common:	*Haemophilus influenzae*
	Neisseria meningitides
	Streptococcus pneumoniae
	*Viruses**
Less common:	Group B streptococci
	Listeria monocytogenes
	Mycobacterium tuberculosis
	Cryptococcus neoformans
	Leptospira spp.

[* Enteroviruses, flaviviruses, measles, mumps, herpes simplex, lymphocytic choriomeningitis and others.]

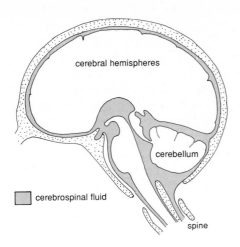

cerebral hemispheres

cerebellum

cerebrospinal fluid

spine

Fig. 11.6 Membranes around the central nervous system. The brain and spinal cord are enclosed in three membranes: **(a)** an outer membrane firmly attached to the skull and spinal column **(b)** an inner membrane closely applied to the nerve tissues and **(c)** a third membrane between these two and resting against the outer membrane. The cerebrospinal fluid fills the irregular spaces between the middle and inner membranes, including the ventricles (cavities within the brain). The cerebrospinal fluid contains salts, glucose, a little protein and other substances, and a very few white cells.

The symptoms and signs of meningitis are: headache, lethargy, vomiting, fever, drowsiness and confusion, stiff neck. The diagnosis is confirmed by 'lumbar puncture', by aspirating cerebrospinal fluid from the lumbar spine for microscopic examination and culture. This procedure should be carried out as soon as the suspicion of meningitis arises; the risk in delay is far greater than the risk of the examination.

Examination of the cerebrospinal fluid normally includes testing for the presence of microbial antigens (p.83). In bacterial meningitis the cerebrospinal fluid shows large numbers of white cells, mainly polymorphs; in viral meningitis mononuclear cells predominate and the cell count is not so high.

In most cases herpes simplex virus causes an encephalitis (inflammmation of the brain tissues) rather than meningitis. This infection is usually fatal and even with antiviral chemotherapy the survivors are usually left with severe disabilities.

BACTERAEMIA AND SEPTICAEMIA

Bacteraemia is the presence of bacteria in the blood. *Septicaemia* is bacteraemia of some duration accompanied by unpleasant consequences such as fever and malaise; there is no clear-cut distinction between the two states. The bloodstream is usually sterile, because there are remarkably efficient mechanisms for removing microbes from it. Most bacteria are less likely to cause disease when injected into the blood than by any other route. Bacteria that enter the blood are removed rapidly by several mechanisms. The blood itself possesses bactericidal systems, the complement system (p.101). Bacteria are removed from the blood by phagocytosis, either by the mononuclear phagocytic system or the neutrophils.

Microbes entering through the skin will encounter macrophages and neutrophils first in the tissue spaces. The polymorphonuclear neutrophils play the major role in combatting extravascular infections, by localising the invasion and destroying the bacteria with the assistance of antibodies and complement. If the bacteria survive this attack, they may spread via the lymphatics and the lymph nodes, finally to enter the bloodstream. From the blood, microbes are filtered out and destroyed mainly in the liver and spleen. Monocytes and macrophages are present in the subcutaneous tissues, the lymph nodes, brain and elsewhere. They line the sinuses of the liver, spleen and bone-marrow (sinuses are dilated vessels in which the blood flows slowly).

Bacteria may enter the blood as the result of a wound, or through a mucosal surface. The mucous membranes of the body bear such heavy loads of bacteria that bacteraemia is likely to occur in any procedure involving a mucosal surface: dental extraction, insertion or removal of a urinary catheter, diagnostic procedures such as bronchoscopy or barium enema, even brushing one's teeth. In the healthy person, these bacteria are cleared from the blood within minutes. Bacteraemia of this sort is called *transient*.

Intermittent bacteraemia is most often associated with large collections of undrained pus (such as subphrenic, intra-abdominal and pelvic abscesses). Continuous bacteraemia commonly means an intravascular source of bacteria — such as the vegetations on a heart valve in infective endocarditis, an infection in a vascular graft, or the organisms colonising an indwelling intravascular catheter or other device (a very common situation in the modern hospital).

In general the number of bacteria in the blood is small and most bacteraemias are intermittent. So it is important to culture an adequate volume of blood (at least 10 mL) and to carry out at least three cultures; more are usually unnecessary. Antimicrobial therapy significantly reduces the likelihood of detecting bacteria in the blood.

In the last 50 years bacteraemia has become much commoner in hospital patients. This is thought to be due to the greater proportion of people with major injuries and other forms of serious illness (e.g. in intensive care units), and the consequent increased use of respiratory support systems and intravascular lines. Gram-negative bacilli are now the predominant cause.

CAUSES OF BACTERAEMIA

Bacteraemia is a manifestation of many different diseases, and almost any bacterium or yeast may be isolated from the blood. Some species (e.g. most *Enterobacteriaceae* and *Pseudomonas*, *Streptococcus pneumoniae* or *Haemophilus influenzae*) are virtually always 'significant'; they do not enter the blood as contaminants during the collection of the specimen. Some organisms such as coagulase-negative staphylococci or *Propionibacterium acnes* are most often skin contaminants, but are occasionally significant. Other species, e.g.

Staphylococcus aureus, are usually important, but may also be found because of contamination.

INFECTIVE ENDOCARDITIS

This is an infection of the lining of the heart, usually involving a valve. A uniformly fatal disease before the antibiotic era, it remains a very serious condition. A clot forms on the surface of a heart valve (usually a damaged valve) and bacteria then become deposited on the clot (transient bacteraemia is a common event) and promote further clotting, so that a 'vegetation' builds up on the valve's surface. Bacteria within the vegetation are protected from the lethal activities of polymorphonuclear leucocytes. It is essential that the antibiotic or antibiotics used to treat infective endocarditis be bactericidal — i.e. capable of *killing* the microbes, not simply inhibiting them, as would normally suffice in the presence of phagocytes. Pieces of vegetation may detach and become emboli, blocking vessels for instance in the spleen, brain or kidney. A heart valve implant predisposes to infective endocarditis, as does intravenous drug abuse. Streptococci cause about 70% of cases of infective endocarditis, *Staphylococcus aureus* about 15%, and the remaining 15% are made up of many different species, including Gram-negative rods, anaerobes and fungi.

NEW INFECTIONS

The infections which we have discussed in this chapter occur commonly in normal individuals, as do many other types: infections of the bone marrow — *osteomyelitis*, of the joints — *infective arthritis*, of the skin and underlying soft tissues — *cellulitis*, of the lymph nodes — *lymphadenitis*. Clinical medicine has taken great strides in the last several decades and many microbial infections can now be treated successfully.

Unfortunately, however, progress in medicine and surgery has presented clinical microbiology with a vast array of new problems. The technical advances in surgery, the sophisticated life-support systems on which many of these techniques depend to keep the patients alive during and after treatment, the powerful drugs which modify the patients' resistance to infection while producing other desired effects, have had the result that a considerable proportion of the patients in many hospitals are surviving despite disabilities that would have been fatal 30 or 40 years ago. The microbiological problems in such patients are largely new, both because we have at our disposal better methods of detecting microbes, and because organisms not previously thought responsible for disease are being encountered in them. We shall discuss these problems in chapter 17.

VIRAL INFECTIONS

A virus can attack a cell only if the cell bears a receptor with which a molecule on the virion surface can react. Viral infections are of two types. In *superficial infections* the cell to which the virus particle attaches on first contact with the host is also the cell in which it multiplies. This is true of the mucosal cells in the respiratory tract and the gut, the two organs most frequently attacked by viruses. Such infections will have symptoms largely referable to one organ system. The incubation period is short, 2-5 days. The clinical course is also brief and the infection is rarely fatal. Transmission is by the aerial or faecal-oral route, never by a biting insect or via a wound.

In *deep infections* the virus attacks an internal organ, such as the liver, heart or central nervous system. The virion either adheres to a surface cell or is deposited in the tissues by a biting insect, needle-stick or other injury. In each case it is usually carried to its final destination by the bloodstream. The incubation period of these infections is usually longer, the clinical course likewise and the infection is more likely to have serious consequences.

In either type of infection the virus particles must reach the target cell, attach to the specific receptor, enter the cell and multiply inside it. Before it enters the cell the virion may be intercepted by antibodies. Antibodies to the influenza haemagglutinin or the measles haemagglutinin prevent attachment to the cell, while clumps of virus particles and antibody may fix complement and be phagocytosed and destroyed intracellularly.

Spread to other susceptible cells may be impeded by interferon. Interferon is important in primary infections of the superficial type; because of the brief incubation period, antibody may come on the scene too late. Antibody, however, probably plays the major role in defence to a second infection with the same agent. In deep infections low levels of antibody are more likely to be effective, because the virus particle has to travel in the blood stream and therefore has a greater chance to encounter the antibody. Because of the long incubation period, there is time for a secondary response, if the host has previously been exposed to the virus.

Once inside the cell, the virus is safe from the effects of antibody. Many viruses can spread to adjacent cells by budding from the cell membrane without becoming exposed to tissue fluids and hence to antibody. Against viruses such as influenza, measles, mumps, rubella and cytomegalovirus, which spread in this way, cell-mediated immunity is important for recovery. T-lymphocytes attack such cells and also release an interferon which prevents multiplication in adjacent cells.

PARASITIC INFECTIONS

Many parasites have ingenious ways of evading the host's defences. trypanosomes and *Plasmodium*, for instance, modulate their surface proteins, so that last week's antibody no longer reacts. Schistosomes cover themselves with host molecules, red cell or MHC proteins, or IgG. Both antibody and cell-mediated immunity come into play. If the organism lives free in the blood, antibody and complement are important in defence. Nematode worms are expelled from the gut by the combined activities of IgG and gut secretions. antibody is important in the defence to malaria and plays some role in inhibiting the spread of *Leishmania* and certain trypanosomes. These latter parasites, and *Toxoplasma gondii*, live inside macrophages and hence T-lymphocytes are important, secreting lymphokines that activate the killing powers of the macrophages.

CHAPTER REVIEW

1   Discuss the relationship between humans and their microbial flora.
2   Describe the modes of transmission of common microbes to humans.
3   What conditions may undermine the body's resistance to invading micro-organisms?
4   Define and give examples of:
    (a)   *symbiosis*
    (b)   *parasitism*
5   (a)   Define a 'carrier'.
    (b)   What is the importance of the carrier state?
6   'Progress in medicine and surgery have caused new problems which modify the patient's resistance to infection'.
    (a)   What is meant by this statement?
    (b)   Discuss some examples of such problems.
7   (a)   Define *bacteraemia*.
    (b)   How does it occur?
    (c)   Why is it important?
8   What microbial characteristics are related to virulence?
9   Describe the two main types of viral infection.

12

ANTIMICROBIAL THERAPY

HISTORY OF ANTIBIOTICS

By the beginning of this century medical knowledge had advanced to the point where doctors were proficient at diagnosis and could predict the outcome of an illness. However they had few means to modify an illness's course. Infectious disease posed the greatest challenge — apart from a few drugs like emetine and quinine, which were active against certain parasites, no drug had a worthwhile effect on microbial infections. No drug then known could cure pneumonia, tuberculosis, osteomyelitis, meningitis or endocarditis.

ANTIBACTERIAL ANTIBIOTICS

Since the 1930s, however, the whole outlook of medicine has changed. In 1936 the *sulphonamides* were introduced — for the first time a drug was rapidly successful in treating a bacterial infection (see following, 'Domagk and the sulphonamides'). In 1940, in a further advance, Howard Florey and a team at Oxford brought *penicillin* into clinical use (this drug had been discovered, and neglected, by Alexander Fleming some 10 years earlier). In 1944 *streptomycin* was isolated from a soil mould and the hunt was on — moulds from all over the world were screened for antibacterial activity, and many more antibiotics were found.

MILESTONES
Domagk and the sulphonamides
The German bacteriologist Paul Ehrlich (1854-1915), the founder of antimicrobial chemotherapy, based his work on the theory

that drugs only acted on microbes if they were *bound* to them. For this reason Ehrlich's successors concentrated on dyes, stains and coloured compounds in their search for chemotherapeutic agents. (In reality, colourless compounds also combine with microbial molecules, but more sophisticated instruments than the naked eye are needed to detect this.)

In the early 1930s another German, Gerhard Domagk (1895-1964) showed that the dye prontosil cured two or three types of infection in animals. Clinical trials soon showed that the drug was also very effective against streptococcal infections in humans, e.g puerperal sepsis (p.178).

The interesting fact soon emerged that in the body, prontosil was split, with the release of a *sulphonamide* and that this was the active compound. This finding explained the fact, already noted by Domagk, that prontosil was inactive in the test tube. (It was extremely fortunate that Domagk had decided to test his compounds by examining their protective effects in experimental infection instead of looking at their ability to inhibit or slow the growth of streptococci *in vitro*!

This sulphonamide was soon followed by others. In 1938 sulphapyridine (May and Baker's 'M and B 693') was shown to cure pneumococcal pneumonia — this was a major advance, since it was the first drug to do so.

Sulphonamides have subsequently been largely replaced by more effective agents, but still find use today in the chemotherapy of certain infections.

Penicillin and most of the agents that were developed until 1960 were *natural* products, produced by fungi and moulds in the soil and elsewhere. But the chemists were also busy, modifying the natural product to endow it with desirable properties: such properties as insusceptibility to the resistance mechanisms that soon appeared in bacteria; ability to withstand the acid of the stomach (a characteristic that allows the drug to be taken by mouth); or slower excretion by the kidney (so that fewer doses are necessary). More recently, fully synthetic drugs such as the quinolones have become important. As a result of all this activity we now have some hundreds of antibiotics with activity against bacteria. (We use the term 'antibiotic' to refer to both natural products *and* synthetic drugs.)

Antiseptics and disinfectants are discussed in chapter 13. They act by disorganising cell membranes or by reacting with and inactivating the proteins, nucleic acids or lipids of microbial cells. These processes are not selective and human cells are also susceptible to their action. Antibiotics kill microbes, bacteria or fungi, but their action is fundamentally different from that of antiseptics and disinfectants. All antibacterial antibiotics act only on *bacterial* cells, *not* on human or other eucaryotic cells (i.e., unlike that of disinfectants, their action is specific). In using antibiotics we are exploiting the differences between bacterial cells and eucaryotic cells (Table 4.1); with antifungal and anti-parasitic agents the targets are the much slighter differences between the biochemical features of fungal and parasite cells and human cells, all eucaryotes.

MODE OF ACTION

Different types of antibiotics act at different sites within the bacterial cell (Fig. 12.1). The cell wall and the ribosome appear to be particularly vulnerable, since many antibiotics act at these sites.

Fig. 12.1 Sites of action of antibiotics on the bacterial cell.

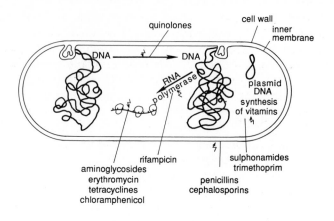

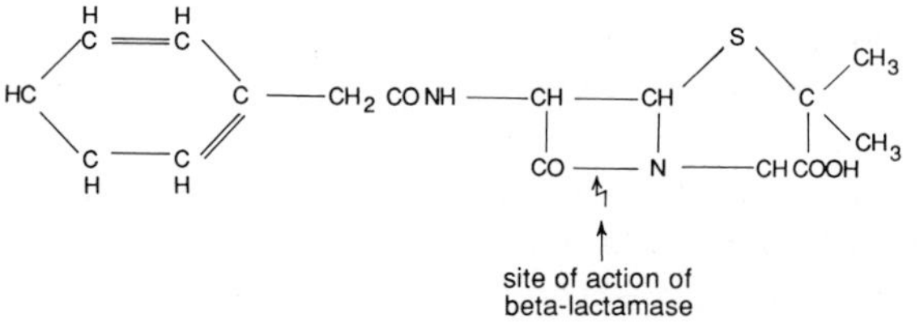

Fig. 12.2 Benzylpenicillin 'penicillin', the first beta-lactam antibiotic. The site where beta-lactamases act is indicated. This four-atom ring is present in penicillins and cephalosporins.

The synthesis of peptidoglycan (p.26) is a key process in cell division. The enzymes involved (the penicillin-binding proteins) are the targets of many antibiotics. The large group of penicillins and cephalosporins — the *beta-lactam* antibiotics, so called because they contain a chemical structure called a beta-lactam ring (Fig. 12.2) — interfere with cross-linking of the peptidoglycan and thus inhibit cell growth and eventually kill the cells. The result may be elongated cells which have not divided because of interference with the formation of a septum (Fig. 12.3) or cells which round up or bulge irregularly. As human cells have no cell wall and hence no enzymes to be targeted by the beta-lactams, they are unaffected.

Superficially, protein synthesis is the same in human and animal cells (Fig. 6.5). In both, the message encoded in the DNA is transcribed onto an RNA 'tape' which is 'played' by the ribosome, and the appropriate amino acids are linked to form a polypeptide. However, bacterial ribosomes are smaller than human ribosomes and their component molecules differ, so that an antibiotic can act on the bacterial ribosome, while leaving the human ribosomes undisturbed.

Aminoglycosides cause the wrong polypeptide to be synthesised, or even stop the synthesis entirely.

Tetracyclines prevent the binding of the transfer RNAs to the ribosome, thus preventing addition of new amino acids to the peptide chain.

Chloramphenicol, erythromycin and clindamycin also disturb protein synthesis on the ribosome in various ways.

Other sites in the bacterial cell are also vulnerable. Rifampicin interferes with the transcription of DNA to RNA. The sulphonamides and trimethoprim both attack the biosynthesis of cofactors required for the production of thymidine nucleotides. The quinolones react with DNA gyrase, an enzyme involved in the coiling and 'packaging' of DNA within the cytoplasm of the bacterial cell.

RESISTANCE TO ANTIBIOTICS

One of the consequences of use (and misuse) of antibiotics has been a steady increase in bacterial resistance. Resistant organisms are widespread, especially in hospitals. Multi-resistant *Staphylococcus aureus* and multi-resistant Gram-negative rods, including *Pseudomonas aeruginosa*, are the most prominent. The predominant organism varies from hospital to hospital and is often a relatively permanent feature of the hospital environment. In many cases it can be shown to be carried by the staff and to be transferred by them. Numerous outbreaks of infection have been due to multiply-resistant Gram-negative rods.

In the Royal North Shore hospital in Sydney gentamicin-resistant *Klebsiella* strains caused a good deal of trouble in 1976-9. Many of these were resistant to ampicillin, tetracycline, gentamicin and several other antibiotics. The resistance genes were often borne on plasmids, some of which transferred resistance to 3, 5 or even 8 antibiotics. The 'antibiotic-rich' environment of the hospital selects for such resistance factors. In the community also, resistant organisms are common, though usually they do not carry as many resistance genes as do hospital strains. In different surveys, 50% or more of healthy persons were found to have such organisms in the faeces.

The most important mechanism of resistance to beta-lactams is the production of beta-lactamases, enzymes which open the beta-lactam ring and destroy its activity. There are many different *beta-lactamases* in Gram-positive and Gram-negative bacteria, some active against penicillins, some against cephalosporins and some against both. A major preoccupation of pharmaceutical chemists is to modify the side-chains of beta-lactams, so that the drugs are no longer susceptible to these enzymes. Methicillin and flucloxacillin are beta-lactamase-resistant penicillins.

However, production of beta-lactamases is not the only mechanism of resistance to beta-lactams. Penicillin resistance in *Streptococcus pneumoniae* and methicillin resistance in *Staphylococcus*

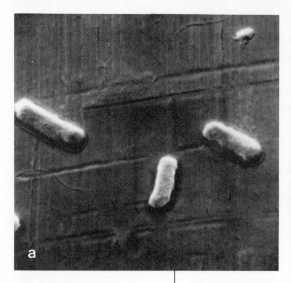
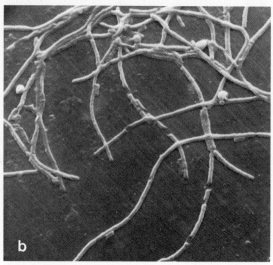

Fig. 12.3 (a) and **(b)** Effect of penicillin on bacterial cells. Note (in **(b)**) the long filaments formed under the influence of penicillin, which has prevented cell-division but not growth.

aureus are due to the production of an altered penicillin-binding protein with a much lower affinity for the drug and hence an insensitivity to it.

Resistance to penicillin is high among staphylococci: even in the community 80-90% of staphylococci are resistant. Resistance to methicillin was first noted in 1960, but in most hospitals it was not a problem until the late 1970s. Until 1975, very few staphylococci in the USA were resistant to methicillin. More recently multi-resistant *Staphylococcus aureus* strains (i.e. strains resistant to methicillin and also to aminoglycosides and other drugs) have appeared in increasing numbers. In Europe, America and Australia these strains have come to represent a major cause of nosocomial infection.

The commonest mechanism of resistance to aminoglycosides and to chloramphenicol is the production of enzymes which inactivate the drug by attaching chemical groups to it, e.g. an acetyl group (CH_3COO-) or a phosphate group. The genes for these enzymes are usually located on plasmids or transposons.

Resistance to tetracyclines is now the commonest antibiotic resistance — it is the only common resistance in streptococci. Most tetracycline resistance genes are on plasmids or transposons. Resistance is due to active transport of the drug out of the cell. Resistance to sulphonamides and trimethoprim is usually due to acquisition of a new enzyme, with which the drug does not combine so avidly, so that the enzyme retains its function. Resistance to the quinolones is due to a mutation in the DNA gyrase (the enzyme that 'packages' the DNA). It appears that there is cross-resistance among the quinolones, i.e. resistance to one is likely to mean resistance to all.

Fortunately organisms resistant to beta-lactams and aminoglycosides are usually not resistant to quinolones and resistance to the latter drugs is not (yet) found on plasmids. But it remains true that a resistance mechanism or mechanisms exist against almost every antibiotic, although some resistances (e.g. to vancomycin), are very rare.

PHARMACOKINETICS

The 'pharmacokinetics' of a drug is a description of what happens to it in the body: how it is absorbed and excreted, how long a useful concentration persists in the blood, what organs it penetrates, whether it enters the cells of the body or remains confined to the extracellular fluids, and so on. Antibiotics may be applied to a body surface (e.g. as eye-drops, or via a vaginal pessary, i.e. by *topical* application), or administered *systemically* (given either by mouth or by injection), so that the drug is present in the blood and other body fluids and is free to enter tissues.

Some drugs are destroyed in the gut or are not absorbed, so that giving them by mouth does not produce a therapeutic concentration in the body and another route of administration must be used. Injections may be given *intramuscularly* (i.e. into muscles) or *intravenously* (into a vein, usually by means of an intravenous drip, an arrangement for administering fluids into a vein on a regular basis). Intravenous administration is preferred if a drug has to be given in large doses or at frequent intervals, e.g. every two to six hours. Administration by injection, i.e. not orally, is termed *parenteral* administration.

Whatever the route of administration, the antibiotic is eliminated from the body more or less rapidly, just as any other drug is. The speed of this process can be estimated by determining the *half-life* of the drug (i.e. the time required for the concentration in the plasma to fall to half its initial value). The beta-lactams have short half-lives, less than 1.5 hours, for gentamicin the figure is 2 hours, for trimethoprim 10 hours and for doxycycline 20 hours — clearly antibiotics vary greatly in this respect. The shorter the half-life, the more often the drug must be given. Most antibiotics are excreted in the urine — in which they reach a much higher concentration than in the blood. Their usefulness in many infections is determined by their distribution within the body. Thus in the cerebrospinal fluid most antibiotics attain concentrations much lower than in the blood and they are therefore of little value in the treatment of meningitis, even though they pass through the inflamed meninges more readily than through the healthy membranes. In chronic staphylococcal osteomyelitis it appears that the organisms can survive within the phagocytes, and drugs which can enter such cells are more effective.

GROUPS OF ANTIBIOTICS

We shall now discuss the main groups of antibiotics from these and other points of view.

PENICILLINS

Penicillin, more correctly termed 'benzypenicillin', is stable in the dry state, like many antibiotics, but *un*stable in solution. It is also destroyed by the gastric acid, and must therefore be given by injection. Penicillin is also excreted fairly rapidly in the urine and must therefore be given frequently. It is inactive against most Gram-negative rods because it does not enter the cells. The related drug *ampicillin* is slightly less active against Gram-positive cocci, but several times more active against *Enterobacteriaceae* and is also acid-stable (i.e. unaffected by the gastric acid, and therefore capable of being taken by mouth). Other penicillins (e.g. ticarcillin) are active against *Pseudomonas*. Large doses of penicillins can give adequate levels in the cerebrospinal fluid.

CEPHALOSPORINS

These drugs, structurally very similar to the penicillins, have attracted a great deal of attention from the synthetic chemists, and dozens of variants have appeared on the market. The earlier cephalosporins showed good activity against both Gram-positive cocci and *Enterobacteriaceae*; the more recent ones have considerably increased activity against *Enterobacteriaceae* resistant to other agents, and some are effective against *Pseudomonas aeruginosa*, but Gram-positive activity has waned. Most cephalosporins need to be given parenterally — a few can be taken by mouth. Most do not penetrate well into the cerebrospinal fluid; some of the '3rd generation' cephalosporins (e.g. cefotaxime and ceftriaxone), are important exceptions.

AMINOGLYCOSIDES

Streptomycin, discovered in 1943, was one of the first antibiotics used. It still plays an occasional role, but has largely been replaced by such drugs as *gentamicin, tobramycin* and *amikacin*. Their main function is in the treatment of Gram-negative infections and they are given by injection. Because they are toxic to the middle ear and the kidney, the dose must be controlled with care, and estimations of the serum concentrations of aminoglycosides are often needed. Cerebrospinal fluid levels are poor.

TETRACYCLINES

These have a broad spectrum of activity — against Gram-positive and Gram-negative bacteria, rickettsias, chlamydias and mycoplasmas, and even some parasites. They can be taken orally or given by injection. They should not be given to pregnant women or children under 12, since they accumulate in (and damage) developing bones and teeth.

Information on the activity of these and other antibiotics is set out in Table 12.1. Note however that the indications of activity cannot be taken too literally. For example 'Ent+++' appears beside ampicillin and beside cefotaxime. This does not mean that the agents have equal activity, but simply that both show good activity against *Enterobacteriaceae*. If the organism is susceptible to both, ampicillin will probably be as effective clinically as cefotaxime. The advantage of the latter is its activity against the not uncommon resistant strains of *Klebsiella, Serratia, Proteus, Morganella* and *Providencia*. Similarly amikacin is no more likely to eradicate a susceptible organism than gentamicin, but resistance to the latter is much commoner.

TABLE 12.1 COMMON ANTIBIOTICS

Generic Name*	*Organisms attacked*
Penicillins	
(Benzyl) penicillin	Gp +++, Ent–, Ps–
Ampicillin ⎫	Gp+++, Ent+++, Ps–
Amoxycillin ⎭	
Methicillin ⎫	Gp+++, Ent–, Ps–
Cloxacillin ⎬	Gp+++, Ent–, Ps–
Flucloxacillin ⎭	
Ticarcillin	Gp+, Ent+++, Ps+++
Piperacillin	Gp+++, Ent+++, Ps+++
Cephalosporins, '1st Generation'[1]	
Cephalothin ⎫	
Cephalexin ⎬	Gp+++, Ent+++, Ps–
Cefazolin ⎭	
Cephalosporins, '2nd Generation'[1]	
Cefamandol ⎫	Gp+, Ent+++, Ps–
Cefoxitin ⎭	
Cephalosporins, '3rd Generation'[1]	
Cefotaxime ⎫	Gp+, Ent+++, Ps–
Ceftriaxone ⎭	
Ceftazidime	Gp+, Ent+++, Ps+++
Aminoglycosides	
Gentamicin ⎫	
Tobramycin ⎬	Gp+, Ent+++, Ps+++
Amikacin ⎭	
Tetracyclines	
Tetracycline ⎫	
Doxycycline ⎬	Gp+++, Ent+++, Ps–
Minocycline ⎭	
Quinolones	
Nalidixic acid[2]	Gp+, Ent+++, Ps–
Norfloxacin[2]	Gp+++, Ent+++, Ps–
Ciprofloxacin	Gp+++, Ent+++, Ps+

Others

Chloramphenicol	Gp+++, Ent+++, Ps−
Erythromycin	Gp+++, Ent−, Ps−
Clindamycin }	
Metronidazole	anaerobes, parasites
Sulphonamides	Gp+++, Ent+++, Ps−
Trimethoprim }	
Nitrofurantoin[2]	Gp+++, Ent+++, Ps−

[*The *generic* names of antibiotics should always be used, not the trade names, since the same antibiotic may have several trade names.
[1] organisms resistant to the '1st generation' cephalosporins will often respond to '2nd generation' agents; fewer organisms are resistant to '3rd generation' agents.
[2] useful in urinary infections only.]

ANTIFUNGAL ANTIBIOTICS

The polyene antifungals — nystatin, amphotericin B and others — are lipid-soluble and contain large ring structures with numerous double bonds. They are believed to act by disorganising the lipid membrane of the fungus. Because of its toxicity on parenteral administration, nystatin is used only topically and orally. Amphotericin B is given intravenously in the treatment of systemic fungal infections; toxic reactions are common and it must be given with caution. Flucytosine is an analogue of cytosine, one of the four bases in DNA and RNA, and apparently acts by interfering with DNA synthesis. It is often used in combination with amphotericin B. A number of imidazoles — ketoconazole, miconazole and fluconazole — are active against fungi, apparently by interfering with membrane synthesis.

ANTIVIRAL ANTIBIOTICS

Chemotherapy of *fungal* infections is made more difficult by the fact that the organisms are eucaryotic, i.e. structurally and metabolically more closely related to human cells than are bacteria. But *viruses* use the *actual* cellular machinery of the human host to replicate, so the task of designing a drug to interfere with this process is even more complex. So far there are relatively few useful antivirals. Acyclovir is an analogue of guanosine, a constituent of nucleic acids, and inhibits viral DNA synthesis. It is active only against herpes viruses (see p.231). Vidarabine is also a nucleoside analogue used in the treatment of herpes infections. The usefulness of azidothymidine in the treatment of AIDS is not yet clear; it appears to delay the progression of AIDS.

MISUSE OF ANTIBIOTICS

Antibiotics are the most effective group of drugs at present available — only tranquillisers are more prescribed. These two groups also share the distinction of being most often *misused*. Over 30 years ago it was estimated that 95% of all antibiotics given were wasted. There has been little improvement since then (see following, 'Common misuses of antibiotics'). Misuse results in the more rapid development of resistance and therefore the need for new agents. It is true that we still have some agents effective against most of the resistant organisms — these drugs, however, are invariably much more expensive than the older agents they replace. Moreover, the fact that a drug is new does not mean that it kills susceptible organisms any more rapidly or any 'deader' than an older drug to which the organism is susceptible. It remains true, for instance, that penicillin is still the drug of choice for streptococci and other Gram-positive species which are susceptible to it.

IN THE WARD

Common misuses of antibiotics

1 The patient does not have an infection.
2 The infection does not respond to antibiotics. The *common cold* is the best example — antibiotics will not cure a cold or prevent you getting a bacterial infection on top of it (this is rare anyway); yet at least 50% of people who consult a doctor because of a cold come away with a prescription for an antibiotic.

   In hospitals antibiotics given for prophylaxis during surgery are often continued for much longer than 48 hours, although there is clear evidence that this is unnecessary. In hospitals, it appears that in about half the instances either an antibiotic is used unnecessarily, or the wrong agent, dose or period of treatment is chosen.
3 The latest 'cephalomiracle' is used ($25-50/g) instead of an older equally effective drug at $1-5/g. This therapy is very expensive and encourages the development of resistance to the latest agents.
4 The patient 'prescribes for himself' an antibiotic left over from a previous illness.
5 In the Third World, antibiotics are sold without prescription — many of them drugs or combinations of drugs which the companies would not be allowed to market at home, because they are toxic or useless.

ANTIBIOTICS AND PHAGOCYTES

It is a mistake to think of antibiotic therapy simply in terms of 'the microbe and the antibiotic': the natural defences of the infected host also play a critical role. Many very effective antibiotics do not kill the target organism, but simply inhibit its growth. Destruction of the organisms depends on the phagocytic cells. The importance of the phagocytes in overcoming an infection being treated with antibiotics can easily be seen when their numbers have sunk very low — either because of disease or the treatment of disease (many anti-cancer drugs produce a shortage of white cells, as well as a shortage of cancer cells, see p.262). If the number of neutrophils in the blood is very small, it is often impossible to cure the repeated infections which assail the patient, however many potent antibiotics are given, and even if the infecting organisms appear susceptible to the antibiotics in laboratory tests.

COMBINATIONS OF ANTIBIOTICS

If two antibiotics are given, the effect may be additive: the result is much as if a larger quantity of one drug were given. Sometimes one drug interferes with the action of the other and in some cases one potentiates the effect of the other. This is termed *synergy* and is important in certain situations. In infective endocarditis the bacteria are locked up inside the vegetations and are not accessible to the phagocytes which would normally co-operate with the antibiotic in killing the bacteria. In this disease, neither a penicillin nor an aminoglycoside is effective alone. However, the combination of ampicillin and gentamicin will kill enterococci in the vegetations on heart valves and achieve cure — the combination is said to be *synergistic*. In the profoundly neutropenic patient, even bactericidal combinations may be unavailing.

IN THE WARD
Administering antibiotics
- Take a careful patient history — enquire about previous antibiotic reactions
- Record all the patient's known allergies
- Tell the patient about the possibility of a reaction
- Handle antibiotics carefully
- Don't spray the room when filling the syringe — you will contaminate the environment and sensitise yourself
- Have adrenaline and cortisone handy in case of an allergic reaction

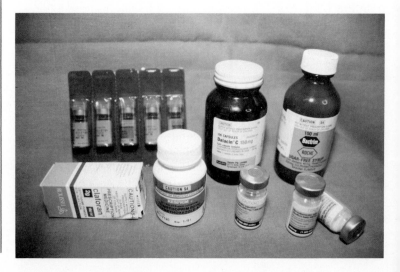

TREATMENT WITH ANTIBIOTICS

Although antibiotics are very powerful agents and relatively safe ones, it is important that they should be used properly.

CHOOSING AN ANTIBIOTIC

The doctor should consider the following aspects in choosing an antibiotic:
- identity of the infecting organism
- activity against the infecting organism
- type and site of the infection
- pharmacology of candidate agents
- patient's age, condition, allergies to antibiotics
- cost

We will now examine these in detail.

IDENTITY OF THE INFECTING ORGANISM

It is most important to know the infecting organism or at least to make a reasonable guess as to its likely identity on the basis of the clinical information and possibly preliminary results. The clinical picture may give a clear indication of the likely pathogen. Acute osteomyelitis of the femur in a 10-year-old boy is most probably due to *Staphylococcus aureus*. Acute pneumonia in a 20-year-old woman who was previously healthy and who is coughing up a fair amount of sputum is most probably due to *Streptococcus pneumoniae*. A similar but less acute clinical picture with cough but little sputum will often be due to *Mycoplasma pneumoniae*, and the likelihood that this diagnosis is correct is increased if it is known that *Mycoplasma* infection is prevalent in the community this winter. (See also following, 'Flea-bites are a bad sign'). The laboratory can often offer help on the basis of rapid tests such as the Gram stain or detection of antigens (see p.83).

IN THE WARD
Flea-bites are a bad sign

On Tuesday five-year-old Paul was quite well. On Wednesday he woke up and vomited. He felt hot and his mother noticed that there were small spots, 'like flea-bites' but in clusters, on the skin of his chest and abdomen. He 'looked strange', his eyes 'seemed to stare' and sometimes he didn't seem to hear what his mother was saying.

She called her local doctor. When he mentioned the 'flea-bites' he told her to take Paul to hospital immediately. In the Emergency room Paul was lucky. The triage nurse was very experienced, knew that he was very ill and suspected *meningococcaemia* (see p.206).

The 'flea-bites' are actually small haemorrhages into the skin and are characteristic of this infection. In a case like this there is no time to wait for the results of laboratory tests. After a rapid clinical examination an intravenous drip was started and within 30 minutes of arriving at the hospital Paul was receiving large doses of penicillin. He recovered. Blood cultures confirmed the diagnosis of meningococcaemia. This disease still kills about one affected child in ten, despite antibiotics and intensive care.

ACTIVITY AGAINST THE INFECTING ORGANISM

If the organism has been isolated, its antibiotic susceptibilities will be determined (see p.163). However this takes a minimum of 5-6 hours and usually longer. In many cases, even if only a provisional identification of the causative organism is available, it will often be possible to form an idea of the likely susceptibilities.

Gram-positive cocci in chains, i.e. streptococci, will be susceptible to most antibiotics except tetracycline, aminoglycosides and quinolones. Gram-positive cocci in clumps will be resistant to penicillin, but will be sensitive to penicillinase-resistant penicillins such as flucloxacillin or oxacillin. A small Gram-negative rod seen in cerebrospinal fluid can be assumed to be *Haemophilus influenzae* and will be best treated with ampicillin + chloramphenicol or with cefotaxime, since 15-20% are resistant to ampicillin. Gram-negative diplococci seen in the same clinical situation will be *Neisseria meningitidis* and the drug of choice is penicillin.

TYPE AND SITE OF THE INFECTION

This factor is important in the choice of antibiotic. One must take into account the distribution of the drug within the body. For example, most antibiotics do not enter the cerebrospinal fluid in appreciable quantities. To achieve adequate treatment of meningitis we can choose a drug such as chloramphenicol or cefotaxime, which crosses the blood-brain barrier fairly readily — or we can give large doses (usually by the intravenous route) of penicillin or ampicillin and maintain adequate levels in the cerebrospinal fluid by ensuring very high blood levels. Aminoglycosides and first generation cephalosporins such as cephalothin are of little use in the treatment of meningitis, since they penetrate very poorly into the cerebrospinal fluid. Infections of the lung do not respond well to aminoglycosides, since these drugs do not reach high concentrations in lung tissue.

PHARMACOLOGY OF THE CANDIDATE DRUGS

This factor will decide the route and the frequency of administration. Drugs which are poorly absorbed from the gut (aminoglycosides, vancomycin, amphotericin B) or which are destroyed by the gastric acid (benzylpenicillin) must be given parenterally. Whether the drug is given intramuscularly or intravenously depends on the size and frequency of the dose and on the seriousness of the disease. In life-threatening infections large doses can be given intravenously with a minimum of discomfort.

PATIENT'S AGE AND CONDITION

If the patient is very ill, the antibiotic will usually be given parenterally, because we can then be confident that the drug reaches the site of infection. Oral absorption tends to be more erratic and the oral route of administration is usually relied on only for less serious illnesses.

Most antibiotics are excreted in the urine; some are excreted into the gut via the bile (in some cases after modification in the liver). In renal disease and in old age the renal function is diminished, so that normal doses of many antibiotics will yield much higher serum concentrations — possibly reaching toxic levels. It may therefore be necessary to reduce the dose or to increase the interval between doses. In the newborn both renal excretion and liver inactivation of drugs are relatively less efficient than in adults, and dosages must likewise be correspondingly adjusted.

The doctor must also take into account any allergic reactions to previous antibiotic therapy and consider whether the other drugs being given to the patient can interfere with the antibiotic he proposes to give. Allergies to antibiotics (and other drugs) must be recorded when the patient is admitted to the ward.

COST

Cost should only be taken into account when drugs of equal efficacy are considered, but it should not be lost sight of. Antibiotics are usually the largest item in the hospital's pharmacy budget; a day's penicillin or gentamicin will cost at most a few dollars per patient, while for cefotaxime or ciprofloxacin costs will be multiplied 20-50 times.

SUSCEPTIBILITY TESTS

One of the most important tasks that the microbiology laboratory performs is to carry out susceptibility tests on isolates thought to be causing infection. The 'gold standard' in susceptibility testing is the determination of the *minimum inhibitory concentration* (MIC) of the antibiotic for the bacterial isolate, i.e. the lowest concentration of the antibiotic which will prevent the growth of the bacterium (see following, 'Minimum inhibitory concentrations'). MICs are established by preparing twofold dilutions of the antibiotic in growth medium and inoculating each tube with the bacterium under test. The first tube in which growth fails to occur contains the MIC. The usual laboratory methods for determining susceptibility offer more or less crude estimates of this.

IN THE LAB
Minimum inhibitory concentration (MIC)
The technique for evaluating an antibiotic's MIC is as follows.
Two rows of tubes are set up. The last tube in row A contains

128 mcg per mL of benzylpenicillin, and the last tube in row B 128 mcg per mL of methicillin.

Proceeding left, each tube contains half the concentration of the drug in the preceding tube; the volume is 1 mL. Now, 1 mL of a dilute culture of the organism to be tested is added to each tube. So the final concentrations of the drug are therefore: 0.125, 0.25, 0.5, 1, 2, 4, 8, 16, 32, and 64 mcg/mL. (See Fig. A.)

The rack of tubes is incubated overnight and 'read' the next morning. In row A, all but the last two tubes are turbid: the first tube in which growth is inhibited is tube 9; the MIC of benzylpenicillin for organism A is 32 mcg/mL. In row B, only the first 4 tubes show growth; the first tube in which growth is inhibited is tube 5 and the MIC for methicillin is 2 mcg/mL.

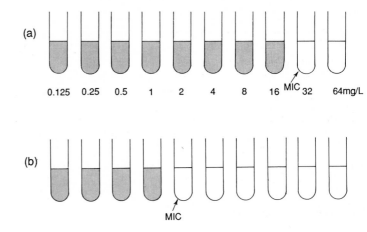

AGAR-DIFFUSION AND AGAR-DILUTION

There are several ways of doing susceptibility tests. The commonest is *agar-diffusion* (Fig. 12.4); widely used agar-diffusion methods are those referred to as Kirby-Bauer, CDS and Stokes. The basis of each of these methods is the same. The bacterium is spread over a plate of antibiotic test medium, and disks containing different antibiotics are put on the surface. The antibiotic diffuses out so that there is a concentration gradient. At some point in that gradient the concentration may be high enough to inhibit the growth of the bacterium and there will then be a zone of inhibition around the disk (Fig. 12.5). The size of the zone can be related to the sensitivity or resistance of the organism by comparison with a control or by consulting a table of zone diameters. The agar-diffusion method has the advantage of flexibility and (apparent) simplicity; to obtain reliable results, however, the tests must actually be performed with skill and care.

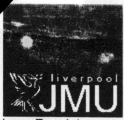

Loan Receipt
Liverpool John Moores University
Library and Student Support

Borrower Name: Al Matrood,Ahmed
Borrower ID: **********5112

Microbiology :
31111007475328
Due Date: 22/03/2011 23:59

Total Items: 1
01/03/2011 14:45

Please keep your receipt in case of
dispute.

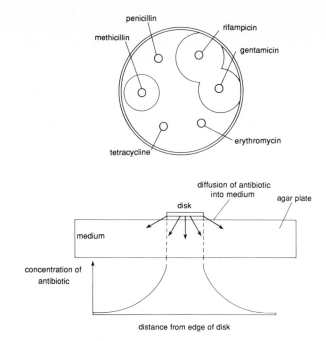

Fig. 12.4 The agar-diffusion susceptibility test. A staphylococcus was spread over the plate, antibiotic disks were applied and the plate incubated. The next day disks containing antibiotics to which the staphylococcus was sensitive were surrounded by a zone free of growth.

Fig. 12.5 Concentration gradient of antibiotic around a disk. From the disk the antibiotic diffuses out into the medium — the further from the disk, the lower is the concentration. Growth is inhibited until a point is reached where the concentration of antibiotic is less than the MIC of the organism.

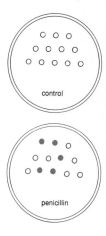

In the *agar-dilution* method antibiotics are incorporated into agar plates, on the surface of which are deposited a number of isolates to be tested (see Fig. 12.6 and Pl. 32). After incubation susceptibility or resistance is judged by the presence or absence of growth on the agar. To vary the repertoire of antibiotics tested is somewhat more difficult than with the agar-diffusion method, since a new plate has to be poured for each drug.

Susceptibility tests are increasingly being carried out by machines: trademark names include AutoBac, CobasBact, MS2, AutoMicrobic System. Most of these provide a more rapid answer (e.g. in 5 hours) but have the disadvantage that the antibiotics to be tested and/or their concentrations are pre-determined by the manufacturer and cannot easily be varied by the laboratory.

How do we decide what is susceptible, and what is resistant ? If we expose them to very high concentrations, almost *all* bacteria will be susceptible to *any* antibiotic. There are limits to the amount of antibiotic that a patient can be given, since some are toxic. So 'susceptible' means in practice 'susceptible to antibiotic levels achievable at the site of infection with clinically-possible doses'. In practice we take the serum level into account when setting the concentrations defining susceptibility and resistance, and if the infection is in a site into which the antibiotic does not penetrate well, the clinician increases the dose.

DANGERS OF ANTIBIOTIC THERAPY

To give any drug entails some risk. While antibiotics are among the safest drugs, they may produce adverse effects at times.

Fig. 12.6 The agar-dilution susceptibility test. The control plate contains no antibiotic; the 'penicillin' plate consists of the same medium plus a standard concentration of penicillin. Comparing the two, we can see that 7 of the 12 bacterial strains were sensitive to penicillin.

- Some are inherently toxic; e.g. the aminoglycosides may cause vertigo, deafness and damage to the kidney, chloramphenicol may depress production of blood cells by the bone marrow.
- Others induce *hypersensitivity reactions*; this is not uncommon with the penicillins and a hypersensitive person may undergo an anaphylactic reaction when injected with the drug.
- Any antibiotic may modify the *normal flora* or lead to colonisation by a resistant organism: Gram-negative rods, *Clostridium difficile*, yeasts.
- Antibiotic treatment of a susceptible organism may result in a second infection by a *resistant* organism, either because the original isolate has responded to the presence of antibiotic by acquiring resistance, or because the treatment has killed off susceptible organism and a resistant organism (from the patient's own flora or the environment) has replaced it.

Some of these undesirable effects can be minimised by using the drugs sensibly. (See following, 'Some golden rules for antibiotic therapy', and 'Rate of microbial killing'.)

IN THE WARD
Some golden rules for antibiotic therapy
- *Don't* give an antibiotic without good evidence of an infection *treatable with the antibiotic.*
- *Don't* forget to stop the antibiotic after five days if the patient is better.
- *Don't* give large doses of powerful antibiotics or combinations of antibiotics unless the patient is very ill. Such therapy is most likely to eliminate the normal flora and lead to further infection.
- *Don't* give inadequate doses of antibiotics. Small doses are more likely to encourage the development of resistant organisms.
- When giving an antibiotic to prevent infection in surgery, *don't* continue therapy for more than 24 hours after the operation — There is no additional benefit.

IN THE LAB
Rate of microbial killing
When microbes are exposed to a lethal influence, whether physical or chemical, a constant proportion is killed in unit time (see table and graph).

Thus if 1 000 000 bacteria are present at time 0, after 1 minute 90% are dead, leaving 100 000.

In the next minute, 90% of these are killed, leaving 10 000 — and so on.

This is what happens under ideal, i.e. theoretical, conditions. In real life, however, various factors may interfere to influence the rate of kill — such as the presence of organic matter, or the protection of the bacteria in clumps or in glycocalyx.

Duration of exposure (min)	No surviving after x min	% killed each min	Cumulative % killed
0	1 000 000	0	0
1	100 000	90	90
2	10 000	90	99
3	1 000	90	99.9
4	100	90	99.99
5	10	90	99.999

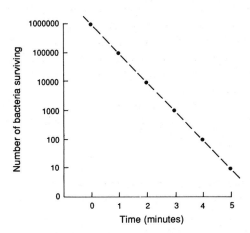

CHAPTER REVIEW

1 (a) List the various groups of antibiotics
   (b) Indicate the site of action of each.
2 (a) What are beta-lactam antibiotics?
   (b) What effect do they have on bacteria?
   (c) What may the bacteria do to overcome this?
3 A consequence of use (and misuse) of antibiotics is resistance. Explain the various mechanisms of resistance.
4 (a) What is meant by the pharmacokinetic properties of an antibiotic?
   (b) Why is a knowledge of these properties important?
5 List the groups of bacteria and the corresponding antibiotic of choice.
6 List some of the drugs used for treating:
   (a) fungal infections
   (b) viral infections
7 (a) What factors should be considered when choosing an antibiotic?
   (b) What are the dangers associated with antibiotic therapy?
8 (a) What are the ways of performing antibiotic susceptibility tests?
   (b) How does one carry out antibiotic susceptibility tests using antibiotic disks?
9 How are antibiotics commonly misused?

13

INFECTION CONTROL IN THE COMMUNITY AND THE HOSPITAL

The main objective of studying infectious disease is to control it, to protect humans from its consequences. We have studied the immune defence system and have seen that vaccination may be used to prevent infection. Antibiotics now play an important role in the treatment of infection. There are other aspects of prevention that we need to look at, equally important in the day-to-day work of the hospital and the community health services. When carrying out medical treatment we must be certain that we do not harm the patient by introducing microbes, hence the importance of *sterilisation* methods. And most fundamental of all, we must find out how infection is transmitted in the hospital and the community, by availing ourselves of the techniques of *epidemiology*. First let us look at methods of sterilisation (and, to a lesser extent, disinfection).

STERILISATION (AND DISINFECTION)

Media for growing microbes of all types must be sterile or as close to it as possible (chapter 5). Furthermore, as we saw in chapter 7, microbes are everywhere in the environment and on all our body surfaces. If a surgeon removes a cancer, he must cut through bacteria-laden skin to reach the organ requiring treatment; if a nurse inserts a needle through the skin in order to give a patient a drug, the needle may introduce bacteria into the patient's tissues. We therefore need a means of preventing the introduction of microbes into the patients while we carry out procedures that hopefully will benefit them.

   Microbicidal agents. Microbes may be killed by:
- physical agents — heat, radiation

- chemical agents — liquids, gases

Sterilisation is the process of removing or destroying *all* living organisms in a substance or on an instrument or other object, including *bacterial spores* (we have seen (p.29) that bacterial spores are capable of resisting many adverse conditions).

Disinfection, on the other hand, means the destruction or removal of microbes likely to cause infection — it is usually a less drastic process and bacterial spores in general escape.

In some circumstances, however, even *sterility* is not enough. *Dead* bacteria in a fluid intended for injection may still cause unpleasant febrile reactions; these *pyrogens* must be removed from intravenous fluids and the water used to dissolve drugs.

APPLICABILITY OF EACH

When is sterilisation necessary, and when can we make do with disinfection?

STERILISATION

Sterilisation is required as follows.
- Fluids for injection, hypodermic needles, surgical instruments and other articles that are to be inserted through the skin or mucous membranes into the tissues *must be* sterile.
- Instruments which are to be inserted into the body via the *respiratory tract* or the *urinary tract* must also be sterile, since these tracts are lined by membranes which are readily injured, so that it becomes easy for microbes to enter the body.
- Laboratory equipment for *growing microbes* (culture media, Petri dishes, test-tubes and such) must be sterile — otherwise the laboratory results cannot be interpreted.
- Laboratory cultures and other materials (blood, laboratory specimens) likely to contain microbes must be sterilised *before discarding*, to prevent possible dissemination of infection.

DISINFECTION

Disinfection is in general a milder process than sterilisation and is used when the material to be treated is too delicate to withstand a sterilisation procedure. Only chemical disinfectants can be used to prepare the skin for an injection or an operation; these reduce the numbers of bacteria present to low levels, but never destroy them all. Disinfection is appropriate for *thermometers, bedpans* or *urinals* used in the wards.

STERILISING AGENTS
PHYSICAL AGENTS
HEAT — DRY AND MOIST

Heat is the commonest sterilising agent.

Dry heat (i.e. heat in an atmosphere free of water vapour) is an effective sterilant. The usual equipment is the hot air oven. The temperature required is 160^0C for one hour or 170^0C for 40 minutes. Remember that the interior of the package to be sterilised will need time to reach this temperature and that sterilisation will not begin until this occurs. It takes 15 minutes for heat to penetrate a package containing a small instrument, and for large parcels the heating time may be several hours.

Moist heat is more effective than dry heat; 'moist' defines an atmosphere saturated with water vapour. All vegetative bacterial cells are killed by exposure to water at 80^0C for 10 minutes and many are killed by a good deal less (e.g. *Salmonella typhi* cannot usually resist 60^0C for 30 seconds). The main effect of heat is to denature the proteins of the cell, i.e. to cause the peptide chain to unfold (p.22).

The spores of organisms such as *Bacillus* are common in the environment and in any materials that have not been specifically treated to remove them. While most bacteria do not produce spores, some of those that do are very dangerous (e.g. *Clostridium tetani*) and even non-pathogens may produce toxic effects if they multiply without restriction in substances that are injected. Even when exposed to boiling water (100^0C at sea level) spores may take almost a day to die, so it is necessary to use higher temperatures to kill them. This is done in an *autoclave* (steam steriliser, Fig. 13.1) which uses steam under pressure. A higher temperature is necessary to vaporise water under pressure and the temperature then achieved is considerably raised. At one atmosphere, i.e. the atmospheric pressure at sea level, water boils (vaporises) at 100^0C. At a pressure of two atmospheres water vaporises at 121^0C. At this temperature spores are killed in 15 minutes, while at 115^0C 30 minutes are required; these are the operating temperatures commonly used.

Fig. 13.1 An autoclave (steam steriliser) is a strong steel vessel capable of withstanding considerable pressure. Steam is admitted while the outlet valve is open, to drive out the air. Then the outlet valve is closed and pressure raised to the desired level and maintained for the necessary period. If the load needs to be dried (e.g.for dressings or drapes) the steam is exhausted from the chamber, which is then heated by steam in the jacket.

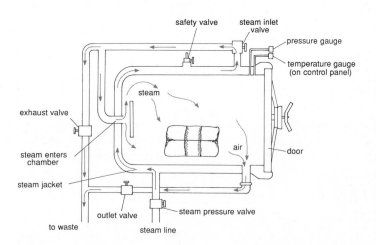

Again, remember the *time* required for penetration of heat: moist heat penetrates better than dry heat, but for a large parcel or a quantity of liquid greater than say one litre, sterilising times should be increased. Hot air ovens and steam sterilisers should be fitted with automatic timers and their operation carefully monitored by automatic recorders; it is also advisable to include a coloured chemical indicator on each item. Paper strips containing bacterial spores can also be used to check the function of these machines.

Boiling: some bacteriological media will not stand this amount of heat, and are simply *boiled*. In deoxycholate citrate agar, which is prepared in this way, one is also relying on the inhibitors in the medium to prevent the growth of organisms that have not been killed.

FILTRATION

Microbes can be removed from liquids or gases by *filtration*. Modern filters are membranes made from cellulose or its derivatives and include millions of pores, of specified diameters (Fig. 13.2). To remove *all* bacteria from a liquid it must be passed through pores 0.22 micron in diameter. This treatment will not of course remove most viruses and mycoplasmas, but they are much less likely to contaminate liquids, since they do not survive in the environment for long periods. Filtration is used for the removal of small particles from intravenous fluids, and for the sterilisation of heat-sensitive solutions: vitamins and growth factors for microbes, serum and some special media constituents, many drugs, e.g. antibiotics. *Blood* for transfusion or for microbiological media must be collected in a sterile state and be kept sterile, since there is no way of sterilising it.

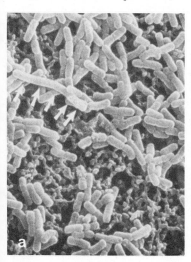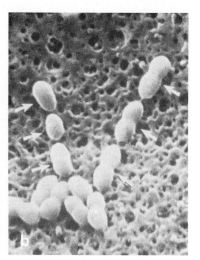

Fig. 13.2 (a) *Leuconostos oenos* and **(b)** *Lactobacillus hilgardii* on membrane filters (electronmicrographs). The pores would clearly not permit such bacteria to pass through, and the filtrate would be sterile.

RADIATION

Gamma rays are produced by the disintegration of certain radioactive substances, and *beta rays* by special equipment. Both types of radiation penetrate well and articles can therefore be wrapped and packed before sterilisation. Radiation targets chiefly the DNA, producing breaks in the DNA strand and changes in some of its constituent molecules. Bacteria and viruses are much more resistant to radiation than higher animals; the sterilising dose of gamma radiation for bacteria is about 1000 times greater than the dose that will kill a human, and the process takes days in the usual installations. Radiation sterilisation has the advantage that most heat-sensitive materials (such as plastics) remain undamaged. However the installations are very large and expensive, so that materials to be sterilised must be sent out of the hospital.

Ultraviolet light is also capable of killing microbes. The rays can only penetrate a thin film of liquid, and are blocked by glass. Although in practice ultraviolet is little used, exposure to sunlight will kill microbes.

CHEMICAL AGENTS

Most microbes will not survive extremes of pH below 4.5 and above 9, nor will they survive high concentrations of salts — hence the use of vinegar or salt for preserving food (pickles, salted herrings). In addition, however, there is a very large number of chemicals which are toxic to microbes. These *chemical disinfectants* can be discussed in groups. (Remember also that the fatty acids in soaps are bactericidal — the effect of hand-washing is not just to remove bacteria mechanically.)

GASES

The gas *ethylene oxide* offers an effective sterilant for materials that cannot withstand exposure to either dry or moist heat at the required temperature. The process requires the presence of water vapour and is somewhat slower than heat sterilisation, taking several hours. Sterilisation must be followed by hours or days of aeration to remove the gas, which is absorbed by porous materials such as rubber or some types of plastic. The sterilisation process must be monitored by spore strips.

ALCOHOLS

Ethanol (the alcohol present in alcoholic drinks) is germicidal when mixed with water; a final concentration of 50-70% ethanol is most effective. Isopropyl alcohol, a 70% solution in water, is a better germicide than ethanol and is much used for skin disinfection (individually wrapped swabs moistened with 70% isopropyl alcohol are available commercially).

PHENOLS

Countless variations on the theme of phenol have been synthesised by the organic chemist. Some of these substances are toxic to humans and may cause chemical burns if strong solutions come in contact with the skin. Many are used for disinfection of surfaces and objects when organic material is also present, since their activity is relatively little affected thereby. They kill Gram-positive and Gram-negative bacteria, and may kill acid-fast bacilli; many viruses, however, are resistant.

Chlorhexidine is very active against Gram-positive organisms and moderately so against Gram-negative organisms. It is dissolved in water or alcohol. Solutions of 0.02 - 0.05% in water are sometimes used for urinary catheterisation and bladder irrigation. Such solutions should be prepared sterile, as certain Gram-negative bacteria can grow in them. Chlorhexidine is used as a sterilant for skin and mucous membranes. A chlorhexidine skin cleanser is used in bathing before surgery.

Hexachlorophene is active against Gram-positive, but not against Gram-negative species. Its main use is in skin disinfection. It must be used regularly for several days to be effective and a single wash is no better than plain soap and water.

ALDEHYDES

Formaldehyde and *glutaraldehyde* are effective against most microbes and even kill spores slowly. Most viruses are susceptible. The vapours are extremely irritant to eye and respiratory tract. Their main use is in sterilising instruments when it is necessary to be confident that all microbes have been attacked and when, for various reasons, heat or chlorine compounds are unsuitable.

HALOGENS

Chlorine compounds. Chlorine gas and various other chlorine compounds are microbicides, active even against spores, amoebic cysts and fungi. All act by forming hypochlorous acid, HOCl. Compounds in this group are sodium hypochlorite and other hypochlorites, and chlorinated isocyanurates. All are active in the form of aqueous solutions and *deteriorate on standing*. These disinfectants corrode many metals — including stainless steel — and give off chlorine gas, which is an irritant. However they have the advantage that the solution remaining after they have acted is not toxic (e.g. $NaOCl \rightarrow NaCl$). Chlorine gas is widely used in the sterilisation of water supplies.

Iodine and *Iodine-containing compounds.* Iodine is insoluble in water. In solution in ethanol or potassium iodide, however, it is a good skin disinfectant, although sometimes people become sensitised (allergic) to it. Iodophors consist of iodine mixed with a detergent which takes up the iodine and releases it slowly. These preparations have largely replaced solutions of iodine, since hypersensitivity reactions are much fewer and stains on skin and garments can be removed by washing. Povidone-iodine is one such preparation. Iodophors are recommended for skin sterilisation: before surgery; when drawing blood and body fluids; or when inserting intravascular catheters and similar procedures.

Hydrogen peroxide is not very suitable as a disinfectant for hospital use, as it is decomposed by the enzyme catalase present in blood and tissues. *Quaternary Ammonium Compounds* (or QACs) are active against Gram-positive organisms and to a lesser extent against Gram-negatives. They do not affect acid-fast bacilli or spores. They are widely used for sterilising surfaces after cleaning.

In the wards the doctor or nurse is not often called upon to make decisions about methods of sterilisation; most of the sterile equipment (needles and syringes, intravenous lines, wound dressing trays and such) is provided prepackaged and appropriately treated by the hospital's central sterilising unit or by commercial suppliers.

However, it is often necessary to disinfect the skin before giving an injection or carrying out some procedure such as lumbar puncture or insertion of an intravenous cannula. And we should all be aware of the practical problems of sterilising certain types of equipment. (For example, the *endoscope* — a narrow, flexible 'telescope' which is inserted to examine internal organs such as the gut or the lung; sterilising it after use requires careful cleaning first of all, then the disinfectant must be drawn through it so that the internal surfaces are all in contact with the agent, and left there for an adequate time.) Sterilisation is such a vital component of medical practice that all doctors and nurses should understand its principles and the limitations of the various methods.

TRACING INFECTION: EPIDEMIOLOGY

It is clearly impossible to prevent the spread of infectious diseases if one does not know how this takes place. *Epidemiology* is the study of the distribution of disease in human populations: how, where, when and in whom it occurs. When an epidemiologist studies a disease, he wants to know at what age(s) the disease occurs, are males and females equally affected, are caucasians, blacks and mongolians equally affected, is it commoner in the poor, in certain occupations or countries, at certain seasons, is it transmissible to others. He is also interested in the biological characteristics of individuals who acquire the disease and in comparing them with unaffected individuals: concentrations of ions, enzymes, antibodies in the plasma, numbers of cells in the blood. Diet, smoking, drink and drugs are also relevant.

The information that the epidemiologist gathers can be combined with data from genetics, biochemistry, microbiology, physiology, and other sources to explain the cause of a disease, to develop strategies for the prevention of disease and to decide what health services are necessary and how they should be organised. In many ways epidemiology is the core science of medicine.

Epidemiologists use many types of data. They may analyse the information on death certificates to find the death-rate from tuberculosis, cancer of the lung or accidental drowning. They may investigate a particular outbreak of disease or they may survey a population to elucidate the occurrence of a disease. The transmission of an infection may be clarified by experiments. We shall look at a few examples of the epidemiologist's work.

COMMUNITY INVESTIGATIONS

In 1846 a Danish physician PL Panum investigated an outbreak of measles in the Faroe Islands off the coast of Denmark. This was the first outbreak since 1781; 6000 of the islanders came down with measles and 170 died. By recording the date of exposure to infection, the time required for the rash to develop *(incubation period)* and by noting when the infection was transferred to others, Panum was able to show the following.

- The disease was transmitted only by direct contact of an infected and a susceptible individual — it did not arise spontaneously. This was an important finding: remember that this study took place well before the acceptance of the germ theory of infection.
- Infection could be transmitted only about the time the rash broke out.
- Immunity to measles was lifelong; no one who had had measles in 1781 came down with it in 1846.

Thus, simply by observing who caught the disease, when and how, Panum was able to amass important basic information about measles. John Snow's studies of cholera in the city of London (see following, John Snow's 'natural experiment') afford us another striking example of the value of such apparently simple investigations.

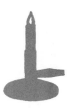

MILESTONES
John Snow's 'natural experiment'
In the 1840s, Londoners drew their home water supplies from the pipes of various private companies.

The Southwark and Vauxhall Company and the Lambeth Company supplied much the same areas in South London. Their water mains often ran in the same streets, so that different houses in one street received their supply from different companies. Both companies took their water from the river Thames, at points where sewage pollution was high.

At this period, epidemics of cholera occurred quite often. In 1849, John Snow noted that deaths from cholera were common in the areas served by these two above water companies. He then noted that by 1854, when another epidemic occurred, the Lambeth Company had moved its intake point upstream to a less polluted part of the river. During this epidemic, Snow ascertained the source of water in houses where persons had died of cholera, and calculated the cholera death rates for houses supplied by each company. The results are as follows.

DEATHS FROM CHOLERA AND SOURCE OF WATER
(LONDON, 1854)

Water supply	No. of houses supplied	Deaths from cholera per 10 000 houses
Southwark/V	40 046	315
Lambeth	26 107	38
Rest of London	256 423	55

The conclusion for Snow was quite clear-cut: if you drank Southwark/Vauxhall water you were over eight times more likely to die of cholera than if you took your supply from the Lambeth Company.

This 'natural experiment' was *controlled:* the fact that the two companies often supplied different houses in the same street ruled out several other possible causes of this difference in mortality rates.

Snow consequently concluded that the disease cholera was spread by some agent present in the drinking water — a considerable achievement, since the *germ theory* of infectious disease was not yet accepted, and the cholera vibrio would not be described by Robert Koch until 1883.

Collecting the epidemiological data is often a huge task. For instance in Framingham, Massachusetts, USA, coronary heart disease has been studied in several thousand people since 1949. The risk-factors evaluated include diet, blood pressure, smoking, exercise, blood level of cholesterol. The subjects have been assessed every two years. All cases of coronary heart disease, stroke etc are being recorded and the analysis will clarify our understanding of the factors contributing to cardiovascular disease.

The case-histories '*Salmonella* for dinner' (chapter 14, p.209), 'Old soldiers meet in Philadelphia' (chapter 14, p.214) and 'A tick in time plagues Lyme: a surprise for the rheumatologists' (p.193) are examples of epidemiological investigations — as are Semmelweis' studies in the Vienna General Hospital (p.178). The important feature of many epidemiological investigations is that they reveal entirely new relationships between diseases and their causes. When Norman Gregg, a Sydney ophthalmologist, noted in 1941 that he was encountering among his child patients an unusual number of congenital cataracts, and asked himself whether this could be due to a recent epidemic of rubella, he made a correlation which revealed a hitherto unsuspected mechanism for the causation of congenital defects. And again, when the taking of thalidomide during pregnancy was shown to cause malformations of the limbs, this observation focused attention on an effect which no drug had previously been shown to bring about.

One epidemiological activity that goes on all the time is the recording of cases of infectious disease by public health authorities. In NSW microbiology laboratories and doctors report all cases of major infections, such as diphtheria, typhoid, *Salmonella* enteritis, Legionnaires' disease, meningitis and about 50 other infections: '*notifiable diseases*'. This information is vital for several reasons. If for example a particular batch of a food is contaminated with *Salmonella*, the occurrence of a cluster of cases of salmonellosis will alert the public health authorities, who can often detect the offending food and bring about its withdrawal from the market, thus minimising the number of persons infected (see following, 'Chocolate bars convicted!'). An unusual number of cases of diphtheria would point to the need for intensifying campaigns to encourage parents to have their children vaccinated; an outbreak of Legionnaires' disease may reveal the need to purify a hospital water supply or decontaminate an air-conditioning system.

IN THE COMMUNITY
Chocolate bars convicted!

In the United Kingdom, several hundred laboratories report on 'notifiable diseases' — and the Communicable Disease Surveillance Centre analyses the data weekly.

In mid-1982 an outbreak of infection due to *Salmonella napoli* occurred in the Midlands and southern England. Investigation showed that imported chocolate bars were responsible.

245 cases were reported, 51 people were admitted to hospital, and of these 20 were severely ill. There is evidence that only a small proportion (3% or less) of cases of salmonellosis are reported — so the actual number of cases in this outbreak was probably about 7000.

Because the infection was discovered fairly promptly, it was possible to recall and destroy four-fifths of the chocolate bars. It is therefore reasonable to suppose that detecting the outbreak at this point prevented close to *30 000 infections*. Epidemiological and laboratory investigations, health-care and social costs (loss of work, pain and suffering, etc) necessitated by the outbreak were estimated at £500 000; prompt discovery of the outbreak and institution of measures to terminate it were estimated to have saved at least a further £1 670 000.

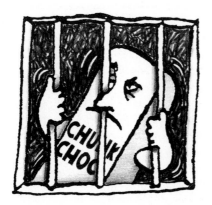

Against this, laboratory investigations and monitoring activities cost only £72 000 — so it will be seen that the epidemiological surveillance paid for itself many times over in prevented infections and other losses to society.

HOSPITAL INVESTIGATIONS

The studies we have just described are examples of community epidemiology. In recent years *hospital epidemiology*, the study of hospital-acquired infections, has become prominent. Infection in hospitals is not new. Until quite recently hospitals admitted patients indiscriminately to their wards, so that the cholera or smallpox victim had a good chance to hand his affliction on. Infection of surgical wounds was almost inevitable and most victims of surgery died from their infections. In the middle of the nineteenth century the mortality rate after amputation of a limb was four times higher in those who were operated on in hospital than at home.

Until the latter half of the nineteenth century, many mothers died soon after delivery of the baby, because of puerperal fever, 'childbed fever'. In the 1840s Oliver Wendell Holmes suggested that the doctors themselves were spreading 'childbed fever' to their patients by means of infected materials they had picked up while performing autopsies or visiting other infected patients (a point of view which, understandably, was not popular with the medical establishment). In Vienna, Ignaz Semmelweis demonstrated the effectiveness of hand washing in this regard. He had come to the same conclusion about the cause of puerperal fever as Holmes, and introduced the practice of washing hands in a crude antiseptic, calcium chloride. The result was a precipitate fall in the maternal mortality rate, as Table 13.1 shows. Unfortunately the head of the clinic did not agree with Semmelweis's ideas on the cause of 'childbed fever' and Semmelweis was not re-appointed — but within a very few years the English surgeon Joseph Lister was successfully putting forward similar ideas on antisepsis in surgery and was using an antiseptic to reduce infection during operations.

TABLE 13.1 MATERNITY MORTALITY IN THE FIRST OBSTETRIC CLINIC — VIENNA GENERAL HOSPITAL (1847-48)

May 1847	12.2%
June	2.4%
July	1.2%
March-April 1848	0

Hospital epidemiology is a relatively new branch of medicine, which developed in response to the worldwide outbreaks of virulent staphylococcal infections in the 1950s. The 1960s saw the appointment of 'infection control sisters' in British and American hospitals and elsewhere, the development of tracing methods in infection control and the elaboration of formal *infection-control procedures* (i.e. detailed instructions for preventing or minimising the spread of infection in the hospital).

NOSOCOMIAL (I.E. HOSPITAL) INFECTION

Despite the major advances in the therapy of infectious diseases, infection in hospitals remains a considerable problem. In the USA it is estimated that approximately 5% of all patients contract an infection in hospital. If doctors say there are no nosocomial infections in their beds, it is almost certain that they are not looking hard enough. A nosocomial infection is a serious matter. The risk of an infected patient dying during an episode of hospitalisation is about double that of a non-infected patient — 6% versus 3%.

The social and economic consequences of hospital infection are also considerable. In one study a disseminated infection (bacteraemia) was found to lengthen hospital stay by seven days; most other infections kept the patient in for an extra four days. Given the current costs of hospital beds, the economics of hospital infections are obviously not trivial. It was estimated in 1980 that in the USA hospital-acquired infections represented an economic burden of 3-10 billion dollars per annum.

Hospital infection is multifactorial in several senses: not only may the same organism be spread in hospital by several different routes (as is clearly the case with staphylococcal infection), but a variety of organisms, each with a different source and mode of spread, may cause infection in a hospital at the same time. There is thus not one single large problem of hospital infection but a *number* of special problems. The infections that occur in hospitalised patients are many and various, but we must distinguish an important group due to organisms that are associated with the hospital — in particular multi-resistant *Staphylococcus aureus*, *Pseudomonas aeruginosa*, and multi-resistant *Klebsiella* and *Enterobacter* species. These have the ability to survive in this environment, of which the most significant feature in this context is the presence of antibiotics and disinfectants in large quantities. Infection with these organisms is by no means confined to the compromised patient.

Nosocomial infections may occur as outbreaks or epidemics or endemically, without obvious clustering in time. A *nosocomial infection* is one arising some days after admission to hospital (the exact interval varies in different studies). Nosocomial infections are produced by microbes brought into hospital by the patient or acquired during hospitalisation and of course may involve not only patients, but staff, visitors, salesmen and the like. The infection may become apparent only after leaving hospital; approximately 25% of operation wounds begin to show symptoms only after the patient has been discharged. Likewise, most breast abscesses in parturient mothers and most infections due to hepatitis B or C or cytomegalovirus in people who have been transfused do not declare themselves until after the patient's discharge. These days the trend is to shorten hospital stay more and more, so we must expect an increasing proportion of hospital infections to be detected only after discharge. And occasionally a patient may bring an infection acquired in the community into hospital and spread it.

Infection may be *endogenous*, i.e. from the patient's own normal flora, or *exogenous*, from an organism that he acquires from another source; in practice, the distinction between *endogenous* and *exogenous* infection may be difficult to make. Table 13.2 summarises the causes of hospital infection in the USA in the late 1970s. Note that half the infections were caused by Gram-negative rods. Forty years ago this table would have looked rather different. Staphylococci then accounted for more than 60% of hospital infections and Gram-negative rods for a much smaller proportion. In the 1980s the major pathogens are little changed from previous decades (Table 13.3).

TABLE 13.2 CAUSES OF EPIDEMIC AND ENDEMIC HOSPITAL INFECTIONS

	% Endemic infections	% Epidemic infections
E. coli	19	3
Enterococci	10	<1
S. aureus	10	12
Pseudomonas	9	4
Proteus	8	<1
Klebsiella	8	3
Enterobacter	4	7
Group A streptococci	2	3
Serratia	2	8
Salmonella	—	11
Hepatitis B	—	8

[From WE Stamm, RA Weinstein and RE Dixon, Comparison of Endemic and Epidemic Nosocomial Infections, in *Nosocomial Infections, RE Dixon* (ed), Yorke Medical, 1981]

TABLE 13.3 MAJOR NOSOCOMIAL PATHOGENS OF THE 1980s

- Multi-resistant *Staphylococcus aureus* 'MRSA'
- Multi-resistant *Staphylococcus epidermidis*
- *Enterococcus faecalis*
- *Pseudomonas aeruginosa*
- *Candida albicans,* other fungi
- Cytomegalovirus

1 Preventable and non-preventable infections

A doctor who examines two patients without washing his hands in between may transfer organisms from one to another and may thus cause an infection which might have been prevented by hand-washing. On the other hand, no current precautions may be able to prevent an infection of an immunosuppressed patient by some member of his own microbial flora (see 'The compromised patient', p.262). From 15 to 40% (estimates vary) of all nosocomial infections are preventable.

2 Sources

Outside of the patient the main sources of infection are the staff and the environment. Infections spread from patient to patient:

- on the hands of the staff
- by the inanimate environment (on equipment, instruments and other fomites)
- in contaminated solutions

Hands The hands are an important means of transmission of infection. The resident flora of the hands consists of diphtheroids and staphylococci (p.73). However, hands are constantly being contaminated by organisms acquired from the patients or the environment. Certain sites on the hands, such as the nail beds, offer special conditions for the growth of microbes and sometimes infection here is difficult to dislodge. And lastly the flora of the hand is constantly being modified by washing, antiseptic soaps and so on.

The numbers of bacteria on the hands are directly related to the frequency of washing. The Association for Practitioners in Infection Control recommends that hands be washed:

- before invasive procedures
- before and after contact with wounds
- before contact with particularly susceptible patients
- after contact with a source likely to be contaminated
- between contact with different patients

Several investigators have assessed the fidelity with which such recommendations are followed. The results are discouraging. In 15 different units in two hospitals, Fox and colleagues observed 90 nurses (unbeknownst to them) for one hour each: nurses failed to wash their hands after contaminating them on 93% of occasions. This is an extreme result. In several other studies, staff failed to wash their hands on 48 to 84% of occasions when it was needed. And all studies agree that *medical staff wash their hands significantly less often than do other health-care staff.*

The duration of handwashing was observed to vary between *one* and *108* seconds, the average being nine seconds in one study and 20 seconds in the other. It is likely that hands can be adequately washed in 10-15 seconds. There is a bewildering choice of handwashing agents and many studies have been carried out on the efficacy of skin antiseptics in reducing the number of bacteria on the hands. For routine handwashing in wards, plain soaps are adequate. Choosing an antiseptic agent that will reduce the bacterial count on the hands by 99% instead of 90% is less important than persuading all staff to wash their hands when they should. The best way to do this is to set a good example.

Inanimate environment (equipment etc). A major source of infection is the inanimate environment, the equipment etc. that is used on or in the patient or surrounds him. Syringes and needles are no longer a major source of hospital infection because of imperfect sterilisation, although they represent a hazard to the staff, who may stick

Fig. 13.3 The 'Centre for Infection Control' in every hospital.

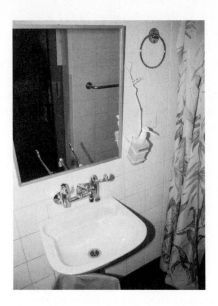

themselves with a blood-contaminated needle and thus acquire hepatitis B or AIDS. The lines that are inserted into blood vessels in order to administer drugs or food and which may remain there for weeks eventually acquire a film of bacteria both inside and outside and this may lead to bacteraemia (or to *apparent* bacteraemia, because the blood cultured was drawn through the contaminated line). Anaesthetic equipment and respiratory support devices have been potent sources of respiratory tract infections. In one study patients on a respirator were found to have a 21-fold greater risk of pneumonia and a 16-fold greater risk of bacteraemia. Such equipment often contains humidifiers or nebulisers, since the gases used, unlike the atmosphere, are essentially free of water. The water-containing reservoirs of these devices are readily contaminated by using unsterile water or by the condensate in the delivery tube running back to the reservoir. Such equipment is difficult to clean and sterilise properly.

All sorts of other equipment have been responsible for infections: cystoscopes, rectal thermometers and barium enema equipment, bed pans, feeding bottle nipples, suction equipment, renal dialysers, endoscopes, artificial heart valves, surgical instruments, padding under casts and so on. The disinfection and sterilisation of this equipment is complicated and may involve, for example, dry heat or steam, ethylene oxide or formalin vapour, formalin-alcohol solution, glutaraldehyde solution, iodophor germicides, hypochlorite, ethanol, phenolic disinfectants — and many other means. It is essential to remember that the best disinfectant or sterilising process will not work if it is not in contact with the material to be sterilised; a small air bubble can quite easily prevent access of the liquid to the interior of an endoscope or other tube.

Contaminated solutions. Some of the most striking incidents of hospital infection have involved contaminated *intravenous products*. In 1970-71 in America about 400 cases of septicaemia due to *Enterobacter* species were documented in the 25 hospitals studied and probably several thousand more occurred throughout the USA. About 13% of these cases of septicaemia were fatal. Bacteria gained entry to the fluids from a new type of stopper and the epidemic ceased when bottles of this type were withdrawn. An episode such as this is very dramatic, but probably far more incidents of bacterial transmission occur sporadically via such means as contaminated eye drops, diagnostic dyes, medicines, and bronchodilators. We do not hear of most of these episodes because no one thinks to culture the material.

There are numerous other possible sources for organisms such as *Klebsiella, Pseudomonas, Enterobacter,* and *Serratia* that are incriminated in these episodes. Most remain without sequel because the body's defences are adept at disposing of small numbers of intruding microorganisms. (Remember that the fundamental premise of medical practice is that human beings are very hard to kill.) Measures to control such infections include the proper design of the hospital in the first place, proper monitoring of sterilisation procedures, good housekeeping, good food-handling practices and the like. There are pitfalls all along the way.

3 Types of infection

What types of infections occur in hospitals? Table 13.4 lists the important ones.

TABLE 13.4 TYPES OF HOSPITAL INFECTION (%)

Urinary tract	38
Surgical wounds	27
Pneumonia	16
Skin	6
Bacteraemia	4
Other	9
	100

(a) Urinary tract infection (UTI). In hospitals this is mainly related to catheterisation and instrumentation. The insertion and removal of a catheter on one occasion leads to infection in about 2% of patients. About 50% of patients with an indwelling catheter on closed drainage become infected in 11-14 days. In community UTI, *Escherichia coli* predominates, being responsible for 60-90% of infections in different series, and *Proteus, Klebsiella, Streptococcus faecalis* and *Staphylococcus epidermidis* are also found. In hospital infections *E. coli* is still common, but other Gram-negative rods such as *Pseudomonas, Klebsiella, Serratia* and yeasts, especially *Candida,* are much more important.

The major route of infection appears to be via the urethra. In the catheterised patient this may be facilitated in various ways. Organisms may be carried in from the urethra on the catheter or may ascend in the layer of exudate that rapidly forms between the catheter and the urethral wall. If drainage is not properly arranged, organisms may multiply in the drainage reservoir and ascend the column of fluid. Short-term catheterisation appears to result in infection with autogenous organisms, whereas patients catheterised for extended periods acquire environmental organisms present ON THE HANDS OF THE STAFF and on the equipment used. In one male surgical ward a single type of *Klebsiella* was isolated from the urine of 36/37 patients.

Do we need to worry about hospital-acquired UTI (apart from its economic consequences)? While catheter-related UTI seems to resolve spontaneously in most cases after removal of the catheter, and long-term sequelae seem to be uncommon, the possibility of *septicaemia* is more serious. Transient bacteraemia commonly follows the withdrawal of a catheter from an infected urinary tract or its insertion into one. The urinary tract is the commonest portal of entry in septicaemia. And even when it is not fatal, septicaemia prolongs hospital stay.

Treatment of catheter-related Infection. The primary act is to remove the *catheter*. It is virtually impossible to cure an infection with the catheter in place and usually its removal is successful treatment without any other measures. Infection in the catheterised patient can only be avoided by scrupulous care in the introduction and management of the catheter. Antiseptic and antibiotic bladder washouts appear to achieve little except comfort of mind for the clinical staff. Prophylactic antibiotics will delay infection only for a few days; instead of the patient being infected after a week or two by a sensitive organism, he is infected after a slightly longer interval by a resistant organism.

(b) Surgical wound infection. Infection has always been the major obstacle to surgical progress. Methods of controlling infection are:

- prevention of access of microbes to wounds by aseptic techniques
- destruction of microbes in wounds by antiseptics and prophylactic (preventive) antibiotics
- improvement in host resistance.

Techniques of asepsis are well developed; their effectiveness can be increased by proper use, but it is unreasonable to look to further great advances. Prophylactic antibiotics have a definite place in the surgery of contaminated sites, but restraint is necessary. The dilemma is that each use of antibiotics in an appropriate situation may benefit the individual patient, but the harmful effects may be both on the individual and on the hospital ecology. The more widespread the use of antibiotics, the more microbes will be resistant to them. Thus, where the risk of infection is low (1% or less), antibiotics should not be used, even if their use would further lower the infection rate. In the prevention of wound infection, host factors are very important. Skilful anaesthesia, apparently by preventing tissue anoxia and maintaining blood flow, helps considerably, perhaps by enhancing the effectiveness of tissue phagocytes. The importance of other factors such as nutrition needs to be assessed.

(c) Pneumonia. Hospital-acquired pneumonia accounts for about 15% of nosocomial infections and is more commonly fatal than most others; it is estimated that about 15% of all deaths in hospital are related to lung infections. Unlike community-acquired pneumonias, more than 60% of nosocomial pneumonias are due to Gram-negative rods (*Pseudomonas aeruginosa*, *Klebsiella* spp., *Enterobacter* spp. and *Escherichia coli*); *Streptococcus pneumoniae*, the commonest cause of pneumonia outside hospital, accounts for only 2-3% of cases *inside* hospital.

The prime contributing factors to nosocomial pneumonia are intubation of the trachea and tracheostomy (*intubation* of the trachea means 'insertion of a tube into the trachea', and a *tracheostomy* is an opening made into the trachea through the front of the neck). Both procedures are carried out in order to provide mechanical respiratory assistance to the patient in respiratory failure, but both interfere with or bypass the normal defences of the upper respiratory tract (p.140). The respiratory equipment itself may supply the infecting organism if it is not scrupulously maintained. Diagnosis of pneumonia in these critically ill patients is extremely difficult, since there are usually several other possible causes for a rise in temperature or other deterioration in the patient's condition.

4 Prevention of hospital infection

How do we prevent the 'preventable' nosocomial infections? This can only be done if we, the clinical staff of the hospital (doctors, nurses and paramedical workers), modify our work practices to minimise infection. Infection risks are known to be associated with:

- insertion and care of urinary catheters
- insertion and care of intravascular lines
- use of respiratory therapy equipment
- deficiencies in surgical technique
- errors in sterile technique, both in the theatre and in the ward
- neglecting to wash the hands

Bringing about these changes in established bad habits is the task of the *infection control team*.

(a) The infection control team and committee. Every hospital should have an *infection control team* (ICT). The team's activities are usually directed by an *infection control committee*, consisting of medical, surgical and nursing staff and including a clinical microbiologist or hospital epidemiologist. The team itself will consist of one or more *infection control nurses* (ICNs); the recommendation is one ICN for every 250 beds, but many hospitals in this country fall short of this standard. In Australia virtually all ICNs have nursing as their primary training: in the USA this would be true of at least 75%.

IN THE WARD
The ideal infection-control nurse

'The infection control nurse needs to possess the qualities of Sherlock Holmes, Mary Poppins, St Francis of Assisi and

Margaret Thatcher' (Prof. F.D. Daschner, University of Freiburg, Germany, at 2nd International Meeting on Bacteriological Epidemiological Markers, Rhodes, Greece, 1990).

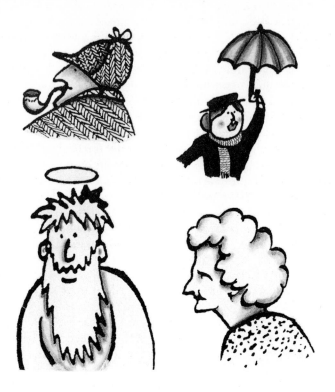

IN THE WARD
Infection control measures
Measures known to be effective:
- Sterilisation
- Handwashing
- Closed urinary drainage
- Intravenous catheter care, non-touch dressing technique
- Preventive antibiotics in contaminated wounds
- Care of respiratory therapy equipment

Measures probably effective:
- Isolation procedures
- Education programs

Measures whose efficacy is doubtful or unknown:
- Disinfection of floors, walls, sinks
- UV Lights
- Laminar air flow, etc.
- Antibiotic prophylaxis in clean wounds
- Routine environmental sampling

HAND WASHING IS PROBABLY THE SINGLE MOST IMPORTANT MEASURE IN THE PREVENTION OF NOSOCOMIAL INFECTION

To practice effectively, an ICN requires a full understanding of:

- nursing procedures (especially in relation to sterilisation and disinfection) and of the use of medical equipment of all types, from urinary catheters to mechanical ventilators and haemodialysis equipment
- isolation procedures and the precautions necessary for handling contaminated equipment and body fluids
- procedures needed for dealing with nosocomial infections and community-acquired infections

A good knowledge of microbiology is also needed. Infection control is learned by on-the-job training, formal education programs and experience.

Because much of the training in the wards is on the apprenticeship system, and because people who have done something in a certain way for 20 years resist the idea of changing their technique, introducing new methods which carry lower risks of infection is not easy. The ICT can achieve this aim most easily by ensuring that improved equipment is used (e.g. a closed urinary draining bag that cannot easily be contaminated), but unfortunately many infection problems do not admit of such a simple solution. So the ICT has to observe the deficiencies and risks of current patient-care practices, and arm itself with information about more appropriate techniques.

The infection-control practitioner plays several important roles in the hospital:

1. collection of epidemiological data: infection rates in wounds, in catheterised patients and such
2. compilation of protocols for infection-control procedures
3. education of nursing and other staff in infection control
   (See box 'The ideal infection-control nurse'.)

(b) Infection control.

(i) HAND WASHING IS PROBABLY THE SINGLE MOST IMPORTANT MEASURE IN THE PREVENTION OF NOSOCOMIAL INFECTION. It is impossible to repeat this message too often. *Even the Senior Surgeon should wash his hands after visiting each patient in the ward — though it may be difficult to convince him of this!* Hands should be washed after touching any patient or any object that might be contaminated. Before surgery, in isolation units and with newborns, antiseptic soaps are recommended. Elsewhere ordinary soaps, bar soap, granules, liquid and leaflets are quite adequate. In our opinion ordinary soap has one considerable advantage over some of the germicidal washes that are provided at considerable expense — it is much more readily accepted; people are more likely to use soap than a drying germicide solution which leaves the hands uncomfortable.

(ii) Universal precautions. Before AIDS, hospitals had sets of procedures to prevent the transmission of infection in hospital; basically these were applied to patients known or suspected of carrying a particular type of infection; 'Blood and Body-fluids' precautions, 'Enteric' precautions, 'MRSA' precautions. While the risk of catching AIDS as a health-care worker is very low, the consequences of

doing so are so serious that 'universal precautions' are now recommended for the blood and body fluids of *all* patients (see following, 'Universal precautions for blood and body fluids'). It is likely that failure to apply these principles would leave a hospital open to *legal action* if a staff member contracted AIDS in the course of duty.

These precautions can be justified on several grounds. Present tests do not identify all patients with AIDS or, for that matter, any of several other infections. And patients in whom the infection is not suspected will not be tested. Furthermore an individual has the right to refuse the test. The precautions offer reassurance to healthcare workers and heighten awareness of the risk in other infections also. The appropriate precautions will of course still be applied where necessary, e.g. in treating the patient with hepatitis A or MRSA.

(iii) Infection prevention. Precautions are determined by the likely routes of dissemination, e.g. hepatitis B is largely spread by blood or serum, many bacteria are transferred on the hands of the staff and by environmental contamination, and *Salmonella* is spread in faeces. For the problem of hospital infections there are no miracle solutions in sight; simple precautions conscientiously observed must remain our mainstay. It is unlikely that better antibiotics or more elaborate equipment will contribute much to the prevention of these infections. Probably around two thirds of them are endogenous and not preventable at present; techniques of selective decontamination of the gut, aimed at eliminating most of the Gram-negative aerobes which are important in endogenous infections, may prove capable of reducing the number of these infections in special groups, e.g. in the intensive care unit. Nevertheless preventable infections occur in 1-2% of all patients admitted to hospital and these infections represent a considerable expense and a major threat to life and the success of the treatment.

> WASH YOUR HANDS
> SHOW THE DOCTOR THE SINK

5 Role of the microbiology laboratory

The results of laboratory cultures will draw attention to about 80% of infections subsequently judged to be nosocomial. Outbreaks of infection with a particular pathogen, an especially resistant strain or unusual organism, may be observed. The laboratory is also often involved in such events as environmental sampling, and the investigation of outbreaks. Copies of positive culture results should be seen by the infection control nurse; a computerised record system should generate daily reports to facilitate infection control. It is essential to detect the transfer of infection from one patient to another, and for this purpose it is necessary to identify any significant isolate accurately. It is no doubt possible to treat the patient if you know no more about the organism than that it is Gram-

UNIVERSAL BLOOD & BODY FLUIDS PRECAUTIONS

Prevent Exposure of Skin and Mucous Membranes to all Blood and Body Fluids!

IF IN CONTACT	RISK OF SPLASHING	ALWAYS WASH HANDS
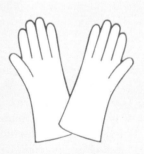	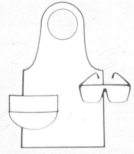	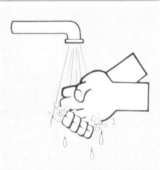
Wear gloves when in contact with blood and body fluids.	Use plastic apron, protective glasses or protective masks where there is risk of splashing.	Wash hands before and after contact with patient and after removal of gloves!

negative and that it is resistant to ampicillin and susceptible to cephalothin and gentamicin. But if all urinary isolates are reported as 'coliforms', a cluster of *Serratia* or *Klebsiella* infections in catheterised patients in the same ward may be missed. If the report is '*Pseudomonas* species' instead of '*Pseudomonas cepacia*', the ability of this organism to multiply in antiseptic solutions may not be remembered.

6 Antibiotics and nosocomial infections

Antibiotics have now been used for 50 years. During the same period the major role in hospital infections has passed from Gram-positive cocci to Gram-negative rods. This change is probably partly connected with the use of antibiotics, and also with the great alterations in medical technology, in the nature of patients and their susceptibility to infection. Antibiotics are widely used in hospitals. Twenty-five to 35% of all patients receive antibiotics and in about half of these cases the aim was prevention of infection, 'prophylaxis'. Most studies of antibiotic use in hospitals have concluded that about half of the antibiotic therapy was misguided. The more antibiotics are used, the more likely it is that resistant strains will appear and persist in the hospital. (The misuse of antibiotics is discussed on page 158.)

OCCUPATIONAL HAZARDS OF HOSPITAL WORK

Hospitals can be dangerous to patients — but what about the *staff*? Risks to the health of the hospital staff range from the psychosocial stress inherent in professions making 'life-and-death' decisions to many and varied physical diseases — back injuries caused by lifting heavy patients (or violence inflicted by disturbed ones), or exposure to radiation, toxic chemicals and infections.

1 Infectious disease

Within the hospital, infections may spread from patient to patient, from patient to staff and from staff to patient. Obviously any infectious disease may be acquired outside the hospital, but several infections need to be discussed in more detail.

(a) Hepatitis B. This presents a special risk for personnel who come in contact with blood or blood products, which have the highest concentrations of virus, though saliva and semen are also infective. Hospital personnel have carriage rates of hepatitis B antigen and antibody (HBsAg and HBsAb) which are two- to fourfold higher than those of the community. There is a higher risk for those who work in operating theatres, pathology laboratories, haemodialysis or intensive care units and in any other unit where exposure to blood is likely. Injuries due to contaminated needlesticks are common.

Precautions.
- *Label 'carrier' blood with an 'infectious risk' sticker*
- *Don't recap needles*
- *Dispose of needles into suitable receptacles*
- *Make sure you are vaccinated against Hepatitis B*

(b) *Rubella*. Outbreaks of rubella can cause serious problems in hospitals, involving both staff and patients. Close to 40% of Australians are susceptible to rubella (in this country vaccination has not been offered to males). Vaccination is desirable for *all* hospital personnel; staff in obstetric services should have documented immunity, i.e. a positive test for rubella antibody or vaccination (the belief that a previous rash and fever was due to rubella is often wrong).

(c) *Mumps*. In adults inflammation of the testes or ovaries is a not uncommon complication of mumps, and pediatric staff are advised to accept vaccination.

(d) *Viral respiratory infections*. Outbreaks of influenza may affect both patients and hospital staff (in some episodes more than 30% of those exposed were infected). Vaccination is recommended for staff caring for the critically ill, since they may transfer the infection to their patients. Respiratory syncytial virus often cause outbreaks among patients and staff in pediatric units; there is no vaccine, immunity is poor after infection, and control depends on 'good housekeeping' (gowns, handwashing and so on).

(e) *Herpes simplex virus*. This is readily spread by contact with infected secretions; a common form of infection is herpetic whitlow, which involves the 'ball' of the thumb or finger. This may be very painful and usually lasts one to five weeks. Wearing gloves when exposed to secretions and conscientious handwashing will prevent infection.

(f) *AIDS*. The virus is transmitted in blood and blood products and the risk factors are discussed on p.259. The patient may not know, or may not say, that he has AIDS, so universal blood and body-fluid precautions should be used with all patients — not just the 'yellow stickers'.

(g) *Tuberculosis*. Hospital staff run a greater risk of acquiring tuberculosis than the general population. The undiagnosed case is the most dangerous (p.204). Modern diagnostic procedures, such as fiberoptic bronchoscopy (examination of the respiratory passages by means of a flexible illuminated telescope) or therapeutic measures (e.g. applying suction to a tracheostomy) can create infective aerosols and thus enhance transmission. In one study, of 13 staff present during the bronchoscopy of one such patient, 10 acquired a positive tuberculin reaction. However, once antituberculous therapy is started, the patient rapidly becomes non-infectious and no special precautions are then necssary. All staff should be tuberculin-tested on joining the hospital; if the result is negative, they should be re-tested at regular intervals afterwards.

(h) *Gastroenteritis*. The outbreaks are most often due to *Salmonella* spread in contaminated food or by infected food handlers. Staff who have culture-positive diarrhoea should not work until symptoms subside and cultures are negative. The outbreak should be controlled by proper isolation nursing, handwashing and food handling.

(i) *Staphylococcus aureus*. This organism often causes nosocomial infections. Staff who are carriers may disseminate the organism

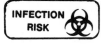

INFECTION RISK

HIGH RISK

HEPATITIS RISK

from the nose or from an infected dermatitis. A boil or other local infection may be the source and the staff member should not work until this has healed. Elimination of staphylococci from the nose has always been difficult; there are, however, favourable reports of the new topical antibiotic mupirocin for this purpose.

(j) Other infections. These can be due to such organisms as cytomegalovirus, *Bordetella pertussis* and streptococci. They occur more rarely. *Legionnaires' disease* may be caused by a contaminated water supply or air-conditioning system, but these outbreaks usually involve patients, rather than staff.

2 Prevention

Vaccination is recommended against several infectious hazards of hospital work:

- hepatitis B virus
- rubella
- mumps (pediatric staff)
- influenza (critical care staff)
- and diphtheria, tetanus and poliomyelitis (if not given in childhood)

Serial tuberculin-testing is important in the detection of tuberculosis acquired 'on the job'.

```
PS:        WASH YOUR HANDS
      SHOW THE DOCTOR THE SINK
```

IN THE WARD
Gloves are not a 'universal answer'

Gloves are worn as part of *Universal Precautions*. Nevertheless, it remains advisable to wash one's hands after a procedure in which gloves are worn.

It is becoming clear that gloves have defects. More than one pair in 10 will be obviously damaged when taken out of the box. Even if they appear *un*damaged, some will have faults: they will leak when filled with water, they will permit HSV to pass through and staff may develop herpetic whitlow. (These defects appear to be found more often in *vinyl* than in latex gloves.)

It is not possible to remove all microbes from soiled gloves by washing them after use.

Precautions:
> *Inspect your gloves after you put them on.*
> *Change your gloves before attending to another patient.*
> *Do NOT wash gloves and reuse them.*
> *Wash your hands after removing gloves.*

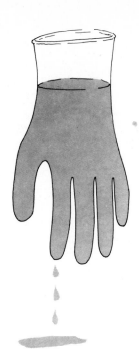

IN THE COMMUNITY
'A tick in time plagues Lyme': a surprise for the rheumatologists

Old Lyme is a small town in eastern Connecticut, USA. In November 1975, a mother living in this community of 5000 people informed the State Health Department that 12 children had been diagnosed as having *juvenile rheumatoid arthritis*; four of these children lived close together on the same road.

Subsequently another woman told staff of the Yale Rheumatology Clinic that she, her husband, two children and several neighbours all suffered arthritis.

Such an outbreak of arthritis was very unusual, and the Yale University School of Medicine began to investigate.

Over the next two years, in Old Lyme and two adjacent communities, investigators saw over 90 children and adults who apparently had the same disease. This involved swelling and pain usually in one joint, but sometimes in more than one; most often the knee was affected, patients often suffered from fever and malaise. The first attack lasted for a week or so, but recurrences were common.

A number of patients remembered that about four weeks before the attack they had notiiced a small reddish lump, which came to be surrounded by a circular red rash — this was thought to be an insect bite, and indeed one patient actually remembered having been bitten by a tick.

The cases occurred in geographic clusters. Half the affected residents in Old Lyme lived on two adjoining country roads, as did half the patients in the other community. None of the affected persons lived in the town centres. But persons who lived close together did *not* get their illness at the same *time*: members of the same family were affected in different years, as were people who lived on the same road. Illness was commoner in June to September (i.e. summer to autumn).

These findings suggested that the source of infection was associated with the countryside, and with a certain season of the year. It apparently did not spread from person to person within the same household. The investigators concluded that the pattern of spread of the disease indeed suggested infection transmitted by an arthropod such as a tick.

In 1983 a previously unrecognised spirochete was isolated from both patients and ticks, and it is now clear that Lyme disease is caused by *Borrelia burgdorferi*, a spirochete transmitted by ticks. A similar disease, in which neurological symptoms are more prominent, occurs in Europe.

Lyme disease has now been reported from the USA, Europe (including Scandinavia), and the Soviet Union, China, Japan and Australia.

CHAPTER REVIEW

1 (a) What is *epidemiology?*
   (b) What sorts of information does an epidemiologist collect?
2 Discuss the importance of handwashing.
3 (a) Define *nosocomial infection*.
   (b) How significant is this problem?
   (c) Can it be prevented?
   (d) What are the main types of nosocomial infection?
4 (a) Explain the modes of transmission of microorganisms into the bladder.
   (b) What measures may be taken to reduce nosocomial urinary tract infections?
5 List and explain the preventive measures that may be taken for controlling surgical wound infections.
6 Explain the importance of:
   (a) the infection control practitioner
   (b) the microbiology laboratory
   in prevention and control of hospital-acquired infection.
7 Several members of the staff of your ward complain of recent attacks of diarrhoea. As an epidemiologist, how would you investigate these cases: what questions would you ask?

14

BACTERIA AND THE INFECTIONS THEY CAUSE

In the next four chapters we shall examine the common microbial pathogens: their characteristics and how they are detected by the laboratory, their natural habitats and the ways they are transmitted to humans, the diseases they cause, and finally how these diseases are treated and prevented. We shall also mention the response of the major bacterial groups to antibiotics.

In the protected and privileged environment of the so-called 'developed countries', it is easy to remain unaware that infectious disease is still a huge problem in the Third World (see Table 14.1). While bacterial infections are still very significant in these countries (meningococcal infection, tuberculosis, leprosy, cholera and others) viral and parasitic infections are also of major importance. Eradication of these diseases is an enormous task. Lack of money and political indifference are the main obstacles to its accomplishment. Simple public-health measures (e.g. the provision of a clean water-supply and an efficient sewerage system) are more effective than the most modern 'high-technology' medical care.

TABLE 14.1 ESTIMATES OF DEATHS DUE TO INFECTIOUS DISEASE IN THE
THIRD WORLD 1980-81

Infection	Deaths per year
diarrhoeal disease	5-7 million
respiratory infections	4-5 million
malaria	1.5 million
measles	0.9 million
tetanus	0.6 million
tuberculosis	0.5 million
hepatitis B virus	0.5 million

[Adapted from JA Walsh, in *Tropical and Geographic Medicine,* KS Warren and AEF Mahmoud (eds), McGraw-Hill Book Co. New York].

GRAM-POSITIVE COCCI

The Gram-positive cocci that concern us are the *staphylococci* and *streptococci*. *Staphylococcus aureus*, *Staphylococcus epidermidis* and more than a dozen other coagulase-negative species make up the genus *Staphylococcus* (Plate 2).

STAPHYLOCOCCI

Staphylococci are facultative anaerobes, grow singly, or in short chains or irregular clumps, are catalase-positive and have fairly complex growth requirements, needing a medium that includes amino acids, vitamins and other substances. Most will grow in a medium containing 7.5% NaCl, a concentration that few other species will tolerate. Many show beta-haemolysis on blood agar. Whenever a staphylococcus is isolated in circumstances indicating that it may be contributing to disease, it is tested for the ability to produce coagulase, an enzyme that causes plasma to clot. *S. aureus* is the only species capable of making this enzyme (see following, 'Coagulase tests').

IN THE LAB
Coagulase tests
Staphylococci release many enzymes and toxic proteins, such as haemolysins, DNAase and enterotoxins. The characteristic which best distinguishes the major disease-producing staphylococcus, *Staphylococcus aureus*, from 12 or more other species, is the ability to produce an enzyme that causes plasma to clot. This *coagulase* occurs in two forms: bound and free.

To detect bound coagulase a *slide coagulase test* is performed. A colony or two of the suspect staphylococcus is emulsified in water and then a loopful of plasma is added. If the bacterial suspension clumps, bound coagulase is present.

In the *tube coagulase* test, a tube of broth containing plasma is inoculated with the staphylococcus. If a clot forms on incubation the test is positive.

Problems with this test usually arise when unsuitable plasma is used. Commercial kits are now available in which plasma components are linked to particles which clump when mixed with a suspension of *S. aureus*. These kits give better results than the standard coagulase tests in a proportion of laboratories.

Most laboratories classify staphylococci as coagulase-positive or coagulase-negative, but do not further subdivide the latter group, simply reporting them as 'coagulase-negative staphylococci' or as 'Staph. epidermidis'. By means of biochemical tests another 12 or more species can be distinguished. It is becoming more important to identify them accurately, since coagulase-negative staphylococci are playing a greater role in infections.

Staphylococci have as their habitat the body surfaces; they are present in the nose (p.74), on the skin, in the vagina and in the gut (Fig. 14.1). Coagulase-negative staphylococci are part of the normal skin flora and are the commonest staphylococci isolated from skin, *S. epidermidis* occurring most widely. They are readily shed and thus are transferred to other persons or inanimate objects. They are resistant to drying and to changes in temperature and therefore can survive for a considerable time in the environment.

S. aureus causes a wide variety of infections, ranging in severity from boils and impetigo to wound infections, pneumonia, osteomyelitis and endocarditis (Fig. 14.2). Bacteraemia may lead to abscesses at distant sites. Untreated, many staphylococcal infections have a high mortality. Of the coagulase-negative staphylococci, one species, *Staphylococcus saprophyticus*, is the second most frequent cause of urinary tract infections in young women. Most of the others are capable of causing infections only when the individual's defences are impaired (p.262), and especially when plastic devices are implanted (prosthetic heart valves, intravascular cannulae and artificial joints). Some *S. epidermidis* strains produce a polysaccharide slime that appears to help them adhere to plastic.

This 'foreign-body' effect is not confined to coagulase-negative staphylococci; the number of *Staphylococcus aureus* needed to set up an infection in the skin is reduced 1000-fold by putting a surgical stitch in the skin. Infections related to plastic implants may not begin for weeks or months after the operation. It is usually impossible to cure the infection without removing the device.

Toxins elaborated by *S. aureus* are responsible for three other diseases. *Staphylococcal food poisoning* may occur when food contaminated with an enterotoxin-producing strain is left out unrefrigerated. The disorder is due to the ingestion of preformed toxin, not to the multiplication of staphylococci in the victim, and symptoms come on rapidly. *Scalded skin syndrome*, in which the skin peels off, is due to another toxin. And in *toxic shock syndrome*, *S. aureus* elaborates a third toxin. About 80% of cases of toxic shock syndrome are associated with menstruation, and almost all of these with the use of tampons: it appears that the tampon binds magnesium, reducing its concentration in the vaginal secretions; this affects the staphylococcus so that release of toxin is much increased.

ANTIBIOTIC THERAPY

Staphylococcus aureus has shown a remarkable ability to acquire resistance mechanisms against a wide range of antibiotics. By now at least 80% of *S. aureus* isolates in most countries are resistant to penicillin; more often the figure is close to 90%. This resistance is mediated by production of a beta-lactamase, an enzyme that hydrolyses penicillin. Penicillin-resistant strains are sensitive to methicillin, oxacillin and cephalothin. Methicillin-resistant strains (MRSA) are almost always multi-resistant also, i.e resistant to all beta-lactam antibiotics, to erythromycin, tetracycline and amino-

Fig. 14.1 Habitats of staphylococci. Staphylococci are an important component of the normal flora, and are found in the nose (and less often in the throat), on moist skin, and in the gut.

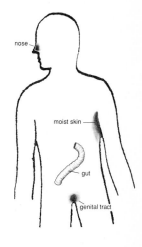

Fig. 14.2 Infections caused by staphylococci: boils and other skin infections, osteomyelitis, endocarditis, pneumonia, wound infections and toxic shock syndrome.

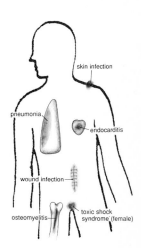

glycosides, but almost always susceptible to rifampicin, fusidic acid and so far always to vancomycin. The basis of methicillin resistance is production of a new 'penicillin-binding protein'. These proteins are actually enzymes involved in the construction of the cell wall and the effectiveness of penicillins and cephalosporins stems from interfering with their function. MRSA are found almost exclusively in hospitals and nursing homes and appear to be carried by patients and staff. Coagulase-negative staphylococci are in general more resistant to antibiotics than *S. aureus*.

STREPTOCOCCI

The streptococci are a large and diverse assembly of Gram-positive cocci, for which a satisfactory classification has not been worked out. Various groups are recognised on the basis of:

- type of haemolysis, alpha, beta or none
- polysaccharide cell-wall antigens (Lancefield group antigens)
- capsular polysaccharides, in pneumococci
- biochemical attributes.

When grown on blood agar many streptococci, but not all, attack the red cells, causing either alpha- or beta-haemolysis (p.92). In the streptococci, beta-haemolysis is due to the presence of two toxins — streptolysin O and streptolysin S. The presence of beta-haemolysis is a useful pointer when examining throat or vaginal specimens, but when streptococci are isolated from other sites their haemolytic reaction is of relatively little help in determining their significance. Many of the streptococci can be classified into groups by the presence of polysaccharide antigens (Lancefield group antigens A, B, C and so on) which form part of the cell wall and which are detectable by antisera. Such antisera are regularly used in the identification of streptococci.

A 'practical' classification of streptococci is:

- the pyogenic streptococci
- the pneumococci
- the viridans streptococci
- the enterococci

The *pyogenic* or 'pus-producing' *streptococci* are all beta-haemolytic and possess a Lancefield antigen, A, B, C or G. The term *Streptococcus pyogenes* is applied to the beta-haemolytic group A strains. Most group A strains produce streptolysin O and hence most patients recovering from infections with this organism have antibodies to streptolysin O. Group A streptococci also produce several DNAases and other enzymes; antibodies to DNAase B are often found after infection. Estimations of the titres of these antibodies are used in the diagnosis of streptococcal infection: the anti-streptolysin O titre or ASOT and the anti-DNAase B titre.

The *pneumococci* form a well-defined species, *Streptococcus pneumoniae*, easily separated from other streptococci (Plate 13). *S. pneumoniae* causes alpha-haemolysis. It has a typical colony shape, like the pieces in the game of draughts. Pneumococci have a capsule, made up of polysaccharide. More than 80 immunologically distinct capsular polysaccharides are known; these can be identified by specific antisera.

The *'viridans' streptococci*, or 'green' streptococci, are so-called because they are usually alpha-haemolytic. They include two fairly well delimited species, *Streptococcus sanguis* and *Streptococcus mitior*, and a number of other groups. There is a non-haemolytic group which contains important pathogens such as *S. milleri*, a species which has its own characteristic polysaccharide antigen. The *enterococci, Enterococcus faecalis* and *E. faecium*, (formerly named *Streptococcus faecalis, Streptococcus faecium*) are closely related to the streptococci, and contain the group D antigen. *E. faecalis* is often beta-haemolytic.

Streptococci are part of the normal flora of humans. In general streptococci groups A, C and G and pneumococci are usually considered to be present in the throat as transients, since carriage rates differ from community to community and one can often show that the strain was acquired from another individual. The 'viridans' streptococci and others are part of the normal flora of the mouth, throat, vagina and gut.

Group A streptococci are a common cause of sore throat (pharyngitis) and tonsillitis, skin infections (impetigo, also caused by *S. aureus*) and infections of the soft tissues (Fig. 14.3). Pharyngitis may occasionally lead to acute rheumatic fever (inflammation of the heart and joints), while pharyngitis or skin infections may lead to acute glomerulonephritis (an inflammation of the kidney). In rheumatic fever and glomerulonephritis streptococci are not found in the involved tissues; the pathological process appears to be some form of immune reaction, not yet understood. Because of this risk, an attempt should be made to detect group A streptococci in pharyngitis, so that penicillin can be given. Groups C and G are occasionally responsible for sore throat and other infections.

Group B streptococci often colonise the gut and/or the genital tract and are acquired by neonates, in whom they may set up life-threatening infections, meningitis and septicaemia. (See following, 'A sick baby'.) Neonates may also be infected in the nursery. Fever in the mother after delivery (postpartum fever) is often due to group B streptococci. Enterococci are normally present in the gut. The most serious infection which they cause is endocarditis; they are also responsible for urinary infections and post-operative infections. Alpha-haemolytic and non-haemolytic streptococci may cause endocarditis or deep abscesses ('deep' meaning 'in an internal organ such as lung or liver'). *S. pneumoniae* remains the leading cause of community-acquired pneumonia; it is also associated with sinusitis, otitis media and meningitis. (See following, 'A fatal motor-cycle accident'.)

IN THE WARD
A sick baby
Mrs Margaret Franklin's pregnancy had reached only the 36th

Fig. 14.3 Infections caused by streptococci: pharyngitis and tonsillitis, impetigo, pneumonia, endocarditis and abscesses in internal organs. A reaction to streptococcal infection is responsible for myocarditis (inflammation of the heart muscle) and glomerulonephritis (a type of inflammation of the kidney).

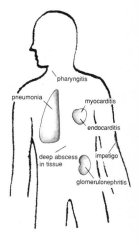

week when her membranes ruptured and she came into premature labour. Baby Franklin weighed 2.2 kg. He was his mother's second child.

He appeared well at birth, but after 36 hours was noted to be lethargic, his respirations were laboured and 'grunting' in nature, he was not feeding well and his temperature was 39°C. Blood cultures were performed. A lumbar puncture showed no increase in white cells and no bacteria were seen.

The clinical findings indicated a serious bacterial infection and he was given large doses of ampicillin and gentamicin as soon as the diagnostic procedures were completed. The next day group B streptococci were grown from his blood and from an ear swab (this site is swabbed because it is less likely to be contaminated after birth). Ampicillin and gentamicin are effective in combination against this organism, and baby (now Wayne) Franklin survived. For this he could thank the fact that he had received prompt antibiotic therapy and that he was not very premature — more than half the babies under 1500g die when they acquire this infection.

The group B streptococcus lives in the gut and colonises the vagina in a proportion of women. Infection of the fetus *in utero* leads to the clinical picture described here. Infection may also occur during birth, and then signs appear after about three weeks.

IN THE WARD
A fatal motorcycle accident

At the age of 20, Paul Mercier sustained internal injuries when he and his motorcycle collided with a fence-post. One consequence of this accident was the loss of his spleen.

One evening, 10 years later, he developed symptoms which he interpreted as 'the flu'; he felt ill, had a high temperature (39°C), and had fits of the 'shivers'. He was sufficiently unwell to visit his local doctor, who agreed with his diagnosis of 'viral infection' and prescribed aspirin and tetracycline. The following morning, however, Paul was much worse, and his girlfriend took him to hospital. Although he was immediately admitted to the Intensive Care Unit and given large doses of penicillin intravenously, he died 12 hours later.

This case represents a tragedy of errors. The spleen plays an important role in removing organisms from the bloodstream. Loss of the spleen brings with it the risk of overwhelming infection — *Streptococcus pneumoniae* is the commonest cause.

If you lose your spleen, several precautions are worthwhile.
1 Remember that you have an increased susceptibility to infection, and be a little readier to see a doctor when you get ill.
2 Have *'splenectomy'* tattooed on the inside of your forearm; this will remind you to tell the doctor whenever you get sick and, even if you are too ill to tell them, he or she will see it when they examine you.

3 Accept multivalent pneumococcal vaccine.

All these precautions should have been explained to Paul after his motorcycle crash.

The local doctor can hardly be blamed for not diagnosing *septicaemia* instead of *viral infection*. The antibiotic prescribed was pointless if the diagnosis was incorrect — but many other doctors would have done the same. The dose was unfortunately quite inadequate to have treated Paul's infection.

ANTIBIOTIC THERAPY

Unlike the staphylococci, streptococci have remained quite susceptible to most antibiotics. Penicillin is still the drug of choice for most infections not caused by enterococci. Isolates of *S. pneumoniae* occasionally show moderate resistance to penicillin; in rare cases strains are found to be highly resistant to this drug, so that it is no longer effective. The only other antibiotic to which resistance is often noted is tetracycline. Enterococci show much more resistance to antibiotics. Fortunately resistance due to beta-lactamases is extremely rare in streptococci.

GRAM-POSITIVE RODS

Bacillus species form a varied group of spore-forming rods, almost all motile. They are saprophytes, commonly found in dust and soil. In the laboratory they are typically air-borne contaminants. In general they have very little pathogenicity. *B. anthracis* causes the uncommon infection anthrax and *B. cereus* may cause a type of food poisoning.

The *coryneform* bacteria or diphtheroids (bacteria looking like the diphtheria bacillus, *Corynebacterium diphtheriae*) are small to medium-size Gram-positive rods, often bent and sometimes club-shaped, arranged singly, or in 'palisades' (side by side) or 'Chinese letters' (Plate 14). Historically the most notable member of the genus is *Corynebacterium diphtheriae*; until the twentieth century this organism was responsible for many deaths. It grows well on the usual media as pleomorphic rods. Disease is due to absorption of a toxin. The ability to make this toxin is borne by a bacteriophage and is not an integral property of the organism, which only produces disease when the bacteriophage has become integrated into its genome, i.e the DNA of the bacteriophage has become part of the bacterial chromosome. An isolate may have the morphology and biochemical characteristics of *C. diphtheriae*, but lack the ability to produce toxin. It is therefore essential to demonstrate the production of toxin as part of the identification.

In diphtheria there is inflammation in the throat and formation of a membrane which may choke the patient, while absorbed toxin attacks chiefly the heart and peripheral nerves (Fig. 14.4). The bacteria do not invade the tissues beyond the throat. The site of

Fig. 14.4 Mechanism of illness in *Corynebacterium diphtheriae* infection. The microbe multiplies on the surface of the throat and does not invade the body. Its toxin is absorbed and damages the heart and the central nervous system.

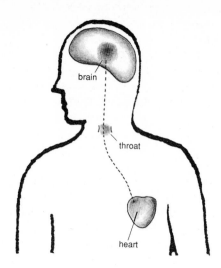

infection may also be the skin. Diphtheria is now a rare disease. A vaccine made from the toxin gives a high degree of protection. In 1932 in the USA about 60 000 deaths were due to diphtheria; there were five deaths in 1982. Of course diphtheria will remain rare only if children continue to be immunised.

There are several other species of *Corynebacterium* that are uncommon causes of pharyngitis or of generalised infection. As well, there are a large number of varieties not yet properly sorted out. Aerobic, microaerophilic and anaerobic types occur. Their habitat is any body surface, including the vagina and the gut, and they represent a major component of the flora on the human skin and mucous membranes.

Recently a new type of diphtheroid has been associated with infection. These *JK diphtheroids* are rather unreactive when examined biochemically, but their distinguishing feature is resistance to many of the common antibiotics. They were isolated from patients who suffered from immunosuppression because of treatment for cancer or because of organ transplantation and, in addition, had received several antibiotics.

The genus *Listeria* includes one major pathogen, *Listeria monocytogenes*, a small motile Gram-positive rod looking like a diphtheroid. It is sometimes mistaken for one and dismissed as a 'contaminant'. It grows on the usual media and produces beta-haemolysis. *L. monocytogenes* is ubiquitous; it has been isolated from many species of animals and from soil. The reservoir is not known, but may be the asymptomatic human carrier. It is estimated that at least 1% of persons carry *Listeria* in the gut. It produces a severe intra-uterine infection, a meningitis and/or septicaemia in the neonate, and meningitis in adults, usually when they are immunosuppressed. One route of exposure to *L. monocytogenes* is contaminated food products. There have been outbreaks of infection associated with contaminated cheese, salads and 'fast foods'.

L. monocytogenes is an intracellular parasite and the immunity which follows infection is cell-mediated.

ANTIBIOTIC THERAPY

Most of the Gram-positive rods discussed above are susceptible to the 'Gram-positive' antibiotics (pp.155–7).

MYCOBACTERIA: TUBERCULOSIS AND LEPROSY

The genus *Mycobacterium* contains numerous saprophytes, some of which occasionally cause disease in humans, and two important pathogens, *M. tuberculosis* and *M. leprae*. The mycobacteria are aerobic or micro-aerophilic, non-motile and non-sporing. The cells may branch or form filaments. The individual cells are thin and slightly curved (Plate 15). The characteristic feature of the mycobacteria is the possession of a lipid coat. This makes the cells difficult to stain and hence their Gram reactions are neither positive nor negative, but colourless. Once stained they retain the dye firmly, so that it is not removed by strong acids or by acid alcohol. The cells are described as 'acid-fast' and the technique of staining is the Ziehl-Neelsen or ZN stain. The abbreviation 'afb' (acid-fast bacilli) is often used in clinical medicine as shorthand for 'tubercle bacilli'. The main pathogens which are acid-fast are the organisms causing tuberculosis and leprosy.

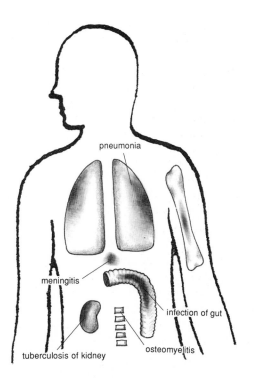

Fig. 14.5 Infections caused by mycobacteria. Mycobacteria most often cause pneumonia, but may also invade the kidney, the gut, the bone marrow or the central nervous system (resulting in meningitis).

Most mycobacteria, including *M. tuberculosis,* will grow on fairly simple media; some will form visible colonies in 24 hours, but most grow much more slowly and cultures for *M. tuberculosis* are normally incubated for at least 8 weeks and often 10 or 12. *M. leprae* will not grow in any bacteriological medium.

Most of the mycobacteria are saprophytes, found in soil, water and on plants. Humans constitute the reservoir of *M. tuberculosis* and *M. leprae.* Tubercle bacilli are spread in droplet nuclei and the initial site of infection is the respiratory tract. Prolonged contact is usually required for infection and a short exposure carries little risk. Adequate air-conditioning largely prevents infection. Fomites play no part in the transfer of infection and bed clothes and eating utensils need no special treatment. If patients cough into tissues, attendants need not wear masks. *M. leprae* grows only in the tissues of humans (and in the armadillo) and the source of infection is an infected patient. The bacilli are present in large numbers in nasal secretions. Prolonged contact is necessary for infection.

TUBERCULOSIS

M. tuberculosis is the cause of tuberculosis or 'consumption', a disease which accounted for 30% of all adult deaths in nineteenth century Europe. Antibiotics have almost eliminated it in Western Europe, USA and Australia and there is now some danger of the diagnosis being overlooked in these countries. Yet half the world's population is still infected with *M. tuberculosis* and it is the commonest infectious cause of death reported; the annual death-rate is estimated as 2.6 million. Africa, Latin America and Asia have high rates of tuberculosis. In parts of Asia and the Pacific the annual number of cases per 100 000 population is 200 or more (in Australia-USA-Europe it is less than 15). In the developed countries doctors must always remember that immigrants are much more likely to suffer from tuberculosis; so are drug addicts and alcoholics.

The chief manifestation of tuberculosis is respiratory tract infection (pulmonary tuberculosis), which leads to destruction of tissue and formation of cavities in the lungs. Once the infection reaches the bronchi, the sputum contains mycobacteria in small or large numbers. (See following, 'In the Ward — A nasty cough'). Only persons who are excreting acid-fast bacilli, 'open cases', are infectious, so other types of infection (e.g. osteomyelitis or miliary tuberculosis), in which the spread is via the blood, present no risk of contagion. *M. tuberculosis* can also cause meningitis, kidney disease, infection of the gut or skin infections (Fig. 14.5). Occasionally other saprophytic mycobacteria cause disease; persons infected with HIV are at special risk from all types of mycobacteria.

IN THE WARD
A nasty cough
When the ambulance brought Albert Pearson to Emergency, it was not difficult to understand why.

He had been found slumped, semi-conscious in a doorway. He had obviously been drinking, and was very thin — his temperature was 38.8°C. He didn't contribute a good history even when he woke up, saying that he was sick and had 'chest trouble', by which he meant a bad cough.

On examination, there were a lot of 'rattles' in his chest and he was coughing up about 50 mL of sputum a day. His chest X-ray showed a picture which was thought to represent patches of pneumonia and chronic bronchitis, and he was given ampicillin.

Albert began to look and feel better; though this was presumably due to regular meals and a warm bed, because his temperature stayed up, and he coughed and coughed. After about 10 days it occurred to the Registrar called to see him one night that alcoholics are likely people to get tuberculosis. The following day a specimen of sputum showed 'acid-fast bacilli +++' and anti-tuberculous treatment was immediately begun.

Albert's future remains rather uncertain, however, since it is unlikely that he will continue his treatment once *he* thinks he is better (tuberculous patients need a lot of perseverance, since they have to take a goodly number of pills daily for 9–12 months).

Tubercle bacilli survive and multiply inside macrophages. After some time cell-mediated immunity develops, manifested by delayed-type hypersensitivity to tuberculin (a preparation of antigens of *M. tuberculosis*) and by enhanced ability of the macrophages to kill the bacilli (p.115). The presence of hypersensitivity to tuberculin is used in the diagnosis of tuberculosis (see following, 'In the ward', 'The tuberculin reaction'). Most often a primary tuberculous infection heals with little trace, once cell-mediated immunity develops and brings about the destruction of the tubercle bacilli. However live tubercle bacilli remain in the apices of the lungs, and elsewhere and disease may break out years later (especially when the individual undergoes a deterioration of general health, becomes malnourished or is treated with immunosuppressive drugs).

IN THE WARD
The tuberculin reaction

The immune response to infection with *Mycobacterium tuberculosis* includes delayed-type hypersensitivity (p.119) to mycobacterial antigens. Hypersensitivity is detected by the tuberculin reaction (the Mantoux reaction) — tuberculin being a solution of mycobacterial antigens.

In this reaction test, a small quantity of tuberculin is injected into the skin, usually on the inner side of the forearm. Nothing happens for several hours. Then, if the reaction is positive, redness and swelling develop at the site of injection; the inflammation reaches its peak after 48-72 hours and then subsides.

It is important to realise, however, that a positive skin reaction *does not prove that the patient has an active infection at present* — but means that he has been infected by *M. tuberculosis* at *some time* in the recent or remote past. Many such infections were symptomless when they occurred and remain so.

In the developed countries today, a positive reaction, especially in a child or young adult, is suspicious and needs to be investigated — whereas 50 years ago a large proportion of the population was tuberculin-positive. Moreover, unfortunately, in the old or the very ill the tuberculin reaction may be negative even though the patient has *active* tuberculosis.

Since 1946, when streptomycin became available, there has been effective therapy against tuberculosis. The modern drugs, mainly isoniazid, rifampin, para-aminosalicylic acid and ethambutol, can now cure almost all cases. (In general mycobacteria are resistant to the 'usual' antibiotics, beta-lactams, tetracycline, erythromycin, trimethoprim and others). These drugs are active against both intracellular and extracellular bacilli. The minimum duration of treatment is usually *nine* months. Because such a long exposure to a drug gives an organism ample opportunity to develop resistance, anti-tuberculous drugs are never given singly; the regime usually includes three antibiotics. Patients cease to be infectious soon after starting chemotherapy, most likely within two weeks.

LEPROSY

M. leprae causes leprosy, also called Hansen's disease. This is uncommon in developed countries (though in Australia, for instance, cases still occur among the outback Aboriginal population); but there are still at least 10 million lepers in the Third World. Like tuberculosis, leprosy is commoner in immigrants to the developed countries. The attitude of society to leprosy is unjustified, since *M. leprae* is of low pathogenicity and clinical disease usually develops only after long contact. The organism attacks the skin and the nerves, resulting in reddened patches which are anaesthetic (have no feeling) because of the involvement of the nerves. Chronic inflammation of the tissues leads to their destruction. There are several effective drugs, including rifampin and dapsone. Patients under treatment are not infectious. As with tuberculosis, the treatment is prolonged.

GRAM-NEGATIVE COCCI
NEISSERIA

The genus *Neisseria* has two important species, *N. meningitidis* (the meningococcus) (Plate 6) and *N. gonorrhoeae* (the gonococcus). Both are Gram-negative diplococci, delicate organisms which require enriched media for growth and prefer additional CO_2. To isolate *N. gonorrhoeae* from the genital tract, especially the vagina with its dense flora, selective media are required, usually a chocolate agar with antibiotics. For best results specimens should be plated in the clinic and taken to the laboratory immediately.

These two species and several other members of the genus have as their habitat the mucous membranes of humans. In pathogenicity they range from the gonococcus (which must always be considered as causing disease) to commensals (rarely invasive except in the compromised host). Humans are the sole reservoir of *N. gonorrhoeae*, which is a major cause of sexually transmitted disease. It produces both symptomatic and asymptomatic infections of the genital tract — vaginitis, cervicitis and pelvic inflammatory disease in the female and urethritis in the male. Given the opportunity it will also infect the throat or the anal canal. About 20-30% of gonococci are now resistant to penicillin, since they carry a plasmid that codes for a beta-lactamase. In such cases tetracycline or a 3rd generation cephalosporin such as cefotaxime or ceftriaxone is given.

The meningococcus is found in the upper respiratory tract of about 5% of healthy people. It is probably transmitted from carrier to carrier by the respiratory route. It causes, most notably, meningitis and meningococcaemia (a generalised infection in which the organisms are disseminated via the blood). Both diseases are among the greatest medical emergencies; death may occur within a day, despite antibiotic therapy. (See chapter 12, p.161 'Flea-bites are a bad sign'.) The meningococcus is susceptible to penicillin.

Branhamella catarrhalis is a Gram-negative coccus rather hardier than *Neisseria*. *B. catarrhalis* inhabits the human nasopharynx and is normally of low virulence. From sputum it is often isolated in mixed culture, and perhaps with recognised pathogens such as *H. influenzae* or *S. pneumoniae*, so that the result must be interpreted with caution. In the normal host its presence can almost always be disregarded. In the compromised host, however, or the patient with chronic lung disease it must be taken more seriously, since it may cause pneumonia or empyema.

GRAM-NEGATIVE RODS

ENTEROBACTERIACEAE

The *Enterobacteriaceae* are a large group of Gram-negative rods — aerobic and facultatively anaerobic; a facultative anaerobe is an organism that can live both in the presence and absence of oxygen. Many are motile. *Escherichia coli*, *Klebsiella pneumoniae*, *Enterobacter* species, *Proteus mirabilis* and other *Proteus* species and *Serratia marcescens*, *Salmonella* and *Shigella* species are the more prominent members of the group. They are relatively hardy and grow on most media, including those containing bile salts, such as MacConkey agar; the ability to grow on bile-containing media is characteristic of gut organisms. They are oxidase-negative, reduce nitrate to nitrite and ferment glucose, forming acid or acid and gas. Many different biochemical tests are used in their identification.

The *Enterobacteriaceae* have several different types of antigens attached to the cell wall. O antigens, also present in *Pseudomonas* and *Neisseria,* consist of lipopolysaccharide, which is made up of lipid A + core polysaccharide + a chain of sugars; the sugars making up the chain and/or their sequence differ in each O antigen. Chains of sugars are used as marks of individuality in eucaryotic cells also; the specific parts of blood group substances consist of them. There are hundreds of different O antigens. The same O antigen may be found in different species, so that it is necessary to identify an isolate both biochemically and serologically. Lipid A itself is referred to as 'endotoxin'. It has powerful physiological effects, causing fever for example, and is probably connected with the shock that accompanies bacteraemia due to Gram-negative organisms — 'septic shock'.

H antigens are flagellar proteins and hence are present only in motile species. In several species of *Enterobacteriaceae* some strains synthesise a capsule — this property is often important in the pathogenesis of the diseases they cause. Capsular antigens (often termed K antigens) are found in several genera — *E. coli, Klebsiella* and *Salmonella.* O, H and K antigens are important in the identification of the *Enterobacteriaceae,* especially *Salmonella* and *Shigella* species. More than one O or H antigen may be present in the same organism; the combination of antigens makes up the *serotype.* Exact

Fig. 14.6 Infections caused by *Enterobacteriaceae.* Gram-negative rods are responsible for urinary infection, wound infection, pneumonia and gastroenteritis.

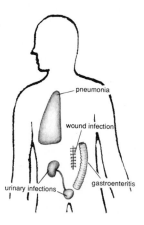

identification is important, for instance, in tracing the source of a food-borne infection. Many of these species carry plasmids, particularly plasmids which bear antibiotic resistance genes.

The *Enterobacteriaceae* are typically resident in the gut. *Escherichia coli* is by far the commonest cause of urinary infection, but *Proteus mirabilis* and *Klebsiella pneumoniae* are also regularly represented (Fig. 14.6).

E. coli sometimes causes a variety of other infections, e.g. meningitis in the neonate, pneumonia, gastroenteritis (p.141), wound infections, abscesses and bacteraemia, especially nosocomial bacteraemia. *Klebsiella, Enterobacter* and *Serratia* are encountered most often in hospital infections, chiefly pneumonia, bacteraemia and urinary infection. *Proteus* species cause urinary infection, both community- and hospital-acquired, and also hospital-acquired bacteraemia.

It is not uncommon to isolate a member of the *Enterobacteriaceae* or a *Pseudomonas* from hospitalised patients. Simply being ill appears to modify the flora of, for instance, the mouth and throat, so that the Gram-positive species are largely replaced by one or more Gram-negatives. This process is assisted by antibiotic therapy. When such a Gram-negative rod is isolated from sputum, urine or a wound, it is often difficult to decide whether it represents infection or simple colonisation, the latter being much commoner. In this case antibiotic therapy is not required.

SALMONELLA

Salmonella and *Shigella* are genera belonging to the *Enterobacteriaceae*. They ferment glucose, but not lactose or sucrose and hence bacteriologists screen diarrhoeal faeces for 'non-lactose-fermenters'. When biochemical tests give a tentative identification of *Salmonella*, this is confirmed by serotyping, using antisera against both O and H antigens. The number of serotypes is very large.

Salmonella serotypes commonly cause food poisoning in humans (see following, 'Salmonella for dinner'). Most are pathogens of animals; salmonellas have been isolated from virtually every animal. Transmission is mostly by the faecal/oral route — i.e. the victim consumes food or water that has been contaminated with human or animal faeces; however in hospitals patients have been infected by improperly sterilised instruments and by fomites. Throughout the world, *Salmonella* food poisoning is commoner in the warm weather. Some 6-48 hours after taking contaminated food or drink, persons become ill with nausea and vomiting, diarrhoea, fever and abdominal cramps (see p.141, infectious diarrhoea). Diarrhoea usually subsides within a week. Only rarely does the causative organism enter the bloodstream, and it can normally be recovered only from the faeces.

IN THE COMMUNITY
Salmonella **for dinner**

Most of the 1700 *Salmonella* serotypes have their primary reservoirs in animals — almost any animal, from chickens to snakes, from cats to parrots. And almost all of them have been studied because they also managed to multiply in the human gut.

About half the outbreaks of *Salmonella* food poisoning are traced to poultry or eggs; meats account for another one eighth. Modern food processing may lead to wide dissemination.

Sometimes the investigative trail is long: 500 cases of typhoid in Aberdeen, Scotland, were traced to preserved meat from the Argentine: the tins had been cooled in contaminated water after processing, and bacteria had entered as the contents contracted.

In 1981 there was an outbreak of food poisoning in a small town in Ohio, USA.

Investigators from the Centers for Disease Control were truly puzzled. There was no obvious link between the victims: they came from different social groups, they hadn't attended any social function together, they didn't eat in the same restaurants or drink at the same bars. It transpired, however, that they *had* all bought their *marihuana from the same dealer* — and the marihuana contained millions of *Salmonella* per gram. It had apparently been adulterated with dried manure — this gave it an unusual kick!

Humans are the only reservoir for *Salmonella typhi* and *Salmonella paratyphi*. Typhoid or enteric fever, due to *S. typhi*, is a severe illness characterised by fever, and less often diarrhoea, abdominal pain and vomiting. *S. typhi* enters the body in food or drink, penetrates the mucosal cells of the small intestine and moves to the lymphoid follicles, where it multiplies in mononuclear cells. From here organisms spread via the lymph to the blood and are removed by the mononuclear phagocytic system. Some organisms multiply in the gallbladder and re-enter the gut in the bile. Thus *S. typhi* can usually be isolated from the faeces only late in the illness. Antibiotic therapy considerably shortens the illness, which otherwise lasts 3-4 weeks. Patients excrete organisms in the stools for some weeks and a few become chronic asymptomatic carriers, excreting the organism for years.

SHIGELLA

Shigella species are unencapsulated and non-motile Gram-negative rods, very closely related to *E. coli*. In diagnosing enteritis, faeces should be processed immediately, as the numbers of *Shigella* fall rapidly with standing, and selective media are necessary. *Shigella* causes bacillary dysentery (dysentery is a diarrhoeal illness with blood and mucus in the stools and painful defaecation). In many campaigns (e.g. the Crimean War (1853-56)), epidemics of bacillary dysentery have probably caused more casualties than can be ascribed to weapons. Humans are the reservoir, transmission is by the faecal/oral route and a small percentage of sufferers become carriers.

ANTIBIOTIC THERAPY

Against members of the *Enterobacteriaceae* numerous antibiotics are active: some of the penicillins such as ampicillin, the cephalosporins, the aminoglycosides, tetracycline, trimethoprim and the quinolones. However many isolates of these species are resistant either intrinsically (e.g *Klebsiella pneumoniae* to ampicillin) or because of the acquisition of plasmids bearing resistance factors (p.63). In some hospitals multi-resistant *Klebsiella, Enterobacter* or *Proteus* strains establish themselves in the environment (which includes the *staff*) and are an endemic cause of nosocomial infection.

NON-FERMENTING GRAM-NEGATIVE RODS

Unlike the *Enterobacteriaceae*, which are mainly inhabitants or pathogens of the gut, the non-fermenting Gram-negative rods are *environmental* organisms. They are obligate aerobes and not fastidious, growing on most routine media, including MacConkey agar. Included in this group are the genera *Pseudomonas, Acinetobacter* and several others less commonly encountered.

PSEUDOMONAS

The natural habitats of *Pseudomonas* species are soil, water and plants. Only *Ps. mallei* is an obligate mammalian parasite, the rest are free-living, nutritionally versatile and undemanding, able to use a wide range of carbon compounds for growth. They are distinguished from most other Gram-negative rods by the oxidase test, which detects a particular type of carrier molecule in the electron-transport chain. In the hospital environment they may be found everywhere, often contaminating food and equipment of all sorts (from sinks to humidifiers) (Fig. 14.7).

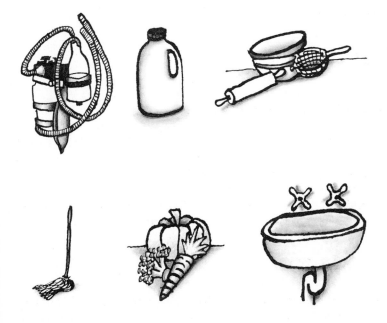

Fig. 14.7 Where *Pseudomonas aeruginosa* may be found in the hospital.

Ps. aeruginosa is the species most commonly isolated from human specimens, followed by *Ps. maltophilia*, *Ps. stutzeri* and *Ps. cepacia*. *Ps. aeruginosa* may occur in faeces, and faecal carriage is increased in hospitalised patients. It is a leading cause of nosocomial infection (see p.179), especially in patients with burns or malignancies or those who are otherwise compromised, and in intensive-care units, neurosurgical, spinal and other units where the patients are likely to have in-dwelling catheters or tracheostomies. Under these circumstances, pneumonia and urinary infection are common. *Ps. aeruginosa* is capable of producing devastating infections.

Ps. cepacia and *Ps. maltophilia* are also widespread in the hospital environment; the former may even grow in disinfectant solutions. These species are often isolated from compromised patients, but it is often uncertain whether they are responsible for disease or are simply colonists. Treatment of *Pseudomonas* infections is complicated by the fact that they are resistant to most antibiotics: the choice is usually limited to a few penicillins such as ticarcillin, one or two of the newest cephalosporins or an aminoglycoside (gentamicin, tobramycin or amikacin).

ACINETOBACTER

Members of the genus *Acinetobacter* are often found in soil and water. *Acinetobacter calcoaceticus* is an aerobic Gram-negative coccobacillus which grows readily on the usual media. It is a frequent commensal in human beings. Of low virulence, it tends to give rise to colonisation of patients much more often than to infection. It is most often isolated from sputum, urine, blood (when intravascular cannulae are present) and from wounds. Factors predisposing to colonisation/infection with *Acinetobacter* are: endotracheal tubes or tracheostomy, previous antibiotic therapy, instrumentation or surgery, wound drains or residence in the intensive care unit. *Acinetobacter* tends to be more resistant to antibiotics than the *Enterobacteriaceae*.

HAEMOPHILUS

The genus *Haemophilus* consists of pleomorphic Gram-negative organisms, appearing as small coccobacilli, often in short chains, and also sometimes forming long filaments (Fig. 14.8). For growth they require X and V growth factors (haemin and NAD), which are provided in chocolate agar. Even when present in large numbers in sputum *Haemophilus* may go undetected because of the overgrowth of commensals, and a selective medium should be used to eliminate the normal flora of the upper respiratory tract. Most isolates of *H. influenzae* are unencapsulated, but some possess a capsule, of which six antigenic types — a to f — are distinguished by agglutination with specific antisera. Most encapsulated clinical isolates are type b.

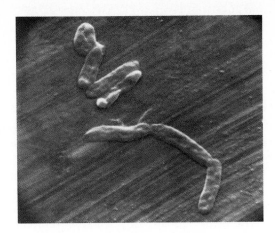

Fig. 14.8 *Haemophilus
influenzae*, a small Gram-
negative rod (scanning electronmicrograph).

Haemophilus species are obligate parasites of humans. Non-encapsulated *H. influenzae* and *H. parainfluenzae* belong to the normal flora of the upper respiratory tract, while encapsulated strains of *H. influenzae* are sometimes present there. Occasionally this asymptomatic colonisation gives rise to disease. Type b strains are almost always those responsible for infection, producing epiglottitis, pneumonia, osteomyelitis and meningitis (Fig. 14.9) — *H. influenzae* is the commonest cause of meningitis in children . Non-encapsulated strains produce sinusitis, otitis media and chronic or acute on chronic bronchitis. Recently *antibiotic resistance* has become a problem in *Haemophilus influenzae*. Fifteen to twenty per cent of isolates are now resistant to ampicillin and 1-2% to chloramphenicol. Because of this, in treating meningitis one now gives ampicillin + chloramphenicol or a third generation cephalosporin such as cefotaxime.

BORDETELLA PERTUSSIS

This is a very small non-motile Gram-negative coccobacillus, difficult to cultivate since it grows slowly and is fastidious. Isolating it requires careful attention to the collection and transport of the specimen and the preparation of the medium. *B. pertussis* is most readily isolated from the upper nasopharynx and specimens from this area are collected with a *pernasal swab* (a fine wire tipped with cottonwool, which is passed through the nostril to touch the back wall of the nose). The swab must be transported immediately to the laboratory, where special media are inoculated.

B. pertussis causes the disease *pertussis* or *whooping cough* (*pertussis* means 'a violent cough'). This is a worldwide disease and still a major cause of childhood illness and death in countries where vaccination is not practised. It is especially dangerous to children aged less than six months. It begins as a 'cold'; a cough develops after several days and progresses to paroxysms of coughing, ending in a characteristic 'whoop' or inhalation of air. Secondary bacterial infection may lead to otitis media, and most seriously to

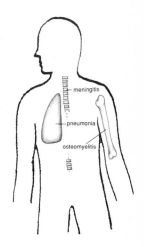

Fig. 14.9 Infections caused by *Haemophilus influenzae*. *H. influenzae* is a common cause of meningitis and osteomyelitis in children, and of pneumonia in adults.

pneumonia. Antibiotics have no effect once the cough has started, except to eliminate the bacteria and make the patient non-infectious. Vaccination is essential to control the infection. Pertussis vaccine has been incriminated as a cause of brain damage; a recent re-examination of the evidence indicates that this is unlikely.

LEGIONELLA

Legionella forms pleomorphic Gram-negative bacilli, motile, unencapsulated and non-sporing. It is more easily seen with special stains (Fig. 14.10). *Legionella* species are nutritionally fastidious in the laboratory, but apparently less so in their natural habitat. They can live and multiply within macrophages and within amoebae in natural waters. Isolation requires special media and may take up to a week. *Legionella* species are primarily saprophytes whose habitat is most forms of fresh water, including rivers, lakes, air-conditioning units and reticulated water supplies for drinking etc. *Legionella* has often been reported from hospital water supplies. Only a few species have so far proved to be dangerous for man.

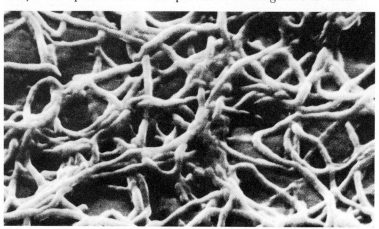

Fig. 14.10 *Legionella pneumophila* grows in long filaments (scanning electronmicrograph).

In disease, *Legionella* is isolated chiefly from the respiratory tract (see following, 'Old soldiers meet in Philadelphia'). Isolation is difficult to accomplish and serological tests are important for diagnosis. *Legionella* species, principally *L. pneumophila* and *L. micdadei*, are a major cause of pneumonia, both in the community and in the hospital; the incidence of infection varies from place to place and from hospital to hospital. It is technically difficult to carry out antibiotic susceptibility tests with *Legionella*. The most effective drug is thought to be erythromycin.

IN THE COMMUNITY
Old soldiers meet in Philadelphia

During six weeks of July and August 1976, 182 people in Philadelphia fell ill: the common symptoms were cough, fever and shaking chills, and most had an abnormal chest X-ray. Most were admitted to hospital and many required oxygen.

Twenty-nine people (16%) died. None of the usual causes for

pneumonia were demonstrated and an intense epidemiological investigation was begun by about 40 medical scientists.

It was discovered that most of the victims had attended an American Legion convention (the equivalent of Australia's 'RSL' for ex-servicemen). The attack rate among those who had stayed at 'Hotel A' was nearly 7% and was also significantly higher among people who had walked along the street outside the hotel.

No restaurant or food vendor was associated with the disease. Illness was more likely among smokers, and among people who had drunk water in the hotel, but was unrelated to drinking alcohol. No function room or group of bedrooms in 'Hotel A' was associated with an increased risk of the disease.

The conclusion from the epidemiological study was that the infection was most likely airborne; waterborne spread was unlikely because cases had occurred in people who walked past the hotel or who had stayed in the hotel but drunk no water.

An equally intense laboratory investigation succeeded in isolating a hitherto unknown Gram-negative bacillus by injecting preparations of lung tissue from fatal cases into guinea-pigs. This organism had failed to grow on the usual laboratory media.

This organism is now known as *Legionella pneumophila* and it has been shown to be a not uncommon cause of illness, often multiplying in the water of air-conditioning cooling towers.

CAMPYLOBACTER

The genus *Campylobacter* (Fig. 14.11) contains a number of species: Gram-negative, thin, spiral organisms which move rapidly. They grow more slowly than the usual gut flora and selective media are necessary for their isolation. *C. jejuni* and *C. coli* cause acute gastroenteritis in man. This is a common disease. It is a zoonosis, and animals are the main reservoir. Most infections appear to be

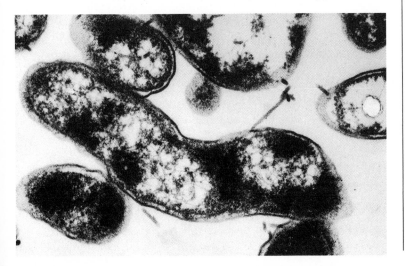

Fig. 14.11 *Campylobacter* are long, curved Gram-negative rods (scanning electronmicrograph).

acquired from contaminated food, especially poultry, which normally harbour campylobacters. In advanced countries *Campylobacter* and rotavirus are probably the commonest causes of infective diarrhoea. 'Travellers' diarrhoea' is also often due to *C. jejuni*. Another campylobacter, *Campylobacter pylori*, which is more difficult to grow, is found in the lesions of gastritis and may well be the cause of gastric ulcers.

VIBRIO

The genus *Vibrio* contains many species found in water, from fresh to salt. They are Gram-negative rods, straight or slightly curved (Fig. 14.12). They grow readily on ordinary media, which may require additional NaCl, since some species will not grow in less than 3% salt. Identification is by biochemical and serological tests. They are oxidase-positive.

Fig. 14.12 *Vibrio cholerae* is a slightly curved Gram-negative rod (scanning electron-micrograph).

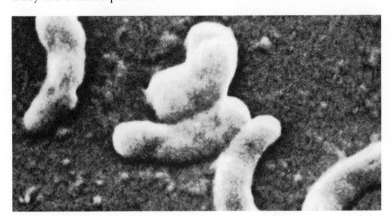

Vibrio cholerae causes gastroenteritis, from mild diarrhoea to fullblown cholera. Epidemic cholera is another of the great plagues — in the world pandemic since 1964, the organism has spread from South-East Asia into India, Africa and the Midddle East, and there have been outbreaks in Europe, the United States and the Pacific. Air travel ensures that no microbiology laboratory lies outside the range of this vibrio. The cholera toxin binds to the intestinal cell membrane and by a complex series of reactions stimulates the secretion of water and electrolytes. In severe cholera there is great loss of fluid and electrolytes in the 'rice-water stools', and the patient may die in a few hours if untreated. In treatment, replacement of fluid and electrolytes (mainly sodium, potassium and chloride ions) is much more important than antibiotics; this is largely true of any severe diarrhoea. Gastroenteritis may also be due to *V. parahaemolyticus* or other vibrios; *V. parahaemolyticus* may contaminate seafood. Vibrios may also cause non-enteric disease, such as wound infections, meningitis and bacteraemia.

SPIROCHETES: TREPONEMA PALLIDUM (SYPHILIS)

Spirochetes cause syphilis, Lyme arthritis and several other diseases.
Syphilis is caused by *Treponema pallidum*, a slender, tightly coiled

organism about 10 microns long (Fig. 14.13). It cannot be cultured and identification depends on detection of the organisms by microscopy in a suspicious lesion. The first manifestation of syphilis is the *primary chancre*, an ulcer which develops at the site where the spirochetes entered the body. After some weeks this is followed by secondary syphilis — in which stage the treponemes spread through the body, the patient develops skin rashes of various types, and is highly infectious. Years later, disease of the arteries or the nervous system may develop; the manifestations of syphilis are extremely varied. Antibiotic therapy has made the late forms of the disease very rare. *Treponema pallidum* has remained susceptible to penicillin, despite the almost universal use of this drug in syphilis.

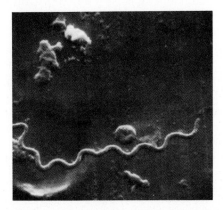

Fig. 14.13 *Treponema pallidum* (scanning electronmicrograph).

Serological tests. Because the treponeme cannot be grown in the laboratory, serological tests are of great importance in the diagnosis of syphilis. The Wassermann reaction (or WR), the RPR test and others detect antibodies to reagin, an antigen apparently produced in the reaction of the tissues to the treponeme, while the *Treponema pallidum* haemagglutination assay (TPHA) demonstrates antibodies to treponemal antigens. The reagin tests become negative with treatment, while the tests for treponemal antigens remain positive for many years.

INFECTIONS WITH ANAEROBES

There are a very large number of species of anaerobes; 400 or more have been distinguished in the gut flora alone. Their exact identification is usually a task for a specialised laboratory. Most of them rarely if ever cause infection. Anaerobes that may be involved in disease are:

- *Clostridium* species
- *Bacteroides* species
- *Fusobacterium* species
- Anaerobic staphylococci and streptococci.

Both the collection and the processing of a specimen intended for anaerobic culture are critical (see following, 'Rules for anaerobic specimens'). Once the specimen reaches the laboratory it

must be processed immediately and the media must be pre-treated
to remove oxygen. Some of the media should contain antibiotics to
inhibit the more rapidly growing facultative anaerobes (e.g.
Enterobacteriaceae).

CLOSTRIDIUM

The genus *Clostridium* consists of Gram-positive spore-forming rods
(Fig. 14.14). The natural habitat is the soil, and most are harmless
saprophytes. *Clostridium tetani*, found in faeces and soil, causes
tetanus. The organism enters a wound, often quite a trivial one,
and multiplies there, but does not spread. Sometimes indeed the
tetanus bacillus cannot be isolated from the patient. The organism
produces an extremely powerful toxin — one gram would probably
kill about a million people. The toxin binds firmly to nerve cells
and interferes with their function, producing cramps and stiffness,
progressing to violent spasms and lockjaw. The clinical picture is
quite characteristic. The mortality is still very high and the disease
remains common in the developing countries. It is completely preventable by vaccination — in the developed countries tetanus is
now as much a 'self-inflicted' disease as is lung cancer. In the
Third World tetanus of the newborn is a serious problem. It is preventable by vaccination of the mother during pregnancy.

Fig. 14.14 *Clostridium tetani*,
showing spores (scanning
electronmicrograph).

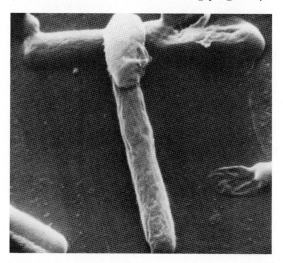

Clostridium botulinum is found in soil. Its toxin, about as powerful
as tetanus toxin, produces the disease *botulism*, the main symptom
of which is paralysis. Most often the disease is due to eating food in
which the clostridium has multiplied because the canning or preserving process has been improperly carried out (e.g. home-pre-
served vegetables, fruit or fish). Again the mortality is high. Both
tetanus and botulism are difficult to treat, because there is no way
of removing the toxin once it has combined with the nervous system.
Antiserum will mop up unbound toxin, but treatment largely consists
of keeping the patient alive while the disease runs its course.

Clostridium perfringens and a few other clostridia cause wound infections. The wound is usually deep and contaminated with soil. The toxins produced by the clostridia break down adjacent healthy muscle and the infection progresses rapidly. In this condition the organism multiplies and spreads in the victim. The disease is termed gas gangrene and is readily fatal.

Clostridium difficile — one of the undesirable effects of antibiotic therapy may be diarrhoea accompanied by inflammation of the colon ('colitis'). The antibiotic therapy modifies the normal flora of the gut, so that *C. difficile* can outgrow the flora and produce its toxin, the result being colitis. The patient may have been a carrier of *C. difficile* or may have acquired it from outside. *C. difficile* may be transferred from patient to patient in the hospital - it is an important cause of nosocomial infection.

IN THE WARD
Rules for collecting anaerobic specimens
Rule 1. Collect specimens only from normally sterile sites — deep abscesses, (e.g. in liver, lung or brain), fluids from body cavities (such as pleural or peritoneal fluid) and tissue biopsies (not including skin). Do *not* collect them from the respiratory tract, the genital tract or any other site normally colonised by a bacterial flora, since these specimens will naturally show large numbers of anaerobes and the results will be uninterpretable.
Rule 2. Exclude oxygen as far as possible while collecting and transporting the specimen. A specimen of pus is best collected and transported in a syringe from which all air is first expelled. If the specimen must be collected as a swab, then this should be transported in a special anaerobic transport container (which contains chemicals to remove oxygen). Pieces of tissue should be placed in similar containers.
Rule 3. Take the specimen to the laboratory as soon as possible — *a good rule for any specimen.*

NON-SPORING ANAEROBES

Most other anaerobic infections are caused by the normal flora. If the barriers that contain the flora are disrupted by injury, by surgical or dental treatment or if the person's defences are compromised by cancer, vascular disease or otherwise, anaerobic infection may result. Such infections are often due to several organisms, both aerobes and anaerobes - the combination seems to act synergistically. Despite their aversion to oxygen, anaerobes occur in about 5% of blood cultures. Anaerobic infections may affect the skin and soft tissues, the head and neck, the lungs, abdomen, female genital tract or the brain. The species likely to be involved are *Bacteroides* (especially *B. fragilis*), *Fusobacterium*, *Clostridium*, anaerobic cocci and others (Fig. 14.15).

Fig. 14.15 *Bacteroides fragilis* is an anaerobic Gram-negative rod (scanning electron-micrograph).

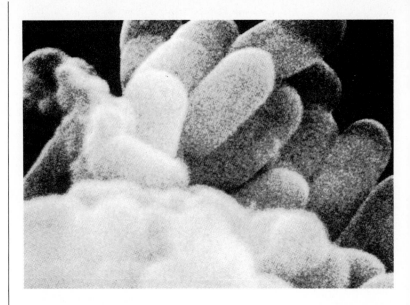

Traumatic wounds, surgical wounds and bites (animal or human!) often contain anaerobes. In the lungs, inhalation of vomitus may lead to the formation of an abscess containing anaerobes. Various infections of the female genital tract (e.g. puerperal sepsis, pelvic abscess, septic abortion and post-operative infections) are chiefly due to anaerobes — *Bacteroides* and Gram-positive cocci. When the wall of the gut is breached by disease (diverticulitis, obstruction or cancer) or by trauma or surgery, both aerobes and anaerobes soil the peritoneal cavity; peritonitis and/or an abscess may result.

ANTIBIOTIC THERAPY

Many of the antibiotics active against aerobes also work against anaerobes. Clindamycin, cefoxitin, chloramphenicol, and some penicillins (e.g. piperacillin, ticarcillin) are active against most anaerobes, as is the 'anaerobe' antibiotic, metronidazole. Benzylpenicillin is effective against some *Bacteroides* spp, and against Gram-positive anaerobes. Clostridia and anaerobic Gram-positive cocci are susceptible to penicillins and cephalosporins.

MYCOPLASMAS

Mycoplasmas, which we can think of as small Gram-negative bacteria lacking a cell wall (Fig. 4.11), are ubiquitous, occurring in many animals, on plants and in the environment. They cause various plant and animal diseases. In man, *Mycoplasma pneumoniae* is a cause of pneumonia and other mycoplasmas are associated with genital disease. *M. pneumoniae* is filamentous and about 0.2 x 0.01 microns in size. It requires a medium containing yeast extract and serum, on which it grows slowly. *M. pneumoniae* causes acute infections of the respiratory tract, most often tracheobronchitis, but also a relatively mild pneumonia (primary atypical pneumonia), the usual symptoms of which are a dry cough, malaise and headache (see following, 'Jaundice with a cough'). Patients rarely need hospitalisation. The organism is resistant to anti-cell-wall antibiotics, penicillins and cephalosporins, since it has no cell wall; erythromycin and tetracycline, which interfere with protein synthesis, are effective clinically. Infection is usually accompanied by the appearance in the blood of 'cold agglutinins', antibodies which cause the clumping of red cells only at low temperatures. This test, however, is not always positive and is being replaced by antibody tests specific for mycoplasmal antigens. In the genital tract several mycoplasmas have been isolated (two commonly), but their exact role in disease is still unclear; it is likely that they are involved in non-gonococcal urethritis, pyelonephritis and pelvic inflammatory disease.

IN THE WARD
Jaundice with a cough

Alana Gardiner, aged 40, began to feel ill about five weeks before she was admitted to Hospital. Initially she felt 'sick', weak and suffered from headache.

Two weeks before admission she had developed a cough without much sputum and felt 'hot'. Her local doctor diagnosed a viral infection and gave her ampicillin and a cough syrup.

Two days before admission she had felt worse, with increased coughing, nausea and vomiting. Her local doctor arranged a chest X-ray; this showed some consolidation in the R upper lung. That afternoon her husband pointed out that she looked 'yellow', and her urine became dark; because of this evidence of jaundice she came to Emergency and was admitted to hospital.

Investigations confirmed the presence of pneumonia and showed that she had anaemia due to breakdown (haemolysis) of her red cells by an antibody. This antibody has the unusual property that, in the test-tube, it causes red cells to clump only at temperatures below 37^{0}C and hence is termed a 'cold agglutinin'. This antibody is characteristic of infection with *Mycoplasma pneumoniae*. In the body the antibody reacts with red cells so that they are rapidly destroyed, producing anaemia and jaundice; the dark urine is due to the excretion of broken-down blood pigments (haemoglobin).

Mrs Gardiner was treated with tetracycline and got better over the following two weeks. (The ampicillin which she had taken previously has no action on *Mycoplasma pneumoniae*, since this organism has no cell wall.)

RICKETTSIAE AND CHLAMYDIAE

Rickettsiae and *chlamydiae* are both small intracellular bacterial parasites (Fig. 4.12).

Rickettsiae are responsible for a number of serious infections: epidemic typhus, scrub typhus, Q fever, Rocky Mountain spotted fever and others. The reservoirs are usually wild rodents, and the vector a tick or louse (Plates 16–18). The symptoms commonly include fever, headache and rash. Epidemic (louse-borne) typhus is one of the great plagues that follow war and famine; in Eastern Europe from 1918 to 1922, 30 million cases occurred. The cause is *Rickettsia prowazekii*, and the vector the body louse. Scrub typhus occurs in Eastern Asia and the Western Pacific. It is a zoonosis transmitted from rodent to rodent by mites and humans are an accidental host. Q fever is due to *Coxiella burnetii*. Infection is by inhalation of airborne organisms (not via an arthropod vector), and the disease is an occupational hazard of abattoir workers, veterinarians, stockmen, and the like. In this disease myalgia is prominent and rash rare; pneumonia, hepatitis and endocarditis are common manifestations; diagnosis is clinical and by serological tests. Isolation of rickettsiae should be attempted only in special facilities, since they are highly contagious. Against the rickettsial infections either chloramphenicol or tetracycline is an effective drug.

The genus *Chlamydia* contains two species, both of which infect humans. *C. trachomatis* has numerous serotypes. It causes trachoma, nongonococcal urethritis and other venereal diseases, perinatal eye and respiratory infections. Trachoma is a chronic conjunctivitis

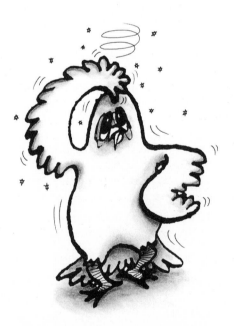

that leads to blindness. Worldwide probably *300 000 000 people* have trachoma. *C. trachomatis* (other serotypes) represents probably the commonest cause of sexually transmitted disease, causing urethritis, cervicitis and acute pelvic inflammatory disease. Around 5% of pregnant women have *C. trachomatis* genital infection, and about two thirds of their infants become infected after vaginal delivery; most get conjunctivitis, but about one fifth get pneumonia.

C. psittaci infects many birds and mammals (*psittaci* means 'of the parrot'); the infection is transmissible to humans by inhalation of dried faeces and such — beware the sick budgerigar! The illness begins with fever, malaise, cough and lower respiratory infection. The disease is diagnosed from the clinical picture and by serological investigations. Tetracycline or erythromycin is the most effective therapy for all forms of chlamydial infection.

CHAPTER REVIEW

1   Describe briefly the infections caused by staphylococci.
2   What antibiotics are active against
   (a)   staphylococci?
   (b)   streptococci?
3   Name some diseases caused by microbial toxins.
4   (a)   What is MRSA?
   (b)   Why is it an important pathogen?
5   List the various groups of streptococci and the diseases that they cause.
6   (a)   What are acid-fast bacilli?
   (b)   What diseases do they cause?
   (c)   What antibiotics should be used against this group of organisms?
7   (a)   What Gram-negative cocci are of clinical importance?
   (b)   Name the two most frequently isolated organisms and the diseases they produce.
8   (a)   List six species of Gram-negative rods, indicating the diseases they produce.
   (b)   Where are these organisms normally found?
   (c)   Which antibiotics are likely to be active against them?
9   Name some Gram-negative rods that are likely to be found in hospitals.
10   (a)   Briefly explain the diseases caused by *Salmonella typhi* and other *Salmonella* species.
   (b)   How are these infections transmitted?
11   (a)   What infections are caused by Gram-negative anaerobes?
   (b)   Which antibiotics should be used to treat these infections?
12   Which organisms often cause urinary infection?

15

VIRAL INFECTIONS

Over 500 viruses are so far known to infect humans. These are grouped into about 20 families. In general, viruses tend to affect only one organ system and to cause only one type of disease. Here we have space to discuss only some of the major types of illness and the viruses which cause them: the respiratory tract infections, hepatitis, and the herpes group of viruses. (Gastroenteritis is discussed on p.141, meningitis on p.144 and AIDS on p.256.) Table 15.1 sets out some features of viral infections.

TABLE 15.1 PATHOGENIC CHARACTERISTICS OF VIRUSES

Virus	Main target	Portal of entry	Also affects
Influenza	RT	RT	
Parainfluenza	RT	RT	
Respiratory syncytial virus	RT	RT	
Rhinoviruses	RT	RT	
Adenoviruses	RT	RT	
Coronaviruses	RT	RT	
Rubella	RT	RT	Skin
Measles	RT	RT	Skin, brain
Mumps	RT	RT	CNS, testes, ovaries
Echoviruses } Rotaviruses	gut	gut	
Hepatitis A, B, C	liver	gut, blood	
Polioviruses	CNS	gut	
Coxsackieviruses	CNS	gut	Upper RT

Herpes simplex	CNS	skin, mucosa, genitalia	
Wart viruses	skin	skin	
HIV	T cells	genitals	CNS

[*Note:* RT = *respiratory tract,* CNS = *central nervous system (brain and spinal cord)*]

RESPIRATORY TRACT INFECTION (RTI)

Respiratory tract infections produce a variety of symptoms and clinical syndromes ('syndrome' means 'group of symptoms'):
- *common cold* upper respiratory tract infection or 'URTI', needs no description
- *pharyngitis* sore throat
- *croup* difficulty in breathing accompanied by 'crowing' inspiration (i.e. when breathing 'in')
- *tracheobronchitis* inflammation of the main airways
- *pneumonia* inflammation of the lung (p.140)
- *sinusitis* inflammation of the sinuses (mucosa-lined cavities in the bones forming the walls of the nose)
- *otitis media* inflammation of the middle ear (the cavity which lies behind the ear-drum).

'COLDS'

Viruses are the cause of most respiratory tract infections. The *common cold* is an infection of the upper respiratory tract (nose and throat); the virus multiplies in the cells of the mucous membrane. The viruses known to be involved include rhinoviruses (the commonest cause), coronaviruses, respiratory syncytial virus, adenoviruses and more. They number well over 100 in total and there are likely to be a lot still undiscovered. The *rhinoviruses* appear to spread in nasal secretions transferred by close contact (nose to hand to hand of second individual to nose), some of the others spread in aerosols. Young children are the main reservoir of cold viruses, acquiring new strains from their schoolfellows and bringing them home to the family. Mild sore throat is common in colds. Colds are commoner in late autumn through to early spring; the reason for this is unknown. It is also interesting to note that cigarette smokers get no more colds than non-smokers, but are more severely ill.

A long-lasting immunity to the particular infecting virus develops after infection. Unfortunately, as there are over 100 different types and as the antibody produced in response to infection is type-specific, one individual can suffer numerous infections. The problems of producing a vaccine against the common cold are obviously formidable.

Fig. 15.1 The influenza virion. Influenza is an enveloped helical virus. It is unusual in that the RNA genome consists of several distinct sections. Inside the envelope lie 8 segments of RNA, each enclosed in its own helical capsid. Haemagglutinin and neuraminidase spikes protrude from the envelope. These proteins are important in the pathogenesis of infection and in its diagnosis.

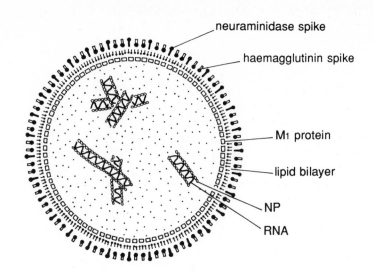

neuraminidase spike

haemagglutinin spike

M1 protein

lipid bilayer

NP

RNA

There is only symptomatic treatment for colds. *Antibiotics should be given only for bacterial pharyngitis, (i.e. where the cause is streptococcal sore throat), and are useless for a 'cold'.* They do not cure the viral infection, nor do they lessen the chance of acquiring a bacterial infection such as sinusitis or otitis media.

RESPIRATORY SYNCYTIAL VIRUS (RSV)

As well as causing 'colds' in older children, this virus causes most of the lower respiratory tract infections in young children (pneumonia and bronchiolitis). RSV is highly infectious — immunity is poor and repeated infections are common in childhood.

Influenza is an Italian word: it was once believed that epidemics occurred under the *influence* of a malign configuration of the stars. The *influenza* viruses, types A and B (Fig. 15.1), *are not responsible for the sporadic illness we call 'flu'*. In true influenza, fever, headache, aches and pains and cough are usually prominent, but the influenza viruses may give rise to any of the other forms of respiratory infection, a 'cold', sore throat, bronchitis, or even pneumonia. And any of the respiratory viruses, rhinoviruses, adenoviruses, respiratory syncytial virus, may cause illnesses with 'flu' symptoms.

However, unlike these respiratory infections, true influenza occurs in epidemics every 1-2 years, usually in the winter, and isolated cases do not occur. (See following, 'Influenza strikes worldwide'). The protein antigens of influenza A change rapidly, so that antibody to this year's strain will only protect for a year or two — and vaccines likewise rapidly become obsolete.

IN THE COMMUNITY
Influenza strikes worldwide

In 1918-1919 influenza swept across the world in the most devastating pandemic of this century. A *pandemic* is a disease occurring across a whole nation, continent, or the whole world). *About 20 million people died,* and a large part of the world population became ill.

In influenza, death is usually due to secondary bacterial pneumonia: the virus somehow undermines the lung defences and *Staphylococcus aureus, Streptococcus pneumoniae* or *Haemophilus influenzae* can set up infection.

There have since been further pandemics — in 1957, 1968 and 1977. These have corresponded to major shifts in the antigens of the virus: new antigens appear, with which antibodies acquired in previous outbreaks do not react. The 1957 Asian influenza pandemic probably arose in central China and from there spread across the world.

Human influenza viruses are related to those of birds — possibly new human strains may arise by exchanging genes with avian strains.

In between pandemics, *epidemics* occur every few years; the viruses causing these infections show minor antigenic changes.

PHARYNGITIS ('SORE THROAT')

In pharyngitis there is soreness and marked redness of the throat, with or without an inflammatory exudate. Pharyngitis is mostly caused by respiratory viruses, but about 20% of cases are due to group A streptococci. It is impossible to decide clinically which infections are streptococcal, so a throat swab should be examined, since antibiotic treatment of a streptococcal pharyngitis shortens the duration of symptoms and prevents the complications (rheumatic fever and glomerulonephritis).

Otitis media occasionally complicates a cold or arises spontaneously. Bacteria are isolated in about two thirds of cases — *Streptococcus pneumoniae* is the commonest cause, followed by *Haemophilus influenzae* and *Branhamella catarrhalis*. *Sinusitis* is most often a bacterial infection complicating a viral cold and has much the same causes as otitis media. Note that these organisms may occur in the normal upper respiratory tract, so that nose swabs and throat swabs tell us nothing about the cause of the otitis/sinusitis.

Infections of the lower respiratory tract include acute *(tracheo)bronchitis* (usually due to the respiratory viruses already mentioned) and pneumonia, which we discussed above (p.140).

HEPATITIS

Hepatitis is an inflammation of the liver. Microbial hepatitis is usually viral and due to hepatitis A virus (HAV); hepatitis B virus (HBV); and hepatitis C virus (HCV). When one of these viruses multiplies in the liver it interferes with the activities of the liver cells, as shown by the abnormal liver function tests and the raised serum bilirubin, which may be detectable as jaundice (bilirubin is the pigment present in the serum in jaundice). The illness typically begins with malaise (the individual feels ill, easily fatigued, and lethargic), nausea and vomiting, headache, and sometimes fever. Liver function tests become abnormal within a few days, followed by the onset of jaundice, dark urine and a raised serum bilirubin.

HEPATITIS A (HAV)

Hepatitis A is a small RNA virus which has not yet been grown in cell culture; experimental work is being done with primates. It is found worldwide and humans constitute the reservoir. The incubation period is about one month. The illness lasts a few weeks and is very rarely fatal. Most infections appear to be subclinical: studies show nearly half the population of the USA has antibodies, although only one tenth of those can recall such an illness.

The virus is shed in the faeces. The virus is highly contagious and can be spread by contaminated food and drink, as well as by close personal contact. Transmission is by the faecal/oral route and this fact presumably explains the high frequency of serum antibodies in the developing countries, which lack adequate housing and sanitary facilities.

Unlike HBV, HAV is only briefly present in the blood, and infection via hypodermic needles or transfusion is rare. Again unlike HBV, persistent infection and carriage of the virus appear not to occur. One infection produces a solid immunity.

As the virus cannot be cultured, diagnosis is clinical and by serological tests for the presence of anti-HAV IgG and IgM. There is no vaccine, one is hardly necessary, since infection rarely leads to death, but human immune globulin protects after exposure.

HEPATITIS B (HBV)

Hepatitis B virus (Fig. 15.2) causes a similar, but more serious illness, with an insidious onset and a prolonged course. Hepatitis A and B cannot be distinguished on clinical grounds. Hepatitis B has a longer incubation period than A; as with hepatitis A, subclinical infections appear to be very frequent. Some 5-10% of patients do not eliminate HBV from their blood or liver and become carriers — most of them are symptomless. In the acute phase of HBV infection all patients are infective, as are chronic carriers with liver disease.

Infection with HBV, for which the only reservoir is humans, is by parenteral transfer — either through the skin or through mucous membranes. The main high-risk groups are infants of carrier mothers, recipients of blood transfusions, drug addicts sharing needles, homosexuals and heterosexuals with many partners, laboratory workers, and dentists. (Fig. 15.3). *Infection can clearly take place by heterosexual intercourse.*

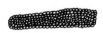

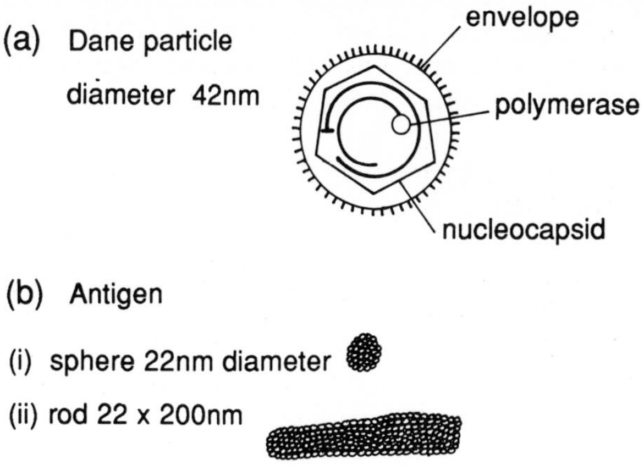

(a) Dane particle

diameter 42nm

envelope

polymerase

nucleocapsid

(b) Antigen

(i) sphere 22nm diameter

(ii) rod 22 x 200nm

Fig. 15.2 HBV particles. **(a)** Dane particle and **(b)** antigen. The Dane particles contain DNA and are infectious; the 22 nm particles and the rod-shaped particles consist of antigen only, and are not infectious.

Blood and blood products are the most obvious sources of the virus, but it is also found in almost any other body fluid: urine, sweat, saliva, semen, vaginal secretions. HBV is quite stable and transmission is possible via toothbrushes, razors, eating utensils and hospital equipment. Ordinary hygiene is sufficient to prevent transmission to or from health-care workers during casual contacts (see following, 'An obstetric afterthought').

IN THE WARD
An obstetric afterthought

Late one Friday afternoon, Ms Georgia Lees presented to the hospital Maternity Unit. She was in early labour. Ms Lees was 22, and this was her first child. She had not seen her local doctor, nor had she attended a prenatal clinic. Ms Lees stated that she was normally in good health.

As she was being (rather hurriedly) put to bed, the nurse noticed that she had several injection marks over the veins in her left arm. On being questioned Ms Lees admitted that she regularly used heroin. She then consented to being tested for hepatitis, but refused testing for AIDS.

The serology laboratory performed tests for hepatitis B immediately (modern automated equipment makes it possible to obtain results within an hour); Ms Lees proved to be a carrier of hepatitis B. She was nursed with the appropriate precautions (universal blood and body fluids precautions). Soon after birth her son, who appeared normal, was given hyperimmune anti-HBV globulin and his first dose of HBV vaccine.

He has better than a 90% chance of not acquiring the virus.

HBV infection is detected by serological tests for the protein surface antigen of HBV (HBsAg), and for antibody to it (anti-HBs).

Test for other antigens and for antibodies to them, e.g. antibody to the core protein, give additional information about the progress of the infection. All blood is now screened for HBV, but even the most sensitive tests available still appear not to detect the virus in 5-10% of blood donations. HBV infection differs from HAV infection in that at some stage the virus DNA may become integrated into the DNA of the liver cells. Chronic infection may lead to permanent liver damage and to cancer of the liver.

HBV represents one of the great public health problems. There are over 200 million chronic carriers in the world. Carriage rates are less than 1% in Western Europe, North America and Australia, 4% in Asia and 7% in Africa. In the developing countries, the commonest means of acquiring HBV is exposure to the blood of an infected mother during or immediately after birth. There is now an effective vaccine (see box p.123, 'Molecular biology and Hepatitis B'). Infection of neonates can be prevented in about 90% of cases if the baby is given vaccine and immunglobulin soon after birth — so it now appears possible to eliminate the virus from the world. It is important that *all* pregnant women should be screened for HBV, since simply testing high-risk groups misses some carriers (see following, 'Who needs Hepatitis B vaccine?').

Boy meets boy

Boy meets girl
(or girl meets boy)

Blood transfusion

IN THE COMMUNITY
Who needs Hepatitis B vaccine?
- newborn babies of carrier mothers
- household and sexual contacts of HBV carriers
- Intravenous (IV) drug users
- prostitutes
- homosexuals
- police and prison warders
- all health-care students and personnel
- municipal and other workers (who may encounter needles while cleaning up rubbish)
- patients at increased risk (e.g. haemodialysis patients and those with coagulation disorders)

IV drug use

Mother and child

Needle - stick injury

Fig. 15.3 Transmission of HBV and HIV.

HEPATITIS C

Blood transfusion also leads to cases of hepatitis in which neither HAV nor HBV can be demonstrated: *hepatitis C* ('Non-A Non-B hepatitis'). Infection is usually symptomless, but permanent liver damage may nevertheless result. Now that a diagnostic test has been developed for hepatitis C virus, more information about it will soon be available.

Human immunodeficiency virus (HIV) and AIDS are discussed on p.256.

HERPESVIRUSES

This family of viruses is responsible for several common infections of humans: herpes simplex, herpes zoster (chickenpox and shingles), cytomegalovirus infection and infectious mononucleosis (Epstein-Barr virus, glandular fever). A common feature of the family is the production of latent or recurrent infections. They are large viruses, 180-200 nanometres in diameter, and the genome is made up of double-stranded DNA. They produce inclusion bodies within the nuclei of the host cells (Plate 20), where the viral DNA is synthesised and virus particles are assembled. The viral particles have a complex structure and contain 25 or more virus-specific proteins (Fig. 15.4).

Fig. 15.4 The virion of herpes simplex virus. The DNA is wound on a protein 'spool' and contained in the capsid. Outside this there is a layer of protein and then the envelope.

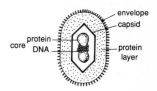

HERPES SIMPLEX VIRUS (HSV)

Herpes simplex viruses are of two types. *Type 1* causes lesions chiefly of the mouth and eye, and is transmitted in upper respiratory tract secretions, while *type 2* attacks the genitals and the anus and is transmitted sexually; however, each can cause infection in the area of the other. The lesions begin as fluid-filled vesicles, which ulcerate and take several days to heal. The infection can be

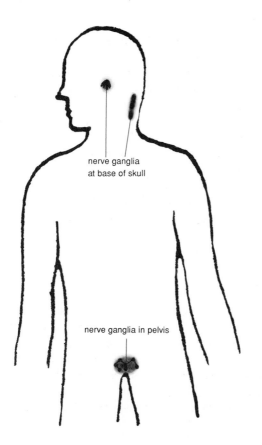

Fig. 15.5 Sites of latency of herpes simplex. After a primary infection the virus becomes latent in nerve ganglia and cannot be detected by culture. Periodically the infection recurs.

detected by growth of the virus in cell culture or by the presence in the specimen of specific antigens demonstrated by ELISA or immunofluorescence.

About 80% of adults have antibodies to the virus and also cell-mediated immunity. A good proportion of these have recurrent herpes. Herpes simplex virus is notable for its latency and ability to recur. The initial infection with herpes simplex type 1 usually takes place in children of 6-18 months and is asymptomatic in most cases, though sometimes vesicles develop in and around the mouth. The virus migrates via the nerves to the nerve ganglia of the region, where it persists (Fig. 15.5). Under many different stimuli — sunlight, heat or cold, unrelated immunological reactions or infections, menstruation and even emotional disturbances — the virus may move back down the nerve and produce a fresh crop of vesicles. Recurrences are usually preceded by tingling or itching in the affected area. The virus is transmitted in the secretions from the lesions.

TREATMENT

Acyclovir is useful in primary genital herpes, but it suppresses recurrences only while treatment continues. No drug currently leads to permanent cure.

VARICELLA-ZOSTER VIRUS

The viruses isolated from *chickenpox* (varicella) and from *herpes zoster* (shingles) are indistinguishable. Chickenpox is usually a mild self-limited disease in young children; it apparently spreads by the respiratory route and reaches the skin via the blood. The rash begins as papules which rapidly turn into vesicles. In adults, varicella can be a more serious and even fatal infection, often manifested as viral pneumonia.

Herpes zoster or *shingles* (Plate 19) is the *recurrent* form of varicella; it occurs in persons with circulating antibody. During the first attack the virus travels from the skin up the nerves to the sensory nerve ganglia, where it lies latent until activated by certain drugs, illnesses or events. In an attack of shingles the virus probably travels back down the nerve to the related area of skin and a crop of vesicles appears in the area supplied by that nerve — hence the localised distribution of the rash in herpes zoster. The rash lasts a few weeks, the pain weeks or months.

CYTOMEGALOVIRUS (CMV)

Cytomegalovirus (literally 'cell-big-virus') is so-called because infected cells grow very large and have massive nuclear inclusion bodies (Plate 20). The virus can be grown in cell culture, but only slowly: isolation may take weeks. The virus appears to be ubiquitous. Like Epstein-Barr virus and poliomyelitis, it is probably encountered by almost everyone if living conditions are crowded and hygiene poor. Surveys show 40-100% of different populations to possess antibodies, according to socioeconomic circumstances; thus antibodies are commoner in Africa and Southeast Asia. The virus is acquired *in utero*, perinatally (during birth or from infected breast milk) or in adulthood, possibly related to sexual spread. Seropositivity is very high in male homosexuals. Blood transfusion may bring infection.

In adults CMV may cause 'glandular fever' (see *Epstein-Barr virus*). The virus may be acquired by contact, sexual or other, with an infected person or by blood transfusion. Infection is common in the immunocompromised (transplant patients, patients with AIDS), where it can cause pneumonia, retinitis, hepatitis and generalised disease — and may be fatal. So far there are no very effective drugs, and vaccines are at an early stage of development. CMV in pregnancy is discussed on p.261.

EPSTEIN-BARR VIRUS (EBV) AND GLANDULAR FEVER

This is the commonest cause of infectious mononucleosis or 'glandular fever' (CMV, *Toxoplasma gondii*, rubella and the initial phase of HIV infection are other possible causes). In most parts of the world, infection occurs during the early years, via the oral route, and the infection is subclinical. In the developed countries, presumably because of better hygiene and reduced traffic in secretions, primary infection takes place in the teens, and about half of those infected show the symptoms of 'glandular fever': swollen and often tender lymph nodes, an enlarged spleen, fever, sore throat and sometimes hepatitis, a rash or other disorders.

Large abnormal lymphocytes, 'mononuclear cells', appear in the blood, hence the term 'mononucleosis'. The symptoms usually clear in a few weeks, but EBV persists even for months in the oropharyngeal secretions. Diagnosis is based on the presence of the 'atypical lymphocytes' in the blood, on antibodies to viral antigens and on the detection of heterophile antibodies (aggglutinins for sheep red cells) by the Paul-Bunnell test or by various kits.

CHAPTER REVIEW

1   (a)   List the main viral causes of respiratory infection.
    (b)   What causes *'the flu'*?
2   (a)   What is viral hepatitis?
    (b)   Explain the differences between hepatitis A, hepatitis B, and non A-non B hepatitis (hepatitis C).
    (c)   Who should hepatitis B vaccine be offered to, and why?
3   What infections do the herpesviruses cause?
4   List the causes of 'glandular fever'.

16

FUNGAL AND PARASITIC INFECTIONS

FUNGAL INFECTIONS

Of the 50 000 or more species of fungi known, less than 200 have caused disease in humans. Most fungi appear to lack the necessary mechanisms of invasion — even the fundamental prerequisite of being able to grow at 35^0C. Infection may be superficial, confined to the skin or mucous membranes; or generalised, involving the deep tissues. According to the clinical circumstances, the same fungus may cause a superficial or deep infection. Superficial infections such as tinea can be acquired by direct contact with infected persons or fomites. Systemic fungal infections are usually acquired from the environment and almost never transferred from person to person. Disease may be initiated by inhalation of fungal spores and hence spread from the lungs; histoplasmosis is an example.

DERMATOPHYTES

One group of fungi, the *dermatophytes*, attacks the skin, nails and hair. They secrete an enzyme which breaks down keratin, a major protein of these structures. Infection of the skin — especially of the feet, but also of the skin on the hands and body — is called *tinea* or 'ringworm' and is most often caused by *Trichophyton, Epidermophyton* and *Microsporum* species (Plates 58 and 59). Infection of the nails, in particular, may respond only slowly to treatment. The yeast *Candida albicans* infects the mucosa of the mouth, *thrush*, and the vagina (see candidal *vaginitis* p.253) and can also cause paronychia, an infection of the nailbed (Plate 21).

SYSTEMIC (DEEP) INFECTIONS

Systemic infections by fungi are uncommon unless the patient's resistance is lowered by illness or drugs. Such infections may be due to *Candida* (Plates 45 and 57), to *Cryptococcus neoformans* and less often to *Aspergillus*. The commonest manifestations of *Cryptococcus neoformans* infection are meningitis and lung disease. This yeast has a large capsule, by which it can be recognised in body fluids and tissues (Plate 5). Antimicrobials active against systemic fungal infections are amphotericin B, 5-fluorocytosine and fluconazole; miconazole or clotrimazole are effective in vaginal candidiasis.

PARASITIC INFECTIONS

The following table lists sources of major parasitic infection.

TABLE 16.1 SOME IMPORTANT PARASITES

Parasite	Numbers of persons infected:
Ancylostoma duodenale Necator americanus }	c. 500 million
Ascaris lumbricoides	c. 1 billion
Entamoeba histolytica	c. 500 million
Enterobius vermicularis	c. 1 billion
Plasmodium spp.	c. 800 million
Schistosoma spp	c. 250 million
Strongyloides stercoralis	50-100 million
Taenia saginata	c. 50 million
Trichuris trichiura	c. 500 million
Wuchereria and other filariae	c. 250 million

HELMINTHS: FLATWORMS AND NEMATODES

Parasites of concern in human medicine may be unicellular or multicellular (chapter 4). In particular, the multicellular ones have complex life-cycles. The *helminths* constitute two groups: the *flatworms* and the *nematodes* (or *roundworms*).

The flatworms consist of the flukes and the tapeworms; most flatworms are hermaphrodite (i.e. they possess both male and female organs).

The flukes are relatively small (a body length measured in millimetres), and have a rudimentary digestive system. In the typical life-cycle there are two hosts. When the egg hatches, the larva penetrates a snail, the *intermediate host*, and in its body develops into a *sporocyst* from which motile larvae, *cercariae*, are liberated. These infect the second, *definitive host*: a human or other animal — the adult worm may inhabit the gut, lung or blood vessels.

The tapeworms have long ribbon-like bodies, which may attain a length of several metres — made up of individual segments, the *proglottids*, each containing male and female reproductive organs.

Tapeworms have no digestive system and absorb nutrients through the surface of the body. In their life-cycle they may have one or two intermediate hosts, as well as the definitive host.

The nematodes or round worms are among the most successful organisms on earth, since they parasitise almost every species of animal and insect and also live free in soil and water. Nematodes have a functioning digestive system. They may parasitise many different organs.

Parasites may be classified in various ways. From a diagnostic standpoint they can be divided into those for which the diagnosis is based on the examination of an excretion (most often faeces, occasionally urine or sputum) and those for which diagnosis demands collection of blood or tissue for examination. Parasitic infections of either class may also be revealed by serological tests. The main technique used in the diagnosis of parasitic infestations is microscopy. The eggs, cysts and trophozoites are very varied in size and shape (Plates 64–71) and are sufficiently individual for the infecting organism to be identified simply by microscopic appearance. A good number of parasites live in the gut, and their reproductive forms pass out in the faeces. Examination of faeces for 'ova, cysts and parasites' ('OCP') is a common procedure in the microbiology laboratory. The faeces are emulsified and either examined directly in a 'wet preparation' or treated so as to concentrate the parasite forms. Stained films also are often helpful.

ASCARIS LUMBRICOIDES (ROUNDWORM)

Ascaris lumbricoides (Fig. 16.10), is 15-35 cm in length. Its distribution is worldwide and humans are the sole host. Adult worms live in the small intestine, their life span being about 18 months. The eggs pass out in the faeces and in moist soil remain infective for months. After ingestion by humans they hatch in the small intestine and pass through its wall into the blood, via which they reach the lungs. Here they penetrate into the alveoli and pass up through the bronchi and trachea to be swallowed again and mature in the intestine. Why they go through this complicated cycle to end up where they started is not known. Parasitisation with *A. lumbricoides* causes malnutrition, allergic reactions and even blockage of the gut by large numbers of worms.

ENTEROBIUS VERMICULARIS (PINWORM)

The pin worm (Plate 62), is a small worm about 1 cm long. Humans are the reservoir and the worms occur throughout the world. The adult worm inhabits the large gut, where it survives two to five weeks. At night the female migrates out the anus to lay her eggs on the perianal skin (Fig. 16.1). The eggs are transferred to a new host on the hands, bedclothes or clothes — in a moist environment they can survive outside the body for up to ten days. When swallowed, the eggs hatch in the gut, the embryos moult and become adults in about 40 days. The most common symptom is anal itching. As the lifespan of the worm is relatively short, prolonged infection means continuous reinfection.

Infestation is diagnosed by the 'sticky tape' test (Plate 65). When the patient awakes a piece of cellophane tape is pressed on the anal skin and then onto a microscope slide, which is examined for the typical eggs.

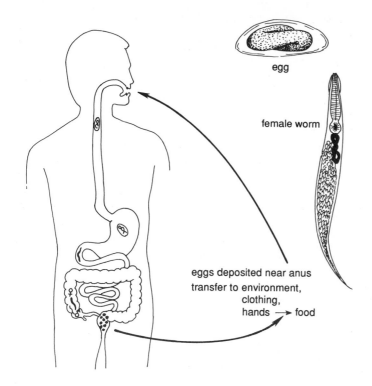

egg

female worm

eggs deposited near anus transfer to environment, clothing, hands → food

Fig. 16.1 The life cycle of *Enterobius vermicularis*. The adults inhabit the gut and the female emerges from the anus to lay eggs on the skin. The eggs easily contaminate hands, clothing and food, and when swallowed hatch in the small intestine. Self-reinfection is very common.

TAENIA SOLIUM (PORK TAPEWORM)

This worm (Fig.16.2) occurs worldwide; it has humans as the definitive host, and pigs as the intermediate one. Humans are infected by eating inadequately cooked pork containing the larvae (cysticerci), which then develop into adults and infest the small intestine of humans. Egg-laden segments of worm (proglottids) are passed in the faeces; the eggs develop into cysticerci in the pig. If the eggs are eaten by humans, the cysticerci can develop in this host also, hatching in the intestine and migrating almost anywhere in the body, with unpleasant results . In the gut the worms have little effect on the health, and patients complain mainly of noticing the motile proglottids.

SCHISTOSOMA

The three species of schistosomes, *S. haematobium* (Fig.16.3), *S. mansoni* and *S. japonicum*, are major parasites of humans, and have been known since antiquity. They occur in Africa and Asia. The worms

Fig. 16.2 (a) *Taenia taeniaeformis* (electronmicrograph). This worm closely resembles *Taenia solium.* **(b)** Life cycle of *Taenia solium.* The adult worm lives in the human gut and may be as long as 9 m (30 ft!), but is usually a restrained 2-3 m. Egg-containing segments (proglottids) pass out in the faeces. If the eggs are eaten by a pig (or a human) they hatch in the gut, pass into the tissues and may develop into the juvenile form (cysticercus) anywhere in the body.

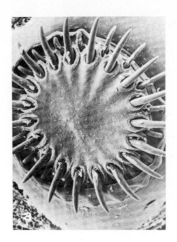

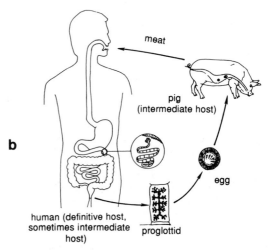

are small: 15-20 mm long. The adults live in veins in the abdomen (Fig. 16.3 and Plate 64). The eggs are laid in these small veins and penetrate their walls to enter the bladder or the gut and escape from the body to hatch in fresh water. The larva then swims off to find and enter a snail, within the body of which it develops into a cyst. After some weeks a further larval form (cercaria) emerges from the cyst and swims about in water. If it comes on a suitable host, it penetrates the skin, enters the blood vessels, and is carried to its favoured site in the abdomen.

Infection is signalled by fever, often allergic symptoms (e.g. a skin rash), abdominal pain, diarrhoea and bronchitis. There is marked enlargement of the spleen and cirrhosis of the liver. Infection with *S. haematobium* involves the bladder and leads to haematuria. Transmission of schistosomes occurs when human faeces or urine contaminates water. Humans become infected by exposure to water containing snails and cercariae; agricultural projects which increase food production may ironically also provide admirable conditions for snails to proliferate and thus do more

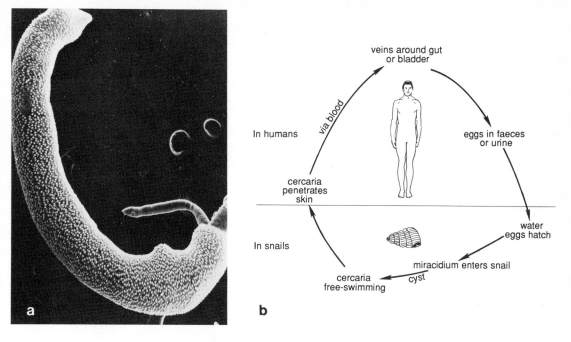

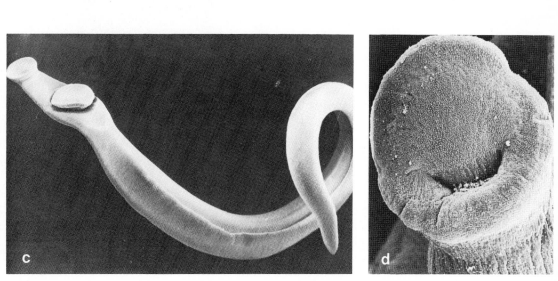

Fig. 16.3 (a) *Schistosoma haematobium*, male and female. The female lives in
a canal in the male's body. **(b)** Life cycle of schistosomes. The adult worms
live in the veins around the gut or the bladder, where they lay their eggs.
The eggs penetrate the bladder or gut wall and are excreted in the urine
or faeces. If they reach water they hatch and the miracidium enters a snail,
where it encysts. The cyst hatches and a free-swimming larva (cercaria)
infects a human by penetrating the skin. It moves to its final adult site via
the bloodstream. **(c)** *S. japonicum* The oral and ventral suckers are seen. **(d)**
S. japonicum Higher magnification of the oral sucker.

harm than good (Plates 22a and b). An adequate sewerage system eleminates the disease, but this is of course unattainable in many parts of the world. Research is being conducted towards the development of a vaccine.

ENTAMOEBA

The genus *Entamoeba* contains several species that are common in humans. The cause of amoebic dysentery, *E. histolytica* (Plate 60), often accompanies war and, like *Shigella*, causes more casualties than the bullets. Its distribution is worldwide. The trophozoites live and multipy in the mucosa of the large intestine, moving about freely, consuming food materials and bacteria and invading the gut wall to produce inflammation and shallow ulcers. Intestinal lesions may be very extensive and perforation of the gut and peritonitis may occur. From the gut, amoebae may pass to the liver or lungs, where they may form an abscess, often of large size. Trophozoites give rise to cysts which pass out in the faeces and can persist in the environment for days. When swallowed by a new host they pass unharmed

Fig. 16.4 (a) *Entamoeba histolytica* A trophozoite surrounded by red cells (electronmicrograph) **(b)** Drawing of *E. histolytica* trophozoite and cyst.

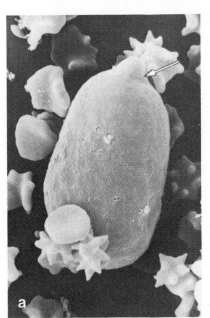

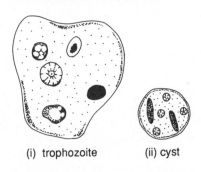

b

(i) trophozoite   (ii) cyst

through the gastric acid and release the amoebas in the small intestine. These are carried down and establish themselves in the large intestine (Fig. 16.4). Symptoms of amoebic dysentery are diarrhoea with blood and mucus, abdominal cramps, fever and malaise.

The disease is transmitted by the consumption of contaminated food or water; cysts can be transported by flies and cockroaches. This infection is common in homosexuals. One small bizarre outbreak was once caused by a contaminated enema machine (colonic irrigation is a form of chiropractic therapy). Infection is usually diagnosed by examining gut contents (fresh stools or specimens obtained by sigmoidoscopy) while they are still warm (so that the actively motile amoebae may be detected), and also by searching for cysts in faeces.

GIARDIA LAMBLIA

Another group of flagellate protozoa includes *Trichomonas* (p.253) and *Giardia* (Fig. 16.5). *Giardia lamblia* (Fig. 16.5) resides in the upper small intestine of man. It exists as a *trophozoite*, or a *cyst*. The

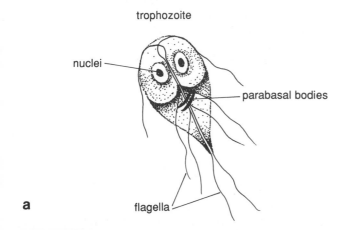

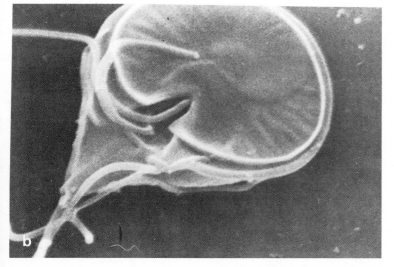

Fig. 16.5 (a) *Giardia lamblia* trophozoite. **(b)** *Giardia muris* (similar to *G. lamblia;* electronmicrograph). Note the ventral sucker disk and the flagella.

trophozoite is the active form — pear-shaped and bearing several pairs of flagella. These mature to form cysts, which are oval, thick-walled and contain two to four nuclei. They are excreted in the stools. Cysts are hardy and survive in water for months. *Giardia lamblia* infection may be acute or chronic and infected persons may variously have no symptoms, a brief acute illness or a chronic relapsing illness. Transmission of the parasite appears to be by contamination of food or water, which may lead to clusters of cases. Giardiasis occurs worldwide (see following, 'A long and busy journey'). The diagnosis should be considered in any patient who has had diarrhoea for a week or more. Stools should be examined and, if this measure produces no result, duodenal contents also.

IN THE COMMUNITY
A long and busy journey

Kylie Jeffreys, a 26-year-old journalist, decided on a world tour with a difference. She caught a merchant ship to Kobe, spent some time in Japan and then moved on to Vladivostock, where she caught the Trans-Siberian to Moscow.

Three days later she developed acute diarrhoea, for which she took various forms of kaolin and pectin. Kylie's symptoms subsided and she lapsed into a chronic diarrhoea, passing frequent stools and feeling bloated with abdominal discomfort.

In Munich she saw a gastroenterologist and had various laboratory tests, including three stools for 'ova, cysts and parasites'. In one of these, several cysts of *Giardia lamblia* were identified and a week's course of metronidazole cured her completely.

Giaridiasis is a common form of traveller's diarrhoea, often caught from drinking water. (In the 1970s many travellers came to grief in Leningrad from this cause — though apparently this was *not* a manifestation of the Cold War.)

TRICHINELLA SPIRALIS

This parasite is unusual in that the juvenile and adult forms develop in different tissues of the same host. Most mammals are susceptible and the parasite occurs worldwide (Fig. 16.6). The juvenile worms are swallowed and after moulting, enter the gut mucosa, where they mate. The female produces juveniles, which are distributed throughout the body by the bloodstream, lodging in muscles and forming cysts which eventually calcify. If infected meat is eaten, the muscle cell and the cyst wall is digested and the worm is freed to repeat the cycle. Many carnivores and their prey are infected in the wild, while humans most often acquire infection by eating undercooked pork. The manifestations of the infestation are due to the penetration of the gut by the adults and by the widespread migration of the juveniles, which may be found anywhere in the body. The infection may be fatal.

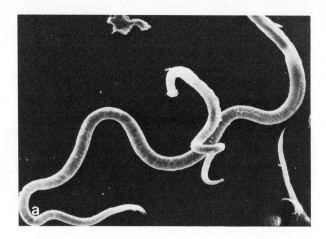

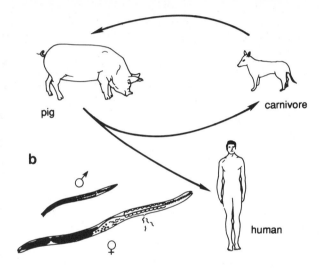

Fig. 16.6 (a) *Trichinella
spiralis*, male and female;
the male is the smaller. **(b)**
Life cycle of *Trichinella
spiralis*. The adults mate in
the mucosa of the small
intestine. The female gives
birth to juveniles, which
migrate to muscles and
form cysts within individual
muscle fibres. Thus the
complete life-cycle takes
place in a single host. When
the meat is eaten the cyst is
digested and the worm liberated to infect another
host. For humans the source
of infection is raw or undercooked meat. (Arctic explor-
ers have died from eating
raw polar bear!)

ECHINOCOCCUS GRANULOSUS (HYDATIDS)

This parasite (Fig. 16.7) causes the disease *hydatids*. It is a very
small tapeworm as an adult — though the juvenile form may be
very large. It is found worldwide. The life cycle in wild animals
involves a carnivore and a herbivore (such as wolf and reindeer,
dingo and wallaby or, in sheep-raising areas, dog and sheep). Dogs
become infected by eating the offal of slaughtered sheep, which
acquired the infection by eating grass soiled with dog faeces.
Humans acquire the eggs by petting dogs, and thus play the role of
the intermediate host, though normally they do not transmit the
infection.

The adult worm lives in the gut of the definitive host. It is only
3-6 mm long, consisting of a scolex and three proglottids (plate 23b).
The proglottid ruptures to release the eggs, which infect the intermediate host. The egg hatches in the small intestine, penetrates the
mucosa and is carried by the bloodstream to various sites in the

body. The usual sites of development are the liver and lung and, less commonly, the brain. Here the parasite grows slowly into a large hydatid cyst (plate 23a); 'large' in some organs may be a volume of several litres (see following, 'A country woman has problems'). In such a case the infection is obviously serious and may be fatal. Surgery is often necessary to remove the cysts. The infection is detected by serological tests.

Fig. 16.7 (a) *Echinococcus granulosus* adult. The scolex has a double row of hooklets and there are four suckers (two visible). **(b)** Life cycle of *E granulosus*. The adult tapeworm lives in the gut of the carnivore and is quite small, 3-6 mm long. The ova are excreted in the faeces and ingested by sheep or other herbivores. The egg hatches in the gut and the larva penetrates its wall and develops in the tissues, mainly in the liver or lungs. The resulting cyst may be very large. When these organs ('offal') are eaten by the carnivore, the protoscolex attaches to the gut wall and develops into the adult tapeworm. Humans are usually infected by petting or working with dogs.

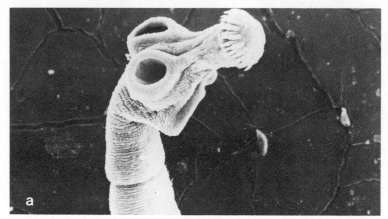

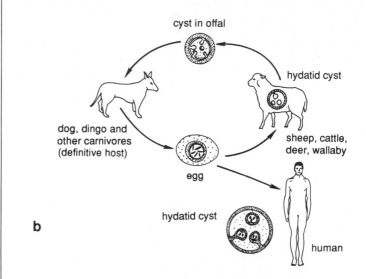

IN THE WARD
A country woman has problems
Marilyn Murphy, an overweight but otherwise healthy and active woman of 70, lived on a sheep property some 30 kilometres from Dubbo.

Four weeks before she entered Dubbo hospital, she became ill, developing a cough with some yellow sputum, and a fever which at times reached 39°C and was accompanied by heavy sweating and bouts of right-sided abdominal pain. This illness had been treated with ampicillin for five days, with little effect.

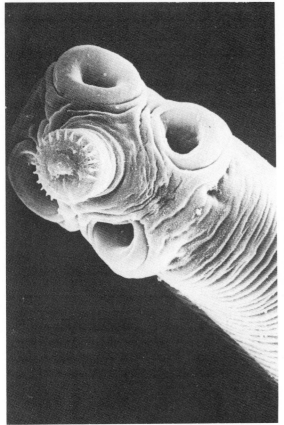

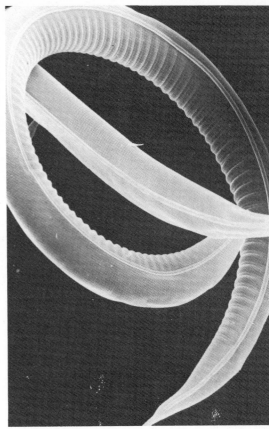

Fig. 16.8 *Hymenolepis nana* scolex, a rodent parasite which sometimes infects humans (electronmicrograph).

Fig. 16.9 *Trichostrongylus colubriformis* larva, a nematode which sometimes infects humans (electronmicrograph).

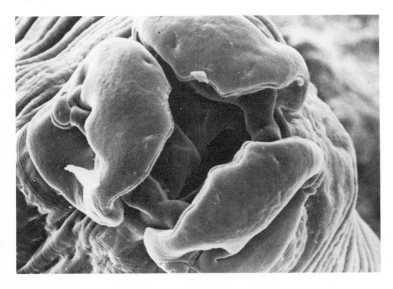

Fig. 16.10 Lips of *Ascaris lumbricoides*, a common nematode parasite of humans. The lips are lined by minute teeth. (Electronmicrograph).

Dubbo hospital described her as an obese lady who appeared acutely ill and in pain. She was tender in the right upper abdomen. Her temperature was 38.9^{0}C, her white cell count was 18 x 10^9/L; the number of leucocytes ('white cells') in the blood is normally less than 12 x 10^9/L and a raised white-cell count occurs in many infections. Mrs Murphy was given antibiotics with no improvement and after three days she was transferred to a Sydney hospital.

There the clinical findings were found to be unaltered. Blood cultures taken soon after admission grew *Proteus mirabilis*. CAT scans (a very sophisticated and expensive form of X-ray) showed that she had a large mass in the R lobe of the liver; this contained fluid and gas and was assumed to be an abscess.

At operation more than two litres of evil-smelling pus were drained from the abscess. Examination of this showed Gram-positive cocci and Gram-negative rods, fragments of the wall of a cyst and several of the *hooklets* characteristic of hydatids, *Echinococcus granulosus* (Plate 23a).

Hydatids is easily acquired in rural areas (see p.243). The size of Mrs Murphy's cyst indicated that it had probably been growing for years and had probably become infected fairly recently. No other cysts were seen or felt during the operation and Marilyn should have no further trouble.

We now come to parasites which are only detectable by examining blood and tissues.

TOXOPLASMA

Toxoplasma gondii (toxoplasmosis) is an obligate intracellular protozoon, which is parasitic on almost all mammals (Fig. 16.11). The trophozoites multiply intracellularly in the gut of the cat and develop into cysts which are excreted in the faeces for a few weeks. The cysts infect other species when eaten, and the trophozoites spread through the tissues and form cysts — especially in the brain and the muscles. These cysts remain for the life of the animal and are infectious if the meat is eaten. Humans are infected by eating raw or undercooked meat, probably by ingesting cysts also (possibly acquired from pet cats) and transplacentally when the mother becomes infected during pregnancy. In countries where meat is often eaten raw, almost all the population has antibodies to *Toxoplasma*.

Infection *in utero* may lead to abortion, stillbirth or birth defects (p.261). While infection later may sometimes cause 'glandular fever' (p.233), it is usually asymptomatic. Antibodies to this organism occur in 20-70% of individuals, the mean worldwide being 30%. As infection is so common, it is necessary to perform serological tests (such as detection of IgM) that indicate recent infection. Treatment is usually unnecessary, but effective drugs are available for use in severe cases. In immunocompromised individuals infection may flare up and cause serious disease and death.

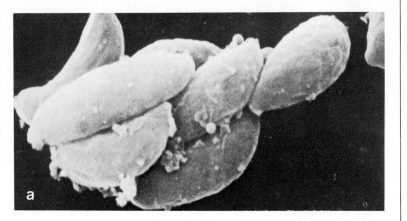

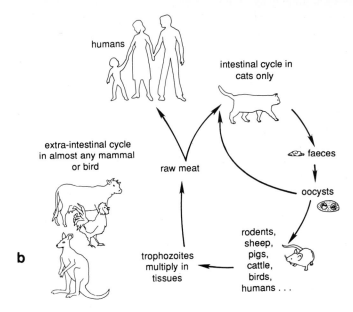

humans

intestinal cycle in
cats only

extra-intestinal cycle
in almost any mammal
or bird

raw meat

faeces

oocysts

rodents,
sheep,
pigs,
cattle,
birds,
humans . . .

trophozoites
multiply in
tissues

Fig. 16.11 (a) *Toxoplasma gondii* A number of the parasites — the body is curved on one side and flattened on the other (electronmicrograph). **(b)** Life cycle of *T. gondii*. The final host is the cat. The parasite multiplies in body tissues, including the wall of the gut, whence the oocysts reach the exterior. The oocysts may infect not only felines, but many species of animals. However, in these *T. gondii* multiplies in the tissues, oocysts are not excreted and the infection is only transmitted when the meat is eaten raw or rare.

PNEUMOCYSTIS CARINII

Pneumocystis carinii is a rather mysterious parasite, which some scientists class as a protozoon and others call a fungus. It is found in the lungs of humans and other mammals. It appears to be ubiquitous and most people acquire antibodies to it. Spread is probably by the aerial route. Special stains are necessary to reveal the parasite in lung tissues; it has trophozoite and cyst forms. The cysts are spherical or oval and contain up to 8 sporozoites. How they reproduce is not known. The infection only occurs when there are predisposing factors such as immunosuppression or malnutrition; there were outbreaks among debilitated infants in Europe after World War II. *Pneumocystis carinii* pneumonia is very common in AIDS; in the X-ray a diffuse general infection of both lungs is seen. Without treatment this is almost always fatal. Sulphamethoxazole/trimethoprim or pentamidine are effective against *Pneumocystis*.

PLASMODIUM (MALARIA)

Malaria is an infection caused by four protozoa of the genus *Plasmodium* (Plates 24 and 73): *P. falciparum*, *P. vivax*, *P. malariae* and *P. ovale*. Humans are infected by mosquitoes. The parasites have a complex life-cycle during which they multiply both in humans and in the mosquito. The mosquito bites the human and injects saliva containing the sporozoites, which soon vanish into liver cells and multiply there. (Only *P. vivax* and *P. ovale* have an eclipse phase in the liver.) Seven to ten days later the parasites break out of the liver cells and enter red cells in the blood. Here they go through further stages ending up as merozoites, forms which can infect fresh red cells. After a number of such cycles some merozoites develop into male and female sexual forms. These enter the mosquito's stomach with a blood meal and conjugate. The resulting zygotes multiply in the cells of the stomach wall and, as sporozoites, migrate to the salivary glands whence they infect humans.

Malaria commonly presents with chills and fever, followed by sweating. Fever may recur at regular or irregular intervals, or be continuous. The spleen is usually enlarged. Infections with *P. vivax* and *P. ovale* may recur over years. *P. falciparum* infections do not relapse, but may progress rapidly, the parasites reaching enormous numbers in the blood and death occurring from cerebral complications.

Malaria is still endemic in most of Africa, Central America and the Caribbean, South America, most of Asia and Oceania. More than a million children die each year from cerebral malaria in sub-Saharan Africa alone. In other parts of the world malaria should be suspected when fever occurs in travellers to endemic regions; it should not be forgotten that malaria can be transferred by transfusion or by the contaminated needles of drug addicts. The diagnosis is made by examining the blood for parasites; repeated examinations may be necessary. There are effective drugs for malaria — chloroquine and primaquine. However resistance to chloroquine has appeared in various regions and other drug combinations are then needed. Travellers to endemic regions should take antimalarial prophylaxis and use other measures to avoid mosquito bites. In the endemic regions malaria is *effectively out of control* since the mosquitoes became resistant to DDT (other control measures are too expensive).

TRYPANOSOMA (SLEEPING SICKNESS)

Trypanosoma brucei causes African trypanosomiasis or sleeping sickness. The host is any one of a number of mammals, including humans, and the organism is transferred by the bite of the tsetse fly. The trypanosomes live and multiply in the blood and tissue fluids of the host and are actively motile. Their surface proteins undergo antigenic variation (see p.137), thus enabling them to elude the immune defences of the host.

LICE AND MITES

Certain *ectoparasites*, lice and mites, may infest humans, and in tropical countries are responsible for a great deal of disease. In
developed countries such infestations are less important, but the
possibility must always be borne in mind. Periodically there are
outbreaks among schoolchildren. Lice infestations may assume
epidemic proportions in wartime or in crowded conditions; the
human body louse is the vector of epidemic typhus and trench
fever (p.222). The body louse is 2-4 mm long, flattened, oblong and
possesses 8 legs (Plate 17). The head louse is virtually the same,
the pubic louse (crab louse) resembles a crab in shape. The head
louse attaches its eggs ('nits') to the scalp hairs (Plate 18).

Scabies is due to the itch mite, *Sarcoptes scabiei*, a tiny creature
about 0.3-0.4 mm across, with a rounded body and 6 short legs. It
burrows into the skin and lays its eggs. The itching is intense. The
typical linear burrows can be seen and the organisms are detected
microscopically (Plate 25). These parasites are transferred by close
personal or sexual contact. Various insecticides can be used to
eliminate them; garments should also be treated.

PROBLEMS OF CONTROL

There are many other parasites capable of causing infection in
humans — we have discussed only a few of the most important.

Parasites represent an enormous problem in world health, as
will be clear from a study of Table 16.1. Furthermore, it is common
for individuals to simultaneously carry several different parasites.
As the people exposed to parasitic infections are in general poor
and uneducated, control is very difficult. The situation is getting
worse in many countries: Brazil had 560 000 cases of malaria in
1988, a five-fold increase in 10 years.

Effective drugs are now available for the treatment of many of
these infections; thus mebendazole is active against *Ascaris* and
Enterobius, metronidazole against *Entamoeba*, *Giardia* and
Trichomonas. Most could be effectively controlled by social measures: better hygiene, proper disposal of faeces, clean water supplies.
In the absence of such public-health measures, reinfection is so
common that drugs have relatively little effect. Many countries
cannot afford either form of control — some governments can spend
only the equivalent of US$4.00 per head per annum on the entire
health system.

CHAPTER REVIEW

1   List three fungal infections and state their significance.

2   (a)   Discuss the importance of parasitic diseases in the developing nations.

       (b)   List 5 parasites important on a world scale.

3   (a)   What is malaria?

       (b)   What is the reservoir and the mode of transmission of this disease?

       (c)   In what regions of the world is this disease found?

17

SOME SPECIAL TOPICS IN INFECTIOUS DISEASE

1 SEXUALLY TRANSMITTED DISEASES (STDs)

Sexually transmitted diseases ('venereal disease', or 'STDs') are very widespread and have become much commoner in the last 40 years. It is estimated these infections exceeded 8 000 000 cases in the USA in 1987 — i.e. about one person in 30 was afflicted. STD may manifest itself in the genitals as one or more ulcers, a rash, or a discharge. Our increasing versatility means that the throat and the anus may also be affected sites. Rashes may occur elsewhere on the body. Some sexually transmitted diseases — AIDS, gonorrhoea, syphilis, herpes simplex, hepatitis B — may give rise to a generalised infection or an infection at a distant site.

COMMON INFECTIONS AND CAUSES

Common infectious causes of a genital ulcer are:
- herpes simplex virus (HSV)
- syphilis
- chancroid
- lymphogranuloma venereum

Common causes of vaginitis are:
- *Candida* species
- *Trichomonas vaginalis*
- *Gardnerella vaginalis*

Common causes of cervicitis (inflammation of the uterine cervix) are:
- *Neisseria gonorrhoeae*
- *Chlamydia trachomatis*

- herpes simplex virus

Common causes of a urethral discharge (urethritis) in the male are:
- *Neisseria gonorrhoeae*
- *Chlamydia trachomatis*
- *Ureaplasma urealyticum*

Symptoms in the genital region may also be due to ectoparasites: nits, crabs and scabies.

GENITAL ULCERS

Genital ulcers may be single or multiple. The four principal causes — HSV, primary syphilis, chancroid and lymphogranuloma — all cause ulcers which can be readily confused with one another, so microbiological confirmation of the cause is needed. Herpes simplex virus (p.231) typically produces groups of vesicles which progress to ulcers. A history of antecedent vesicles is important evidence that HSV is to blame. Ulcers are located on the external genitals and are painful — sometimes extremely so. They are of uniform size and the vagina is rarely involved. In *primary syphilis* there is most often a single ulcer *(chancre)* — usually not painful. Typically the inguinal lymph glands are swollen. In *chancroid* (an uncommon infection due to *Haemophilus ducreyi*, a small fastidious Gram-negative rod), a single ulcer is usual, located on the penis in men and on the external genitalia in women. *Lymphogranuloma venereum* is caused by certain serotypes of *Chlamydia trachomatis* and is almost always transmitted sexually — a single painless ulcer heals rapidly and is followed by enlargement of the inguinal lymph glands. This infection is unusual in developed countries, but endemic in Africa, Asia and South America.

IN THE STD CLINIC
A quiet morning
Tallulah Jarvis, age 18 and a 'sexually active woman' complains of itching and vaginal discharge of two weeks' duration. She was treated six months ago for a similar problem, due to 'yeast'.

Microscopy of the discharge shows motile trophozoites of *Trichomonas vaginalis* in moderate numbers *and* yeast cells and hyphae, presumably *Candida albicans.*

Tallulah is given metronidazole and clotrimazole and a peptalk about finishing the treatment.

Peter Purdie, age 29 and a 'sexually active man' complains that 'the stuff you gave me last time was no good — me discharge is back'.

A month ago his urethral discharge, diagnosed as gonorrhoea, was treated with a large injection of penicillin. He has no sign of gonococci in the discharge this time. A specimen of the discharge is taken to be examined for *Chlamydia* and he is given 10 days supply of tetracycline and told to make sure he takes all the capsules or he will 'be back'. Chlamydial urethritis is commoner than the gonococcal variety, and does not respond to penicillin. (This diagnosis will be confirmed by the laboratory next day.)

Algernon Murphy, age 35, has an itchy, red rash on his private parts. This started about three weeks ago, and is spreading. It itches 'like fury'.

Algernon has treated it with three ointments out of the bathroom cupboard (including some antibiotic cream that a mate of his left behind) — but it's getting worse.

Examination of pubic hair with a hand lens shows nits and a crab louse.

He is given an 'anti-louse' lotion to apply immediately and again after seven days, and is advised to boil his underwear.

VAGINITIS

Vaginitis is a common condition, manifesting itself by vaginal discharge, pain and irritation, dysuria (painful or difficult urination) and dyspareunia (pain during intercourse). The nature of the discharge and other clinical features cannot be relied on for diagnosis and the pathogen should be demonstrated. The common microbial causes are listed above.

Trichomonas vaginalis. The trophozoite form of *Trichomonas vaginalis* is pear-shaped, about 10 x 7 μm in size. It has an undulating membrane and five flagella. It ingests bacteria and red cells, its metabolism is anaerobic and it can utilise various carbohydrates. The organism does not form cysts. It multiplies by longitudinal fission and sets up colonies on the mucosa of the vagina, urethra or prostate. Infection is diagnosed by examination of wet films, in which the trophozoites can be seen moving in a characteristic jerky fashion; no other trichomonads or protozoa occur in the vagina. It is sometimes seen in urine when cell counts are carried out. The organism can also be grown in special media, but this takes several days.

T. vaginalis is found worldwide. The trophozoite is transferred during intercourse. Infection is acquired by about 3 000 000 American women each year and by a high proportion of their sexual partners. Infection is commonest in women with multiple sexual partners, and detection of trichomoniasis should always lead to screening for other sexually transmitted diseases. In men the disease is often self-limited and most infected men are completely asymptomatic. In about 25% of women in whom it is detected there are no symptoms, while the remainder complain usually of discharge, and less frequently of irritation or soreness, of dysuria or dyspareunia. Whether the patient has symptoms or not, the organism should be eliminated, since such persons constitute a reservoir of infection and many of them will develop symptoms themselves in time. Metronidazole is an effective treatment.

Candida albicans, a yeast, is probably the commonest cause of vaginitis (Plate 26). Pregnancy, diabetes or antibiotic treatment predispose to this infection, which is not usually transmitted sexually. There is intense itching, the discharge is usually thick and whitish and in it epithelial cells and yeast cells can be seen. Small numbers of *Candida* may be found in the vagina in the absence of symptoms.

Gardnerella vaginalis causes a common form of vaginitis often termed 'nonspecific vaginitis' (NSV), characterised by discharge and vaginal odour; there is little inflammation in and around the vagina and dysuria and dyspareunia are unusual. Direct microscopy of discharge in a wet preparation shows 'clue cells' — epithelial cells studded with small coccobacilli; these can also be seen in Gram stains. Few polymorphs are present. The normal vaginal secretions contain predominantly a large rod, *Lactobacillus*; in NSV this is replaced by the small coccobacilli. The infection appears to be acquired sexually. *G. vaginalis* is easily grown from the discharge. However it occurs in small numbers in asymptomatic women and its isolation does not therefore prove that the patient has NSV. Furthermore, there is some evidence that the disease is due to cooperation between *G. vaginalis* and various anaerobic bacteria. Diagnosis is based on both clinical and laboratory findings.

Vaginitis may also be due to a foreign body such as a forgotten vaginal tampon. Most other causes of local infection, staphylococci, streptococci, *Enterobacteriaceae* or mycobacteria do *not* cause vaginal infections or vaginal discharge.

CERVICITIS

Cervicitis or inflammation of the uterine cervix often occurs independently of vaginitis. *Neisseria gonorrhoeae* produces an acute inflammation of the cervical canal and is most often isolated from this site in acute gonorrhoea. An endocervical swab is the best specimen for diagnostic purposes. *Chlamydia trachomatis* can be isolated from the cervix of most women whose partners have chlamydial urethritis. In a good number of such women the cervix appears quite normal. Neither gonococcal nor chlamydial cervicitis can be excluded by physical examination. Most women with gonococcal or chlamydial cervicitis have no symptoms, but about one third note some discharge. Note that *Neisseria gonorrhoeae* and *Chlamydia trachomatis* do not cause a frank vaginitis.

Pelvic inflammatory disease (PID) is an infection involving the upper genital tract. Infection generally extends from the vagina to involve the cervix and the endometrium (the lining membrane of the uterus) and then the tubes and ovaries. An acute infection may lead to pelvic peritonitis. Chronic infections are likely to end in a scarred blocked tube and an increased risk of ectopic pregnancy (pregnancy in which the fertilised ovum is implanted in the tube or even in the peritoneal cavity) — the outcome is very often infertility. PID is increasingly common. The main causes of PID are *Neisseria gonorrhoeae*, *Chlamydia trachomatis* and *Mycoplasma hominis,* but especially in chronic infection many different organisms may be isolated from the pelvic organs. As most of these may readily occur among the flora of the vagina, vaginal or cervical swabs reveal little of significance unless *N. gonorrhoeae* is isolated.

IN THE WARD
An 'unhappy event': ectopic pregnancy

Mrs Jean Hefferan, age 34, came to Emergency on Sunday morning. For the previous two days she had had the 'flu'. In the early hours of Sunday she had awakened with 'crampy' abdominal pain. When she tried to get up she felt giddy. While dressing she noticed some vaginal bleeding.

She was eight weeks pregnant, and apart from the 'flu' was in good health.

In Emergency she was found to have a rapid pulse and a slight fever (38.2⁰C). Her abdomen was tender on the right side, but no lump could be felt. Her blood white cell count was slightly raised. Her urine showed normal numbers of white cells and there was no indication of infection. The urine pregnancy test was positive. She was admitted to hospital.

Mrs Hefferan continued to complain of abdominal pain — now more severe — and fainted when she got out of bed. Of the many possible causes of her illness, appendicitis and ectopic pregnancy appeared the most likely.

At operation it was found that an ectopic pregnancy (i.e. a pregnancy in an inappropriate place) was present. The fertilised ovum had implanted in the right Fallopian tube. Here it had insufficient space to develop and eventually the tube ruptured, causing abortion and bleeding into the abdominal cavity. The tubes showed signs of chronic inflammation suggestive of chlamydial infection; there were antibodies to *Chlamydia* in the serum.

Mrs Hefferan was not aware of any previous chlamydial infection; her 'flu' was unrelated to her other problems.

Ectopic pregnancy is now occurring much more often, largely because of the frequency of chlamydial infection — chronic inflammation of the tubes leads to scarring and blockage, so that the ovum cannot pass. In 1978 over 10% of pregnancy-related deaths in the USA were due to this disease.

Herpes simplex. Primary infection with herpes simplex virus usually involves the cervix, but this is true only of a small proportion of recurrent infections. Cervical infection usually leads to visible cervicitis, which may or may not be accompanied by ulcers on the external genitalia. The cervical discharge is usually mucoid. Herpetic cervicitis is a significant risk to the infant during birth (p.262).

URETHRITIS

Urethritis is estimated to afflict 4 000 000 American men each year and a large but unknown number of women. Urethral discharge, the commonest symptom, is more obvious to men. Dysuria is often associated. In acute urethritis a Gram-stained film of the discharge will show polymorphs. Gram-negative cell-associated diplococci may be seen - an observation strongly suggesting gonococcal infection, and justifying treatment in the absence of a positive culture. However nongonococcal urethritis (NGU) is at least as common as gonococcal and probably more so; it is usually transmitted sexually. Patients are more likely to complain of dysuria than of discharge. The main cause of NGU is *Chlamydia trachomatis*, which causes 30-50% of cases; of the remainder, most are probably due to *Ureaplasma urealyticum*, a primary infection with HSV or *Trichomonas vaginalis*.

TREATMENT OF STDs

- *Candida* infections — there are several effective drugs: e.g. clotrimazole, miconazole or nystatin applied vaginally.
- Trichomoniasis. A number of drugs are available; metronidazole or tinidazole is most often used.
- *Gardnerella vaginalis* infection. Metronidazole is effective.
- *Neisseria gonorrhoeae*. See p.206.
- Syphilis. See p.216.
- Herpes simplex. See p.232.
- *Chlamydia* infection. Doxycycline or erythromycin is effective.

AIDS

In 1981 the Centres for Disease Control called attention to the fact that several hitherto rare disorders — in particular *Pneumocystis* pneumonia, severe herpes simplex infection, Kaposi's sarcoma (a rare malignancy) and *Candida* oesophagitis — were occurring both much more frequently and also in individuals who had previously been healthy. Most had had fever, weight loss and fatigue for some time before the first major illness. It speedily became clear that this was an epidemic of a new kind — an epidemic of *immunodeficiency*. Unlike the forms of immunodeficiency usually encountered previously, the defect in *immunity* was acquired, not congenital, and was not due to drugs. The disease was named the *acquired immunodeficiency syndrome* or AIDS. By 1983 a virus had been isolated, and AIDS is now known to be caused by human immunodeficiency virus (HIV) — actually a group of closely related viruses.

CLINICAL PICTURE

The human viruses are similar to certain African monkey viruses, from which they are thought to be derived in the relatively recent past (decades or centuries ago). Why the virus has spread so dramatically in the last decade is not clear. It is estimated that in 1990 some five to 10 million people are infected with HIV (1-1.5 million in the USA and 30-90 000 in Australia). Figure 17.1 shows the rapid increase in cases of AIDS in the USA since 1981.

No. of cases

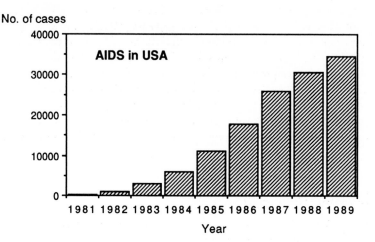

Fig. 17.1 Number of cases of AIDS in the USA since 1981.

HIV infection progresses slowly. Primary infection may be symptomless, but within six weeks of infection about 50% of people suffer an acute illness resembling 'glandular fever' and lasting up to three weeks. Features may include fever, muscle pain, lymphadenopathy, splenomegaly, diarrhoea and rash. There may be a fall in the numbers of neutrophils and lymphocytes in the blood (neutropenia, lymphopenia) and later 'atypical mononuclear' cells may appear. HIV antigen may be detectable in the serum during this period. Antibodies to HIV take from a few weeks to months to appear.

HIV attacks T-lymphocytes, binding to the CD4 protein in the cell membrane and entering the cell. HIV belongs to the retroviruses (Fig. 17.2, so called because the virion contains a reverse transcriptase, an enzyme that synthesises a DNA copy of the RNA which makes up the genome of the virus). These copies are made in the cytoplasm and move into the nucleus, where they are integrated into the nuclear DNA and transcribed to RNA by the host cell's RNA polymerase. Some of the resulting RNA molecules are incorporated into new virions and others function as messenger RNA to ensure synthesis of viral proteins (Fig. 17.3). Other cells carry CD4 proteins in smaller numbers and are also susceptible to HIV, including monocytes and macrophages and certain brain cells. Thus infection with the virus leads to the destruction of several cell types essential for the immune response and produces a variety of immunological abnormalities: lymphopenia (a decrease in the numbers of lymphocytes in the blood), decrease in CD4+ lymphocytes, depressed or absent delayed-type hypersensitivity and raised serum immunoglobulins.

Fig. 17.2 Structure of a retrovirus. The envelope consists of a lipid layer from which protein spikes protrude. Inside the envelope is the icosahedral capsid. This contains 2 molecules of single stranded RNA, to each of which a molecule of the enzyme reverse transcriptase is linked.

Fig. 17.3 HIV replication. (1) Virus merges with cell membrane and loses its envelope, releasing the capsid (2). The reverse transcriptase synthesises DNA from the RNA template (3). The DNA integrates into the host cell chromosome (4) and is transcribed into messenger RNA (5). The mRNA is translated into reverse transcriptase, envelope protein and capsid protein (6). These proteins plus RNA are assembled into new virus particles (7).

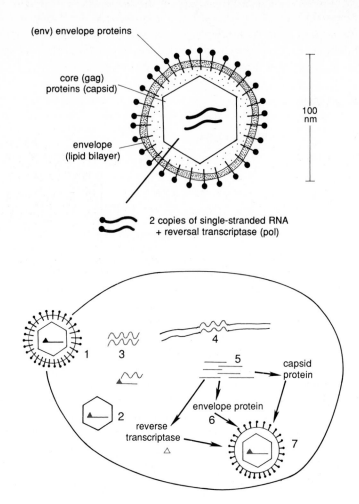

Many infected persons remain clinically well for months or even years after infection, even though HIV antibodies can be demonstrated in their serum. They are not immune to HIV. The next stage of the infection is persistent generalised lymphadenopathy (enlargement of the lymph glands); the person is otherwise well. AIDS-related complex (ARC) is a definite illness lasting three or more months, with one or more of the following features: weight loss, fever or night sweats, lethargy, oral candidiasis or a decrease in T_4 cells.

Fully-developed AIDS is characterised by one or more serious infections which may be related to the respiratory tract, the gut or the central nervous system (CNS). A diffuse pneumonia is common, almost always due to *Pneumocystis carinii*. In the CNS the virus can cause an inflammation progressing to dementia, and *Toxoplasma gondii* may cause abscesses or *Cryptococcus neoformans* lead to meningitis. Cytomegalovirus infection of the retina may cause severe loss of vision. Diarrhoea is common in AIDS patients; many different enteric organisms may be found in the faeces — *Entamoeba*

histolytica, Giardia lamblia, Salmonella and *Shigella,* and in addition
other organisms rarely associated with diarrhoea in normal persons, *Cryptosporidium* (Plate 63) or cytomegalovirus. *Candida albicans*
may cause oral thrush or oesophagitis. Mycobacterial infections are
common, including the otherwise very rare mycobacteraemia.

MODES OF TRANSMISSION

1 *Sexual.* In the USA, Europe and Australia most AIDS cases are
among homosexuals (in Africa AIDS occurs mainly in heterosexuals). Transmission is most likely with receptive anal intercourse.
Asymptomatic carriers are more infectious than AIDS patients, in
whom the number of cells capable of producing virus is reduced.
Transmission in heterosexual intercourse is more likely from male
to female than vice versa. Kissing is not known to transmit the
virus.
2 *Via infected blood.* Transfusion of infected blood is very likely to
lead to infection and in most Western countries all blood is now
screened for HIV. Some haemophiliacs were infected by infusion of
contaminated coagulation factors. Now the main risk of infection
by contaminated blood is among intravenous drug users who share
needles.
3 *Congenital infection.* HIV crosses the placenta, so the child of an
infected mother has a high risk of acquiring AIDS *in utero.*

It should be noted that close social or familial contact does not
transmit AIDS. If there is no sexual relationship, then living with,
associating with or treating an AIDS patient or an HIV carrier
presents only the *very slight risk* of needle-stick injury or exposure of
injured skin to infected blood. Transmission to health-care workers
is very rare. A needle-stick injury carries about a 1% risk of transmission, i.e much lower than for HBV. Transmission requires a
break in the skin or mucosae.

LABORATORY DIAGNOSIS

HIV infection is detected by the presence of antibody to the virus;
it may be some months after infection before antibody appears.
Attempts to grow the virus are made only in specially equipped
laboratories.

TREATMENT

Azidothymidine (AZT) prolongs life; no drug yet discovered cures.
The many other infections of AIDS patients are treated as usual.

PREVENTION

1 *Less promiscuity.* DON'T SLEEP AROUND. AIDS can be caught from
'straights' as well as 'gays'.
2 *Use condoms.*

3 *Don't share needles.* IV drug abusers are especially likely to carry the virus.

4 *Screening donors* and *donor blood* almost eliminates the risk from blood transfusion.

5 *Vaccines.* No vaccine is at present available or in prospect — developing one is clearly a very difficult task. There are a number of different strains of HIV. Neither antibodies nor cell-mediated immunity to HIV appear to be protective; antibodies and virus are normally both present in the blood of infected individuals. Located in the genome of the lymphocyte, the virus is protected from the usual immune defences and from current antiviral drugs.

2 INFECTION AND PREGNANCY

In a pregnant woman infection with most common pathogens is not transmitted to the fetus. The placenta forms a barrier to the intra-uterine spread of most organisms and any adverse effects are due to the (little understood) consequences of severe illness. But a few microbes do succeed in reaching the offspring; this may occur either *in utero* or at the time of birth. Table 17.1 lists the main organisms responsible for these perinatal infections.

TABLE 17.1 MICROBES CAUSING INFECTION RELATED TO PREGNANCY

In utero	At birth
rubella, CMV	HBV, HIV, CMV
Listeria monocytogenes,	herpes simplex,
Toxoplasma gondii	*Listeria monocytogenes,*
herpes simplex,	Streptococcus group B
Treponema pallidum,	*Chlamydia trachomatis*
HIV	

Intra-uterine infections produce different results at different stages of the pregnancy. In the first weeks resorption of the fetus or miscarriage is the rule. Later congenital malformations may result or a continuing infection may be set up, manifest at or after birth. Infection of the fetal membranes appears to play a role in their premature rupture, leading to delivery of the fetus before full term. Infection at the time of birth is due to exposure of the infant to blood and secretions containing the microbes.

CONGENITAL MALFORMATIONS

About 3% of all newborns have a major malformation at birth. The cause of 65-70% of these is unknown, and most of the rest are genetic — i.e. due to a chromosomal defect. About 3% of malformations are due to intra-uterine infection and are therefore potentially preventable. Maternal infections which may give rise to fetal defects are rubella, CMV, toxoplasmosis, syphilis and HIV. In the developed countries syphilis is now a very rare cause of congenital infection, since screening for syphilis is routinely performed in pregnancy.

1 RUBELLA (GERMAN MEASLES)

This is a mild infection due to an RNA virus. It is spread by the respiratory route, and before the extensive use of the live attenuated vaccine, epidemics used to occur regularly. The main symptoms are rash and lymphadenopathy; complications are rare. Most infections are subclinical. However infection of the fetus *in utero* can lead to fetal death, premature delivery or congenital defects. Infection in the first two months of pregnancy causes abortion or multiple congenital defects in about 50% of fetuses; in the third month about one third develop a single defect — congenital heart disease, cataract, deafness, mental retardation. There is still danger in infection until the twentieth week. Other defects that may arise include jaundice, fits, diabetes mellitus, microcephaly, behaviour disorders and speech defects. Before the vaccine came into use, congenital rubella was relatively common — a single epidemic in the USA once resulted in 30 000 affected children. Vaccination has virtually eliminated this disease; in 1982 in the USA there were only 5 cases of congenital rubella.

2 CYTOMEGALOVIRUS (CMV)

If a pregnant woman acquires a primary CMV infection there is about a 50% chance that the baby will be infected, most often during birth and less commonly *in utero*. Previously infected women are less likely to infect the child, but there is still a considerable risk, because virus is shed from the cervix with increasing frequency as pregnancy proceeds; the risk is very high if virus is being shed at delivery. Most of the infected children do not show obvious symptoms, but more subtle effects are common. Mental defect, deafness or damage to sight may occur. CMV is the commonest infective cause of mental deficiency. At present there is little that can be done to prevent the disease; work on a vaccine is underway.

3 TOXOPLASMOSIS

A woman who acquires a primary infection with *Toxoplasma gondii* during pregnancy is likely to bear an affected child. The risk to the infant is greatest in the first trimester (i.e. the first three months of pregnancy). Unlike rubella, *T. gondii* does not cause malformations in the fetus and the damage is due to continuing infection, which may be evident at birth or may only manifest itself months or years later. The possible outcome may be microcephaly, hydrocephalus, mental retardation, blindness, epilepsy, anaemia, jaundice, pneumonia — the list is not complete. Infection is diagnosed by serological tests. Treatment with pyrimethamine and sulphonamide appears to be effective.

4 HERPES SIMPLEX

Herpes infection in the newborn is usually acquired during passage through an infected cervix (p.255), but may arise *in utero* by spread from maternal genital lesions. If the mother is excreting virus at delivery the risk of infecting the infant is high. A primary maternal infection is more dangerous for the infant than a recurrent one. The outcome may range from a symptomless infection to an overwhelming illness.

Herpes simplex, rubella, CMV and *Toxoplasma gondii* may all rarely give rise to a similar clinical picture of congenital infection with jaundice, enlargement of liver and spleen, bleeding disorders and abnormalities of the central nervous system, usually leading to death.

3 THE 'COMPROMISED' PATIENT

A patient may be 'compromised' (i.e. the patient's defences may be undermined) by: (a) *naturally-occurring illness* or (b) two important forms of modern *medical treatment* — the administration of immunosuppressive and cytotoxic drugs, and the insertion of foreign bodies.

One of the body's most important defences is provided by the white cells. The *cytotoxic* drugs used to kill cancer cells attack cells which are rapidly dividing; in this category must also be included the cells of the bone marrow. Hence anti-cancer therapy leads to a sharp fall in the numbers of neutrophils in the blood, a state termed *neutropenia* or *granulocytopenia*. Once the neutrophil count falls below $500 \times 10^9/L$ the number of infections rises sharply; if the patient has less than $100 \times 10^9/L$ neutrophils, they are around 10 times as likely to acquire an infection of some sort.

In transplantation of organs the combinations of drugs given to suppress the patient's ability to reject the graft interfere with the immune system in general, as well as leading to neutropenia. In particular, cellular immune dysfunction may result, so that the patients acquire infections due to intracellular pathogens (mycobacteria, *Listeria monocytogenes*, some viruses, fungi and protozoa). Less often antibody formation is depressed.

The infections that arise in compromised patients are almost entirely endogenous, i.e. the causative organisms are already present as part of the normal flora or by reason of a previous infection now latent. Changes in the normal body flora often occur under the stress of illness or hospitalisation. The normal flora has often been modified by antibiotic therapy, so that the upper respiratory tract is colonised by *Enterobacter, Klebsiella, Proteus,* or *Pseudomonas,* while in the gut *Enterobacter* and *Pseudomonas* have often increased at the expense of *Escherichia coli.* Infections of the respiratory and urinary tracts and soft tissues predominate, together with bacteraemia. Most prominent among the latent infections stimulated into activity under these conditions are herpes simplex, CMV, vari-cella-zoster and toxoplasmosis.

In particular the respiratory tract is at risk. The normal defences of the respiratory tract (see Fig. 11.4) may be impaired in various ways. If the patient's consciousness is depressed (Plate 29), the gag reflex is lost and pneumonia may ensue because organisms in the upper respiratory tract can pass down the trachea. Intuba-tion of the trachea or a tracheostomy carry a similar, but heavier risk. In fact, insertion of any foreign body into a vessel or tissue carries with it an infection risk. Indwelling vascular catheters may lead to bacteraemia. An indwelling urinary catheter usually brings with it urinary infection after a week or two, even if catheter care is absolutely scrupulous.

4 'NEEDLE-STICK' INJURIES

A needle that has been used for an injection is contaminated with blood and may therefore transfer various infectious agents. Any member of the health-care team — nurse, doctor, physiotherapist or ward cleaner — runs a risk of accidentally stabbing him or her-self with a blood-contaminated needle. Indeed of course, as IV drug users may discard needles anywhere, the risk extends to the municipal worker collecting rubbish or the passerby on the beach. The most serious infections likely to be transmitted are hepatitis (B and C) and AIDS. While any patient known to carry one of these agents should be managed with especial care, the diagnosis may not be known and therefore *universal blood and body fluid precautions should always be observed*.

HBV

Any member of the health-care team should know his or her HBV status. Anyone who is immune need not fear getting HBV from a 'needle-stick'; anyone who is *not* immune should undergo vaccina-tion. So this paragraph applies only to those who have no immun-ity or who do not know their immunity status.

The HBV status of the 'donor' of the needle should be estab-lished immediately. If he or she is a carrier of HBV, the recipient of the 'needle-stick' becomes infected in 5-10% of cases and should be given hepatitis B hyperimmune serum as soon as possible, pref-erably within 24 hours or less. If the needle is 'anonymous', (e.g. protruding from a bag of rubbish), the risk of contracting HBV is obviously less, since only a small proportion of such needles will carry virus. It would be wise, nevertheless, to accept hyperimmune serum.

HIV

If a staff member receives a needle-stick, the HIV status of the 'donor' and of the staff member should be established immediately (consent to this procedure can almost always be obtained).

The risk of acquiring HIV infection appears to be much lower than that of acquiring HBV — around 1%. This is fortunate, since prophylactic treatment with zidovudine (azidothymidine, AZT) will probably not always succeed.

CHAPTER REVIEW

1 List the sexually transmitted diseases.
2 Which microorganisms cause genital ulcers?
3 (a) List the causes of vaginitis
   (b) Describe the symptoms and signs.
4 (a) What is pelvic inflammatory disease?
   (b) How does this infection arise?
   (c) What are its consequences?
5 (a) What does human immunodeficiency virus (HIV) cause?
   (b) Describe the modes of transmission, signs and symptoms of this infection.
6 (a) Define rubella.
   (b) Why is this 'mild' infection important?
   (c) Explain the role of vaccination in reducing the spread of this condition.
7 What microbes may cause congenital abnormalities in the newborn?
8 What does the term 'compromised patient' mean?
9 Which groups of people are at risk of catching AIDS?

GLOSSARY

Abscess: a localised collection of pus.

Acetyl-coenzyme A (acetyl-CoA): coenzyme A is a carrier molecule which accepts the acetyl group when pyruvic acid is oxidised and transfers it into the citric acid cycle. (*See* citric acid cycle).

Acetyl group: $CH_3 - C = 10$.

Acid: a substance that when dissolved in water dissociates into hydrogen ions H^+ and negative ions.

Acid-fast stain: a differential stain used to detect and identify some types of bacteria, especially mycobacteria.

Acquired immunity: immunity which develops in response to a stimulus, e.g. an infection.

Active immunity: immunity depending on the production of antibodies or sensitised cells by the host animal; contrasted with passive immunity.

Active site: the region of an enzyme which combines with the substrate.

Active transport: energy-dependent movement of a substance across a membrane from a site of low concentration to one of high concentration, i.e. against the concentration gradient.

Acute infection: an infection which runs its course in a relatively short period.

Adenine: an organic base found in DNA, RNA and elsewhere.

Adenosine triphosphate (ATP): a chemical compound which contains energy-rich bonds and serves as the main 'energy currency' of the cell. It breaks down into adenosine diphosphate and phosphate ion, releasing energy.

Adherence (adhesion): the 'sticking' of a microbe to a body surface or other surface; this is an important phase in the initiation of infection.

Aerobe: a microbe that grows in the presence of oxygen. A strict aerobe requires oxygen. See anaerobe.

Agar: a polysaccharide made from seaweed and used in solidifying bacteriological media.

Agglutinate: to stick to one another, clump (of particles, red cells, etc); the result is agglutination.

'Alcohol': = ethanol,
$$H-\overset{\displaystyle H}{\underset{\displaystyle H}{C}}-\overset{\displaystyle H}{\underset{\displaystyle H}{C}}-O-H$$

(the reason for the intoxicating effect of beer, wine etc).

Algae: photosynthetic microbes; the blue-green algae are procaryotes and the others eucaryotes.

Alkali: a substance that, when dissolved in water, dissociates into OH^- ions and positive ions.

Allele: one of two or more alternative forms of a gene, only one of which is present in a chromosome.

Allergy: an undesirable immune response due to hypersensitivity. (See hypersensitivity.)

Amino acid: an organic acid occurring in proteins and elsewhere. It has the structure
$$R-\underset{\displaystyle NH_2}{\overset{\displaystyle |}{C}}-COOH$$
where R may be any one of various chemical groups.

Aminoglycoside: a type of antibiotic; examples are gentamicin, amikacin and streptomycin. The aminoglycosides are active against Gram-negative organisms, including *Pseudomonas* species, and some Gram-positive species.

Amino group: a chemical group consisting of nitrogen and 2 hydrogens, $-NH_2$.

Amoeba: a eucaryotic organism that lacks a rigid cell wall and moves by pseudopods.

Anaerobe: a microbe that grows in the absence of oxygen. A strict anaerobe will not grow in the presence of oxygen, a facultative anaerobe grows in the presence or absence of oxygen.

Anaphylaxis: one of the forms of hypersensitivity.

Anion: an ion bearing a negative charge.

Antibiotic: a substance which is toxic for certain microbes; the first antibiotics to be used were produced by microbes, but many are now partly or wholly synthesised by the pharmaceutical chemists. = antimicrobial agent.

Antibody: a protein which appears in the body fluids of an animal after contact with a foreign molecule, 'antigen', and which combines specifically with that antigen.

Anticodon: the set of three nucleotides on the transfer RNA molecule. The anticodon is paired by the ribosome with the corresponding codon in the messenger RNA and the amino acid carried by the tRNA is linked into the peptide chain.

Antimicrobial agent: *See* antibiotic.

Antiseptic: a chemical used to reduce the numbers of microbes on body surfaces.

Antiserum: a serum that contains antibodies to a particular antigen.

Antitoxin: a serum containing antibodies to a toxin, either as a result of natural infection or, more often, in response to injection of toxoid.

Arthropod: an animal which has a hard outer 'skeleton' and jointed legs; examples are insects, ticks and lice.

Aseptic: free of contaminating microbes.

Atom: the smallest unit of matter capable of taking part in a chemical reaction.

Atomic number: the number of protons in the nucleus of an atom.

Atomic weight: the weight of the atom; it corresponds almost exactly to the number of protons and neutrons in the nucleus.

Attenuated: a microbe that is *attenuated* has lost its virulence and may be suitable for use as a vaccine.

Autoclave: a machine in which materials can be exposed to steam under pressure and therefore at a temperature higher than that of boiling water.

Autogenous: arising within the individual.

Autotrophic: autotrophic organisms can obtain from atmospheric carbon dioxide most or all of the carbon they require to synthesise their component molecules.

Bacillus: any rod-shaped bacterium; also the name of a genus of bacteria, Gram-positive rods which are often found in soil and dust.

Bactericidal: capable of killing bacteria.

Bacteriophage: an 'eater of bacteria', a bacterial virus which enters a bacterial cell and multiplies within it by directing the bacterial metabolic machinery to manufacture bacteriophage components.

Bacterium: a procaryotic microbe.

Base: an ion or molecule capable of accepting a hydrogen ion. Bases normally produce OH^- ions when dissolved in water.

Base pair: two nitrogenous bases linked by hydrogen bonds in the double-stranded DNA molecule. Adenine-thymine and guanine-cytosine are the only two possible pairings.

Basophil: a white cell of the blood, so called because it takes up basic dyes; in the usual stains for blood films, basophils have large black granules. *See* Plate 10.

B-cell: one of the two main cell types of the immune system, chiefly involved in the production of antibodies.

BCG strain of tubercle bacilli: an attenuated strain that is used as a vaccine against tuberculosis.

Binary fission: division of one cell into two daughter cells, the usual method of reproduction in bacteria.

Biochemistry: the science dealing with chemical processes in living organisms.

Biosynthesis: the synthetic processes carried out by living cells.

Buffer: a chemical that tends to minimise changes in the pH of a solution.

Calvin cycle: the process whereby atmospheric carbon dioxide is converted to carbohydrates, using the energy generated by photophosphorylation.

Capsid: the protein layer enclosing the nucleic acid of a virus.

Carbohydrate: a compound of carbon, hydrogen and oxygen, the hydrogen and oxygen being present in a ratio of 2:1; e.g. glucose $C_6H_{12}O_6$ is a carbohydrate.

Carbon cycle: the series of reactions whereby carbon is converted from CO_2 to organic compounds and back to CO_2 again.

Carboxyl group: $-C=O$. It ionises in solution, $\rightarrow -C=O$
$\quad\quad\quad\quad\quad\quad\quad\quad\;\; |$ $\quad\quad\quad\quad\quad\quad\quad\quad\quad\quad\quad\; |\quad$ and H^+
$\quad\quad\quad\quad\quad\quad 0-H$ $\quad\quad\quad\quad\quad\quad\quad\quad\quad\quad O^-$

Carrier: an individual who persistently excretes a microbe or who has a body surface colonised by a microbe, but who is not obviously ill of this infection.

Catalase: an enzyme that catalyses the breakdown of hydrogen peroxide to oxygen and water.

Catalyst: a substance that increases the rate of a chemical reaction, but is itself unaltered when the reaction is complete.

Cation: an ion bearing a positive charge, e.g. Na^+.

CDS method: a method of testing the susceptibility of bacteria to antibiotics by means of disks, i.e. an agar-diffusion method. It was developed by Prof. Sydney M Bell.

Cell-mediated immunity: a form of immune response carried out by cells.

Cell wall: the rigid outer layer of most procaryotic cells and of some eucaryotic ones.

Centrifuge: an instrument which can spin liquids in containers at high speed, thus depositing particles on the bottom of the tube. It is often used to concentrate bacteria from body fluids for examination.

Cephalosporin: an antibiotic containing a beta-lactam ring; many different types are now available, active chiefly against Gram-negative organisms.

Cercaria: the final larval stage of a fluke (trematode).

Chemical energy: energy generated by, or able to be used in, a chemical reaction.

Chemotaxis: movement of a cell in response to the presence of a chemical.

Chemotherapy: treatment of disease with chemicals; in practice, this means antibiotics.

Citric acid cycle: the process of oxidising acetyl groups to carbon dioxide and water, the final stage of the generation of energy from carbohydrates.

Clone: a group of organisms descended from a single parent by asexual reproduction and therefore exact copies of it. The term is now extended to the production of copies of DNA molecules.

Coccobacillus: a short oval rod, i.e. between a coccus and a bacillus in shape.

Coccus: a bacterium that is a sphere or almost so.

Codon: a set of three nucleotides in DNA or messenger RNA that specifies a particular amino acid.

Coenzyme: a non-protein molecule (often derived from a vitamin) which is needed for the function of an enzyme.

Coenzyme A: a coenzyme that accepts acetyl groups and introduces them into the citric acid cycle and other metabolic processes.

Colonisation: a microbe that establishes itself in a particular environment such as a body surface without producing disease is said to 'colonise' the site.

Colony: when a bacterial cell (or a few cells) multiplies on a solid medium until the group is visible to the naked eye, the group is called a *colony*. A typical colony contains 10–100 million cells.

Commensal: a commensal organism lives in association with another, without benefiting or harming it. Many members of the gut flora appear to be commensals.

Communicable: a disease that can be transmitted from one person to another is communicable (= contagious, = infectious).

Complement: a complex of proteins in the blood; reactions between the component proteins (often after reacting with an antigen-antibody complex) promote the movement of phagocytes and the phagocytosis and killing of bacteria.

Complex medium: a bacteriological medium derived from natural products such as meat or yeast; the chemicals making up such a medium are not known.

Compromised person (host, patient): a person whose normal defences against infection are impaired.

Conjugation: the transfer of genetic material from one bacterial cell to another by cell-to-cell contact.

Conjugative plasmid: a plasmid which bears the genes needed to bring about the conjugation of its host bacterium with another bacterium.

Constitutive enzyme: an enzyme that is produced by the cell, whether or not the chemical on which it acts is present. Compare *'inducible enzyme'*.

Contagious: *See* communicable.

Counterstain: a stain used to enhance contrast in a differential stain.

Covalent bond: a chemical bond in which electrons are shared between two atoms.

Culture: a culture of microbes is the result of inoculating a medium with them and incubating it until large numbers are present.

Cutaneous: relating to the skin.

Cyanobacteria: autotrophic procaryotes capable of photosynthesis.

Cyst: (a) a sac or closed cavity in the (human or animal) body, filled with fluid or other material; (b) a stage in the lifecycle of some protozoan parasites, in which the organism is encased in a tough outer wall.

Cysticercus: a larval stage of some tapeworms, in which a fluid-filled cyst is formed.

Cystitis: a urinary infection confined to the bladder.

Cytoplasm: in a procaryote, everything inside the cytoplasmic membrane; in a eucaryote, everything inside the cytoplasmic membrane, except the nucleus.

Cytoplasmic membrane: the membrane which constitutes the outer boundary of the cell except for the cell wall (when one is present) and which prevents the escape of the large and small molecules making up the cytoplasm of the cell.

Cytosine: an organic base found in DNA, RNA and elsewhere.

Cytotoxic: toxic to cells. Some T-cells are cytotoxic.

Dalton: the unit in which atomic and molecular weights are expressed; for practical purposes it equals the weight of a hydrogen atom.

Dane particle: a complete and infectious hepatitis B virion; it consists of DNA enclosed in a protein capsid.

Defined medium: a medium the exact composition of which is known, since it is made of chemically pure substances.

Definitive host: the host organism in which the adult form of a parasite lives.

Delayed(-type) hypersensitivity: a hypersensitivity reaction carried out by cells and requiring 24 or more hours to be manifest.

Denaturation: (a) of proteins, the loss of folding brought about by heat or chemicals; denatured proteins have lost their normal biological activity. (b) of DNA, breaking the hydrogen bonds that hold two DNA strands together, resulting in their separation.

Deoxyribonucleic acid (DNA): the large molecule in which genetic information is encoded, the genetic material. The component nucleotides contain the sugar deoxyribose.

Deoxyribose: a five-carbon sugar present in the nucleotides of DNA.

Dermatophyte: a fungus that attacks ths skin, hair and nails without invading the deeper tissues.

Differential stain: a staining procedure that can dye some objects in the preparation but not others.

Diffusion: the process whereby the random movement of molecules tends to equalise their concentration in regions initially of higher and lower concentration.

Diploid: a diploid cell contains two copies of each chromosome. The body cells of most eucaryotic organisms are diploid.

Disk diffusion: a method of testing bacteria for susceptibility to antibiotics. *See* Kirby-Bauer, CDS.

Disulphide bond: a covalent bond between two sulphur atoms, —S—S—.

DNA: *see* deoxyribonucleic acid.

Dysentery: a severe form of infectious diarrhoea, characterised by blood and mucus in the stools.

DNA probe: see probe

Ectoparasite: a parasite that lives on the outer surface of the host, e.g. a tick or louse.

Electron: a negatively-charged particle in orbit round the nucleus of an atom.

Electron microscope: a microspcope in which a beam of electrons is used instead of light rays to produce an image.

Electron transport chain: a series of compounds along which electrons pass during the generation of ATP.

Electrophoresis: the separation of molecules by subjecting them to an electric field in which they move at different rates.

Element: a chemical composed of atoms with the same atomic number.

Elementary body: the infectious form of the procaryote *Chlamydia*.

ELISA (enzyme-linked immunosorbent assay): a technique for detecting and estimating antigens and antibodies, in which a coloured compound is formed by the enzyme linked to the detector antibody.

Embolus: material, especially a blood clot, which is carried by the circulation and blocks a blood vessel at a distance from the site where it originally formed.

Encephalitis: inflammation of the brain.

Endemic: if a disease is endemic, cases regularly appear in the population. *See* epidemic.

Endocarditis: an inflammation, especially one due to infection, of the lining of the heart, including its valves.

Endogenous: arising within the body; an *endogenous* infection is caused by the normal flora.

Endoplasmic reticulum: a complicated membrane system extending throughout the cytoplasm of the eucaryotic cell. During protein synthesis, ribosomes are often attached to it.

Endotoxin: part of the outer membrane of Gram-negative cells; it consists of various sugars and a lipid and possesses toxic properties, causing activation of complement, inflammation, blood clotting and fever. = lipopolysaccharide.

Envelope: in some viruses, an outer coat that surrounds the capsid and may be derived partly or wholly from the host cell.

Enzyme: a protein which catalyses a biochemical reaction.

Eosinophil: a white cell of the blood, so called because it takes up the dye eosin; in the usual stains for blood films, eosinophils have large orange-red granules. (*See* Plate 10.)

Epidemic: in an epidemic of a disease, many cases appear in a short time and then the number decreases for months or years.

Epidemiology: the study of the occurrence of diseases, how and when they occur, how they are transmitted, etc.

Eucaryotic cell: one of two chief types of living cells, in which the nucleus is delimited from the cytoplasm by a membrane.

Exogenous: derived from outside the body; compare *'endogenous'*.

Expression of gene: a gene is *expressed* when it is transcribed and translated into a protein.

Extracellular: outside the cell.

Facilitated diffusion: diffusion mediated by carrier proteins across the cytoplasmaic membrane from a region of high concentration to a region of low concentration.

Facultative: an organism which is not restricted to a particular way of life; thus a facultative anaerobe can live in the absence or presence of oxygen.

Facultative anaerobe: *see anaerobe*.

Fermentation: production of energy from carbohydrates in the absence of oxygen. The electrons generated are passed to organic molecules.

Fibrin: When blood clots, a meshwork of fibrin is formed from the fibrinogen in the plasma.

Fix: to prepare a specimen for staining; heating causes most bacterial specimens to adhere to the glass slide and is an adequate preparation for staining, other specimens need to be soaked in liquids such as formalin.

Flagellum: an organ attached to the surface of the cell and used for locomotion.

Flatworm: any of the flat-bodied worms, especially the flukes and tapeworms, which are important parasites.

Flora: originally the plant life of an area or period (*Flora* was the Roman goddess of flowers); bacteria were originally considered to be plants, hence the term is still applied in microbiology to the community of microbes colonising a body region.

Fluke: a parasitic flatworm (= trematode). Adult flukes are important parasites of man — *Fasciola,* the liver fluke, or *Schistosoma.*

Fluorescent antibody technique: a technique for detecting microbes in which the antibody is tagged with fluorescent dyes and thus rendered visible when viewed with a special microscope (*fluorescence microscope*) in which ultraviolet light is used.

Fomites: objects which have been touched by a person with an infectious disease and which may be contaminated with microbes, so that any person subsequently touching them may be infected. Common fomites are towels, bedclothes, furniture and crockery.

Gamete: a male or female sex cell; it is haploid.

Gangrene: Death of body tissue such as a limb, because of interference with the blood supply.

Gas gangrene: Death of body tissue such as a limb, because of infection with *Clostridium perfringens.*

Gene: a 'unit of heredity', a segment of DNA that encodes the structure of a protein.

Generation time: the time required for a microbe to undergo division, producing two individuals.

Genetics: the science of heredity.

Genome: the genetic information specifying an organism.

Genus: in biological nomenclature the *genus* is the larger grouping and is written with a capital; the *species* is the smaller grouping. Both words are modern Latin and are printed in italics.

Globulin: a type of protein which includes antibodies.

Glycocalyx: a more or less diffuse layer outside the cell wall of procaryotes; it consists of polysaccharide, polypeptide or both.

Glycogen: a polysaccharide stored by animals and some bacteria.

Glycolysis: the main path for the generation of energy by breaking down glucose to pyruvic acid.

Golgi complex: an organelle present in the cytoplasm of eucaryotic cells; it is involved in the secretion of proteins from the cell.

Gram stain: a staining procedure that distinguishes two types of parcaryotes, Gram-positive and Gram-negative.

Guanine: an organic base found in DNA, RNA and elsewhere.

Habitat: the part of an ecosystem (environment) in which a creature lives.

Haemolysin: a molecule that lyses red cells. Many bacteria produce haemolysins.

Haploid: a haploid cell contains only one copy of each chromosome. The cells of procaryotic organisms are haploid. Compare *'diploid'*.

Heat-labile: easily destroyed by heat.

Helix, helical: spiral.

Hermaphrodite: possessing both male and female sex organs.

Heterotrophic: heterotrophic organisms (heterotrophs) require an organic source of carbon, e.g. glucose, to synthesise their component molecules.

Histamine: a molecule released by mast cells; it causes inflammation, increased permeability of blood vessels, asthma.

Histocompatibility antigens: cell-surface antigens involved in many aspects of immunological recognition; they are the main antigens recognised in the rejection of grafts. In humans the chief group of such antigens is called the *HLA antigens*.

HLA antigens: *See histocompatibility antigens.*

Hydrogen bond: a type of chemical bond, relatively weak in nature.

Hypersensitivity: an exaggerated or inappropriate immune response, leading to inflammation or tissue damage.

Icosahedron: a solid figure with 12 (vertices) corners and 20 triangular faces.

Immunity: the result of infection by a particular microbe or of immunisation against that microbe.

Immunisation: the process of artificially inducing immunity to infection by a microbe.

Immunoglobulin: an antibody.

Incubation period: the interval between contact with the microbe and the development of the symptoms and signs of infection.

Inducible enzyme: an enzyme present in very low concentration in the cell if its substrate is not available. The presence of the substrate triggers production of more copies of the enzyme molecule.

Infection: entry of a harmful microbe into the body and its multiplication in the tissues.

Inflammation: a response to infection or other injury characterised by swelling, heat, redness and pain.

Innate resistance: resistance which does not depend on previous exposure to microbes.

Inoculum: material (containing bacteria) added to a growth medium to initiate a culture; hence *'inoculate'*.

Inorganic compounds: small molecules present in living creatures and also in non-living materials; they usually do not contain carbon.

Insertion sequence: part of a transposon.

Interleukins: immunological hormones, messenger molecules released during immunological reactions.

Intermediate host: a host organism in which the larval form of a parasite lives; there may be more than one intermediate host.

In vitro: 'in glass', i.e. carried out in the test-tube, in the laboratory.

In vivo: 'in the living', i.e. in the animal (or patient).

Intracellular: inside cells.

Isotope: an atom of an element which possesses the same number of protons and electrons as all atoms of the element, but has a different number of neutrons.

Kirby-Bauer method: a method of testing the susceptibility of bacteria to antibiotics by means of disks, i.e. an agar-diffusion method. It was developed by Prof. WMM Kirby and Dr AW Bauer.

Latent infection: a condition in which the clinical signs of infection are absent and the causative organism may be temporarily undetectable; under certain conditions the infection may again become obvious.

Leucocyte: white blood cell.

Lipid: a fat, a molecule made up of glycerol and fatty acids.

Lipopolysaccharide: a constituent of the Gram-negative bacterial cell-wall, in which chains of various sugars are linked to lipid A. = endotoxin.

Lymphocyte: any one of several different types of cells involved in the immune response. They have a round or oval nucleus and the cytoplasm is usually free of granules. (*See* Plate 10.)

Lymphokines: polypeptides released chiefly by T-cells and activating macrophages.

Lysosome: an intracellular organelle, a bag of enzymes.

Lysozyme: an enzyme that can dissolve the cell walls of certain bacteria.

Malaise: a general feeling of being unwell.

Macrophage: a type of phagocyte. (*See* plate 74.)

Mantoux test: a tuberculin skin test.

Mast cell: a cell involved in the type I hypersensitivity response. In appearance it closely resembles the basophil (Plate 10). It contains histamine and other substances the release of which causes inflammation.

Meiosis: a form of cell division, characteristic of eucaryotic cells; it results in haploid progeny cells (male and female gametes).

Membrane filter: a filter, usually made from a cellulose derivative, which contains large numbers of pores of a specified size.

Messenger RNA: the transcript of the DNA from which a polypeptide is synthesised by the ribosome.

Metabolism: a general term for all the biochemical processes that occur in a living cell.

Microbe: a creature too small to be seen with the naked eye (or only just visible); the term includes bacteria, fungi, protozoa, some of the algae and the viruses. = microorganism.

Micrometre (μm): a unit of length, = 10^{-6} metres.

Microorganism: *see microbe.*

Minimal inhibitory concentration (MIC): the lowest concentration of an antibiotic or other agent that will inhibit the growth of a microbe.

Miracidium: the first-stage larva of a parasitic fluke; it emerges from the egg in water.

Mitochondrion: an intracellular organelle that contains the energy-generating systems of eucaryotic cells.

Mitosis: division of a eucaryotic cell into two diploid daughter cells.

Molecular weight: the weight of a molecule expressed in daltons.

Monocyte: a white cell of the blood, which develops into the tissue macrophage of the mononuclear phagocytic system. See Plate 10.

Mononuclear phagocytic system: a system of phagocytic cells consisting of the blood monocytes, the wandering monocytes and macrophages of the lung and other tissues, and the fixed phagocytes in the liver and spleen.

Mordant: a substance that helps a dye to bind firmly.

Motility: the ability to move.

Mould: a fungus that forms a mycelium which may be seen as a 'furry' growth on the surface of e.g. bread or a fruit.

Mutation: a change in the sequence of the bases in the DNA strand.

Myalgia: pain in the muscles, a feature of many viral infections.

Mycelium: an intertwined mass of filaments *(hyphae)*, typical of the growth of moulds.

Nanometer: a unit of length, $= 10^{-9}$ m (10^{-3} micrometer).

Natural killer cells: large lymphoid cells capable of killing cells with the appropriate receptors on the surface.

Nematode: one of the large group of worms which have an unsegmented, cylindrical body tapering at each end (= roundworm). Some are free-living, in soil and water, others are parasites of plants and animals.

Neutrophil: a white cell of the blood, actively phagocytic. *See* Plate 10.

Nitrogen cycle: the series of reactions whereby nitrogen is converted from atmospheric nitrogen gas to organic compounds and back to gas again.

Normal flora: the community of microbes that colonises a body surface.

Nosocomial: acquired or occurring in a hospital; e.g. a nosocomial infection.

Nucleolus: an area in the nucleus of a eucaryotic cell where RNA is synthesised.

Nucleotide: a constituent of DNA or RNA, made up of a sugar, an organic base and a phosphate group.

Nucleus: (a) the central part of an atom, made up of protons and neutrons. OR (b) the part of the eucaryotic cell that contains the genetic material.

Objective lens: the lens of a microscope which forms the primary image of the specimen.

Obligate: an obligate organism is restricted to a particular way of life; e.g an obligate parasite cannot live free without a host.

Obligate aerobe/anaerobe: *see aerobe, anaerobe.*

Ocular lens: the lens of a microscope which further nagnifies the primary image formed by the objective lens.

Operon: the functional unit in many gene systems, consisting of operator, repressor and structural genes .

Organelle: a distinct structure within the cytoplasm of a eucaryotic cell that possesses a separate function; e.g. the mitochondria, Golgi complex.

Organic: an organic compound is one that contains carbon.

Oxidation: the addition of oxygen to, or the removal of electrons from, a substance.

Pandemic: a worldwide outbreak of an infectious disease.

Parasite: an organism that lives in or on another creature and obtains food and shelter without benefitting the host. Hence *'parasitism'. See commensal* and *symbiosis.*

Parenteral: administered by injection directly into the tissues.

Passive immunity: immunity conferred on the host animal by antibodies made in another host.

Pathogen: a microbe capable of causing disease.

Pathogenicity: the ability of a microbe to invade and cause disease.

Penicillins: a group of antibiotics containing a beta-lactam ring; some are natural products, but most are at least partially synthesised.

Peptide: a chain of amino acids.

Peptidoglycan: a major structural component of bacterial cell walls, consisting of chains of sugars cross-linked by peptides.

Peptones: short chains of amino acids derived from the breakdown of proteins.

pH: the symbol denoting hydrogen ion concentration; the pH ranges between 0 and 14 and its value indicates the relative acidity or alkalinity of a solution.

Phagocyte: a cell capable of phagocytosis.

Phagocytosis: the ingestion of material by a cell either in order to destroy foreign matter or for its own nutrition.

Phase-contrast microscope: a microscope which is fitted with a special illumination system that reveals the structure of living cells without the need for staining.

Phosphate group: phosphorus appears in many biologically important compounds in the form:

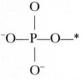

The oxygen atom marked * may be linked to another phosphate group, as in ATP, or to an alcohol, as in a phospholipid, or to another molecule.

Phospholipid: a lipid made up of glycerol, two fatty acids and a phosphate group.

Photophosphorylation: the process of converting solar energy into the chemical energy of ATP.

Photosynthesis: the use of solar energy by green plants and some bacteria to synthesise carbon compounds from CO_2 and water.

Plasma: the liquid portion of blood.

Plasma cell: a cell that develops from a B-cell and that manufactures a specific antibody.

Plasmid: a double-stranded circle of DNA which may be present in the cytoplasm of a microbial cell; it may be able to bring about conjugation between bacterial cells and it may carry genes for antibiotic resistance, for virulence and for various biochemical pathways.

Pleomorphic: varied in shape.

Polymer: a molecule made up of similar subunits.

Polymorphonuclear leucocyte: the blood contains three polymorphonuclear leucocytes, the neutrophil, the eosinophil and the basophil. *See* Plate 10.

Polypeptide: a chain of amino acids, containing at least four and usually more.

Precipitate: the result of a reaction between two soluble substances to form an insoluble material that 'falls' out of solution.

Precipitin reaction: a reaction between antigen and antibody which results in a visible precipitate.

Primary response: the production of antibody in response to the first contact with the antigen.

Probe: a short single-stranded segment of DNA or RNA which is identical in base sequence to a part of a gene, plasmid, ribosome etc, and which can be used to detect the presence of the gene or plasmid, and hence to identify the microbe of which it is a part, or to detect a hereditary defect.

Procaryotic cell: one of two chief types of living cells, in which the nucleus is not delimited from the cytoplasm by a membrane. In general procaryotic cells are smaller and of less complex structure than eucaryotic cells.

Proglottid: a segment of a tapeworm; it contains male and female reproductive organs and eggs.

Prophylaxis: treatment which is intended to prevent disease rather than cure it after it has developed; e.g. prophylactic antibiotic therapy.

Protein: a large molecule, one of the main constituents of living matter; it consists of one or more polypeptide chains.

Protozoa: microscopic single-celled eucaryotic microbes; some are free-living, others are important parasites.

Pseudopod: an extension of the cytoplasm of a cell; pseudopods are formed for the purposes of feeding and locomotion. *See* Plate 74.

Pus: an accumulation of fluid due to infection; it consists of living and dead microbes, phagocytes and tissue cells, together with the fluid that has accumulated in the tissue because of inflammation.

Pyelonephritis: an infection of the kidney.

Replication: the synthesis of copies of a DNA molecule or a virus.

Reservoir (of infection): the permanent source of infection; e.g. foxes are a reservoir of rabies in Western Europe.

Respiration: the generation of energy by the conversion of organic compounds to carbon dioxide and water. The energy generated is stored as ATP.

Restriction enzymes: enzymes that cut DNA strands at points determined by the sequence of the bases and which therefore always yield the same fragments from a given DNA.

Reverse transcriptase: an enzyme that works 'in reverse', synthesising DNA from an RNA template. The human immunodeficiency virus contains a reverse transcriptase.

Ribonucleic acid (RNA): a nucleic acid in which the component nucleotides contain the sugar ribose. The ribonucleic acids of cells are messenger RNA, transfer RNA and ribosomal RNA; in addition the genome of some viruses consists of RNA.

Ribose: a five-carbon sugar present in the nucleotides of RNA.

Ribosomal RNA: RNA which forms part of the ribosome.

Ribosome: the protein-synthesising 'factory' of the cytoplasm.

Root nodule: a small rounded lump on the root of a leguminous plant; it contains symbiotic nitrogen-fixing bacteria.

Roundworm: *see nematode.*

Saprophyte: an organism that lives on dead organic matter.

Scolex: the head of a tapeworm, armed with suckers and often with hooks.

Sense strand: the strand of DNA that carries the genetic message.

Septicaemia: bacteraemia accompanied by symptoms and signs of infection and illness.

Serotype: a strain of a bacterial species which can be differentiated by the antigens present on its surface; these are detected by antibodies (*serological* methods).

Serum: the liquid which remains when plasma clots.

Sign: *see Symptoms and signs.*

Species: *see* genus.

Subclinical infection: an infection which produces no symptoms or signs of disease; most infections are subclinical.

Subcutaneous: beneath the skin.

Subphrenic abscess: a collection of pus below the diaphragm and usually between it and the liver.

Substrate: the substance(s) with which an enzyme reacts.

Symbiosis: an obligate association between two species in which there is mutual benefit.

Symptoms and signs: symptoms are the patient's complaints; signs are the physical evidence of disease.

Syndrome: a set of symptoms and signs that forms a distinctive clinical picture suggesting a particular disease.

Synergy: when the effect of two antibiotics (or other drugs) given together is greater than can be accounted for by the effect of each acting alone, this is said to be due to synergy.

Systemic: involving the whole body.

Tapeworm: a long segmented flatworm parasitic in the intestine.

Teichoic acid: a polymer of an alcohol, phosphate and other molecules found in Gram-positive cell walls.

Template strand: the strand of DNA complementary to the sense strand; both the sense strand and the messenger RNA are synthesised on the template strand.

Tetracyclines: a group of broad-spectrum antibiotics which interfere with protein synthesis.

Thymine: an organic base found in DNA.

Titre (titer): a means of expressing the concentration of an antibody.

Topical: a drug that is applied directly to the affected part (e.g. skin or eye) is applied *topically*.

Toxin: any poisonous substance produced by a living organism, especially a microbe.

Toxoid: a microbial toxin treated (usually with dilute formaldehyde) so that its toxic activity is destroyed, but it is still capable of stimulating the production of antibodies which react with and inactivate the parent toxin.

Trace element: a chemical element required for growth, but only needed in very small amounts.

Transcription: copying the sense strand of the DNA into messenger RNA.

Transduction: the introduction into a bacterial cell, by a bacteriophage, of new genes which are not bacteriophage genes and which are derived from the bacterium in which the phage previously replicated.

Transfer RNA: RNA molecules which carry individual amino acids to the ribosome.

Transformation: the introduction of new genes into a cell by the uptake of 'naked' DNA from solution.

Translation: synthesising a polypeptide chain from the messenger RNA template.

Transposon: a 'jumping gene', a segment of DNA which can move from one DNA molecule to another, or from one site to another in the same DNA molecule.

Trematode: see fluke.

Trophozoite: the normal actively feeding form of a parasite, which is often too frail to survive the conditions involved in transfer to a new host.

Tuberculin test: a skin test used to detect infection by mycobacteria.

Ubiquitous: present everywhere.

Ultraviolet light: invisible light of wavelength shorter than the light at the violet end of the visible spectrum.

Uracil: an organic base found in RNA.

Vaccination: the process of inducing immunity by administering a vaccine.

Vaccine: a preparation of killed microbes, inactivated microbial toxins or microbial antigens used to induce immunity.

Vector: an animal, usually an arthropod (insect or tick) that transfers an infectious microbe from one host to another.

Virulence: the ability to cause disease.

Zoonosis: an infectious disease of animals that may be transmitted to man. Brucellosis, rabies and toxoplasmosis are examples.

INDEX

1 2 3 4 5 6
A B C D E F